Contraception and Abortion
from the Ancient World
to the Renaissance

◆ JOHN M. RIDDLE ◆

Contraception and Abortion from the Ancient World to the Renaissance

◆

Harvard University Press
Cambridge, Massachusetts
London, England
1992

Library of Congress Cataloging-in-Publication Data

Riddle, John M.
Contraception and abortion from the ancient world
to the Renaissance / John M. Riddle.
p.   cm.
Includes bibliographical references and index.
ISBN 0-674-16875-5
1. Contraception—History.   2. Oral contraceptives—History.
3. Abortifacients—History.   4. Medicine, Ancient.
5. Medicine, Medieval.   I. Title.
RG137.5.R53   1992
613.9′4′0901—dc20   91-33682
CIP

✦ CONTENTS ✦

This book is an attempt to make sense out of the historical records related to birth control. As I looked at classical and medieval medical records, I was struck by the number of oral contraceptives and abortifacients mentioned. Historians have tended to relegate antifertility agents not to the proverbial "dust-heap called history," as Augustine Burill called it, but to the realm of nonscience next door. Classical and medieval birth control methods are regarded by us moderns as magic and superstition. Almost universally it is agreed that these agents were not effective because they could not be effective.

Over a period of years I learned that our distant ancestors could distinguish between a contraceptive and an abortifacient (which is no easy task) and that they knew more about reproduction than we have credited them with. If the documents describe real practices, dismissal of the methods they recorded as mere magic and superstition was too simple.

Two recent global surveys asked about the use of contraceptives and family planning (Anderson 1984). As many as 93.5 percent of the women in Bangladesh and as few as 33.2 percent in Costa Rica were certified as nonusers of contraceptives. Persons who indicated that they used herbs were recorded as "not using" contraception. The surveyors did not ask about pharmaceutically induced abortion, probably because of its sensitive nature (if not criminal status) in almost all cultures. They did not inquire about oral early stage abortifacients, because such things were not thought to exist. Even now, the "morning-after" pill, as it is popularly called, is still being developed and is available in only a few countries. Early stage abortifacients still await scientific, medical, legal, and moral approval in most countries.

Were people in the past simply fooled by physicians, witch doctors, herbalists, witches, midwives, village wise persons, and charlatan medicine-show salesmen into taking something that did not work? In developing a partial answer to this question, I mean to set aside the issue of possible psychosomatic factors involved in fertility. When the documents describe magical birth control practices, I shall note their presence in the record but give no analysis. By magic, I mean only something that we moderns regard as nonscientific, such as an amulet or incantation. Such methods may have effects comparable to the placebo effect in the complexity of fertility physiology. To put it simply, a full-term pregnancy cannot be psychosomatic. If a person takes an agent to prevent pregnancy and does not become pregnant, one cannot be certain whether there was a causal link with that agent. On the other hand, if pregnancy does occur, one knows that the agent did not work.

We too easily draw a hard line that separates us from the premodern period. We acknowledge that our ancestors can speak to us about certain values but we dismiss their specific solutions to problems. In this attempt to make sense out of the historical records, I take into account what modern medicine, botany, pharmacy, pharmacology, demography, and anthropology say is a reasonable explanation. Modern studies of the possible effects of plants on human fertility come from a variety of sources: scientific journals and books devoted to medical and pharmacy research; animal science research focusing on antifertility actions of plants on grazing animals; laboratory and clinical testing of traditional remedies (notably in Chinese and Indian journals); anthropological descriptions of population groups that employ traditional antifertility agents.

Some critics of this study will say that I too have committed the transgression of historical positivism because my study uses modern science to validate historical practices—selected ones at that. Yet my mission is not to hand out medals to moderns by finding historical antecedents to modern discoveries. Instead I hope to induce caution and, perchance, second thoughts in those historians and demographers who reject the historical data on the basis that the antifertility agents could not have worked. I am asking no more of my colleagues than to consider the historical record before rejecting it. I believe that what is recorded regarding birth control and family planning largely happened as stated.

As this book was in production, Angus McLaren's *A History of Contraception from Antiquity to the Present Day* (Basil Blackwell, 1990) was published, too late to incorporate his findings into this study. McLaren's perspective is on social history and follows the traditional interpretation that effectual family planning began in the late eighteenth century. I see a different trail of learning, in which premodern people knew important things about birth control that we do not.

The trail of learning also leads back in time. The Greek medical records, preeminently the writings ascribed to Hippocrates, are tangled in linguistic and interpretative problems. Rather than following a strictly chronological approach, I introduce this subject matter through the works of two authors of the first centuries of our era, Soranus and Dioscorides. The Hippocratic writings in turn led back to the medicine of ancient West Asia and Egypt.

Most of the drugs discussed in this book are of plant origin. The identification of plants in historical records is an inexact and tedious task. Even when a plant is cited by the modern taxonomy (as I have attempted to do), the identification is not as precise as it may appear. In an earlier study (Riddle 1985) I explained my methodology for botanical identifications. Behind each plant lies an impressive record of classical scholarship. When the authorities are in substantial agreement, I do not burden the notes with references. When there is reasonable doubt or when I disagree with the conventional authorities, I cite the evidence.

I have frequently cited in the original language texts that are old, rare, or unavailable in most libraries. When Hunain ibn Ishaq translated Greek medical works into Arabic in the ninth century, he apologized to his readers for not being able to translate some technical terms. Occasionally, he would simply transliterate a term into the Arabic alphabet and leave Allah to provide his reader with greater wisdom than he had. By providing the original text, I hope to follow the spirit of Hunain.

Many antifertility recipes are reproduced in this book. Readers should not try to use them. The possibility for error is too great and the risk might be considerable. Although "natural," plant drugs are nevertheless drugs and can have unintended effects.

We tend to believe that quandaries over birth control are recent, brought on by science and technology. In fact the human problems now are much the same as when Juvenal wrote almost two thousand years ago that "we have sure-fire contraceptives." Hundreds of generations have faced many of the same problems we do—saints and sinners, people in distress, kings, queens, merchants, and peasants. Were we wise, we would learn from the past. At the very least, let us be consoled by the realization that our times are not as unique as we think they are.

The initial research for this paper was conducted in 1988 at the Institute for Advanced Study, Princeton, New Jersey, and I acknowledge and value the institute's support. Since then, North Carolina State University has supported the research. Colleagues, especially in history, chemistry, biology, and the medicine and veterinary medicine communities in the Research Triangle Area, have been an invaluable resource.

A number of scholars have read all or part of this manuscript. Others have answered technical questions or provided translations. The number of persons who gave me their time, patience, and expertise is large and so is my gratitude to them. I wish to thank James Banker, William Block, Glen Bowersock, Jane Chance, Giles Constable, Elizabeth Crawford, Jane Crawford, Alexander De Grand, Gerald Elkan, Steven Foster, Christian Habicht, Ann Hanson, Joseph Hobbs, Andrea Lain, Anthony Lavopa, Helen Lemay, Robert Lerner, Cynthia Levin, Keith Luria, Michael McVaugh, Gordon Newby, John Noonan, Michael Novak, Vivian Nutton, Peter Rhodes, Robert Ritner, Steven Rowan, Miri Rubin, Michael Rulison, John Scarborough, Wesley Smith, Mark Sosower, Gerald Surh, Samuel Tove, Steven Vincent, and Ming Jing Wu. The librarians in the National Library of Medicine and the D. H. Hill Library at North Carolina State University were particularly helpful. Especially I express gratitude to Dora Zia for sharing her expert knowledge of computer data resources. Kaye Greenlaw, William Inman, Pat Sullivan, and Paul Petersen assisted me with the editing.

CHAPTER ONE

Population and Sex

Cousin to Young Bride: Why, you little Devil, you would not take Physick to
  kill the child . . . ?
Bride: No, but there may be Things to prevent Conception; an't there?
Cousin: What! the same thing to prevent a Conception as to destroy the Child
  after it is conceived . . . !
Bride: I cannot understand your Niceties; I would not be with Child, that' all;
  there's no harm in that, I hope.

   Daniel Defoe, *Matrimonial Whoredom* (1727 ed.), pp. 138–140

Was it possible for premodern people to regulate their reproduction without resorting to the extremities of dangerous abortions or infanticide or the denial of the biological urge to mate? In the first fifteen hundred years of our era, wars, pestilence, and even food supply did not appear as factors in motivating or discouraging reproduction. Demographers say, not surprisingly, that if a society values a large family, then families tend to be large. Conversely, if small size is considered desirable, human intervention produces a slow rate of population growth or even a decline.[1]

The importance of fertility was recognized by some leaders in premodern communities[2] as well as by historians of the period between the Roman Empire and the Renaissance.[3] From Augustus Caesar through the late empire, Roman emperors were concerned about the declining population. As best we can tell, people did not have many children simply because they did not wish to have them. Despite a variety of governmental encouragements to marry and to have large families and also to raise children born out of wedlock, people often declined to heed such imperial calls. When there were no more emperors to announce state policy, people continued to be less fertile than was necessary to maintain population size.

Henri Pirenne correlated the progressive decline in early medieval population with the reduction of urban populations and spoke eloquently of its drastic consequences.[4] From approximately 1000 to 1320, European population rose considerably, only to see a decline, followed by a relatively constant size for the next several centuries. The population increase of the early eleventh century was followed by a decrease that began even before the catastrophe of the Black Death. Historians, demographers, and anthropologists have studied the causes of the gross and long-term population fluctuations.[5] The Malthusian explanation of the tie between food supply and population size does not readily coincide with the historical data of the Mediterranean and European worlds in the last two thousand years. For example, population in the early Roman Empire was declining, although the period was one of prosperity, with apparently adequate food supply. Even in premodern and contemporary traditional societies, the birth rate can be, in the words of David Herlihy, "extremely sensitive to social conditions."[6]

I consider, however, not the complex issue of possible motivation for slow population growth or decline but the question of what means existed to limit conception and birth. If people had the normal biological urges for sexual intercourse but—for whatever reason—did not wish to increase their numbers, how did they limit reproduction?

Statements from literary, medical, legal, and theological sources, as well as from natural philosophy, speak of measures that people were taking to prevent births. Evidence for birth control will be presented in this book from many of these ancient and medieval sources that have long been available to scholars. Not believing that the agents (primarily drugs) mentioned in the sources were scientifically effective, scholars have either discounted or ignored chemical birth control agents in favor of other explanations for population decline or for reduced rates of growth.

Contrasting Classical Antiquity and the Middle Ages

We have evidence that during both classical antiquity and the Middle Ages people had effective population control measures. But what were those measures? The answers are sharply debated. Can we find a common factor in sexual mores and customs to explain the data? This search is implausible because of the basic differences between the two periods. Let us consider seven factors—the last two, abortion and infanticide, in some detail.

Sexual Restraint

In antiquity, the evidence suggests, sexual restraint was largely ignored; pagan religion normally did not attempt to regulate sexual activity.[7] Free males could do almost anything sexually, even if they had to resort to slaves, with no moral or societal consequences to themselves.

Not so in the Middle Ages. In the late Roman, early medieval, and Byzantine periods, restraint and outright celibacy were important, or so say numerous sources.[8] By the early Middle Ages, pagan and Christian alike had reached consensus in condemning sodomy, adultery, abortion, contraception, mutilation (notably castration), nudity, sexual relations during menstruation and after birth until weaning, and infanticide.[9] But by the time of the late empire, the replacement rate had been dropping or was no better than relatively constant for around four or five centuries, even with the Germanic migrations. Christianity was thus not the primary factor, since the trend began before that religion was established. The changing mores are separated by too many centuries for there to be a causal link between them and the demographic profile. The late Middle Ages (A.D. 1300–1500) witnessed demographic ups and downs at a time when sexual customs and attitudes did not radically change. Sexual restraint or continence, either during antiquity or the Middle Ages, can be rejected as a critical factor simply because, comparing the two periods, one would not expect the stark contrasts to have the same results. During antiquity almost anything was permissible; during the Middle Ages almost nothing went unchecked. Medieval religion, customs, and law all spoke differently from their classical counterparts (as evidence presented later will show). Both periods, however, evidently had some means of effective family limitation.

Marriage Age

Classical antiquity differs in another respect from the medieval period. Besides the contrasting attitudes toward sexual restraint, the two periods differed in their preferred age of marriage. In antiquity, females commonly married around age fourteen.[10] During the Middle Ages, the marriage age for women varied from time to time but generally was later than fourteen.[11] David Herlihy believes that limited fertility is partly attributable to late marriages in the late medieval and Renaissance periods, but he notes that the low birth rate among urban Florentine and Veronese married women may indicate some effective means of birth control. Also poorer households in the same towns had fewer children than wealthy ones. Herlihy observes that in some periods families seemed to sense the advent of difficult times and limited their fertility; there is evidence of a population decline, for instance, prior to the Black Death.[12] In the case of this plague, of course, people did not sense its coming, but they may have responded intuitively to economically deteriorating conditions.

Coitus Interruptus

Scholars agree that evidence in Roman literature for coitus interruptus is virtually nonexistent.[13] One could argue that it was so common and private that our sources do not refer to it. On balance, however, this practice was not likely; the records of the times are sufficiently abundant, and other aspects of sexual behavior are avidly and vividly described. Because there was no reticence to discuss other details of intimate sexual activity, there is no reason to suppose a reticence to discuss coitus interruptus, were it in practice. Especially notable is the absence in detailed medical writers, such as the Hippocratics, Soranus, and Galen.

Coitus interruptus is, and perhaps was, thought to be what was referred to in the Old Testament (Gen. 38:8–10) when Onan incurred the displeasure of Yahweh by releasing his seed on the ground rather than in the womb. The author of this Genesis passage appears to have meant that Yahweh was displeased because Onan refused to conceive a child in the name of his older brother. The passage was not interpreted this way later. Epiphanius (fourth century) construed the sin of Onan as coitus interruptus.[14] The Babylonian version of the Talmud speaks against the practice.[15]

According to Jean-Louis Flandrin, coitus interruptus was "seldom mentioned" in the period between classical antiquity and the fourteenth century, but P. P. A. Biller postulates the extensive use of this method because of the necessity to explain the medieval and Renaissance data and argues that no other explanation of the low birth rate seems plausible.[16] French scholars, especially E. LeRoy Ladurie and Philippe Ariès, argue that, for potentially fertile intercourse, coitus interruptus was the only effective contraceptive means prior to the nineteenth century. Its knowledge and use, however, were narrowly confined to the educated elite until the late eighteenth century. From the region of Hérault, LeRoy Ladurie has published data that reflect when coitus interruptus spread to the masses: "between 1789 (the *terminus a quo*) and 1813 (the *terminus ad quem*)." Euphemistically he calls coitus interruptus "funestes secrets" (baleful secrets).[17] Many scholars, however, accept neither its secrecy nor its usage (and do not speak of its balefulness).

If coitus interruptus was widely practiced from ancient times in West Asia until the modern period, we should expect a critical volume of documentary evidence, but there is a paucity. The effectiveness of this contraceptive measure rests primarily with the will or cooperation of the male, who suffers neither the anguish and danger of childbearing or, for the most part, the care of the infant.

Condoms

There is little if any evidence for usage of a condom or sheath during antiquity to prevent conception.[18] The earliest published description appears in Gabriel Fallopio's *De morbo gallico* (Padua, 1563), chapter 89. It was named for a Dr. Condom, physician at the court of Charles II (ruled 1660–1685), and supposedly used extensively by Casanova (1725–1788), who called it an "English riding coat." The condom as a birth control device emerged in wide usage only after the vulcanization of rubber in 1844.[19]

Nonfertile Intercourse

One means of avoiding pregnancy is to engage in a variety of sexual encounters that cannot be fertile, such as anal, oral, or homosexual intercourse. Certainly such behavior was not rare, and perhaps was common, during classical antiquity.[20] The medieval church roundly condemned such practices, however, and there was a string of biblical citations on which to base the damnations. All the same, Philippe Ariès believes that "perversité sexuelle" may have been the only effective contraceptive means available prior to the modern period.[21] The church's position hardened in canon law when the Roman church encountered and resisted the heretical cults (for example, the Bogomiles and the Cathars) with their doctrines and practices against procreative intercourse.[22] Sexual practices, whether of peasants or of emperors, are sufficiently elusive to escape direct knowledge by historians, given the nature of documentation. Scholars nevertheless must judge the reasonableness of explanatory hypotheses. Ariès's "perversité sexuelle" does not seem sufficient to explain the ancient, medieval, or early modern (1500–1800) data, as well as collateral literary and legal sources.

Rhythm

Two reasons compel us to discount the rhythm method for intercourse as being effective historically in controlling the birth rate. First, the sources seldom indicate its usage; second, ancient and medieval medical and gynecological authorities all agreed that the most fertile period for intercourse was near the end or just after the menstrual period, a misunderstanding apparently widely held.[23] The rhythm method should be dismissed as a substantial factor in limiting family size, but not because it

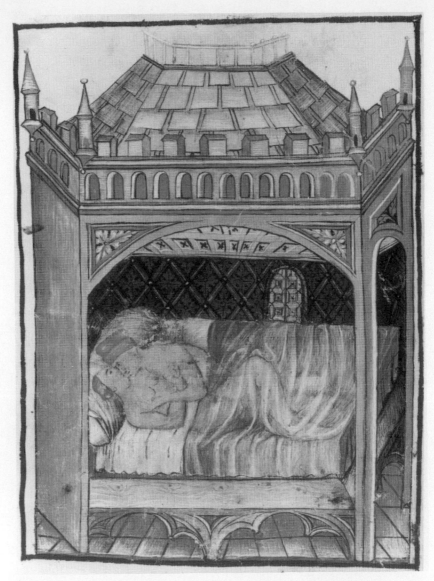

"Coytus": a depiction of sexual union from a fourteenth-century treatise on health. The text says that the purpose of coitus is to preserve the species, but it can be harmful to those with a cold and dry nature. The harmful effects can be offset by eating sperm-producing foods. (Paris, Bibliothèque nationale, nouv. acq. lat. MS 1673, fol. 100v)

was unknown. Instead, on the basis of what we moderns understand about the physiology of the reproductive process, the ancients' practice of the rhythm method would be not only ineffective but counterproductive. Their period for infertile intercourse was part of the period when it would actually have been more fertile.

Vaginal Suppositories

The use of vaginal suppositories (pessaries) is frequently recommended in the medical sources as a means of both preventing conception and causing abortion. Keith Hopkins, who studied contraception during antiquity, believes that some of the suppositories may have been effective because some of the substances are resins that would have mechanically blocked the mouth of the cervix. Other substances in the prescriptionary formulas may have altered the acidity or alkalinity (pH) in the vaginal chemistry and therefore acted as spermicides.[24] More recently Danielle Gourevitch, who has studied medieval gynecology, suggested that suppositories may have had only limited efficacy.[25] No one who has commented on this subject asserts that this means of birth control was sufficient to account for the demographic profiles. It is believed only that vaginal suppositories could have had some degree of effectiveness and thus were a contributing factor.

Abortion

Abortions were always available.[26] The degree to which they may have limited population historically is not clearly known. Late-term abortions induced by drugs or by manipulation were often dangerous to the mother, and the Greco-Roman medical literature cautioned and sometimes counseled against it.[27] The well-known line from the Hippocratic oath regarding abortions was, despite its fame, not generally followed by ancient physicians. For that matter, not only do we not know who swore to its principles, it is also not entirely obvious what the oath means. The oath did not prohibit one who swore to its tenets from administering an abortion. It prohibited the administration of an abortive suppository, or pessary. Following a statement that the physician will neither administer a poison nor advise its use, the next line reads: ὁμοίως δὲ οὐδὲ γυναικὶ πεσσὸν φθόριον δώσω. It has been translated, "Similarly I will not give to a woman an abortive remedy" and "Neither will I give a woman means to procure an abortion." Closer to the literal meaning, however, is ". . . give a suppository to cause an abortion."[28] Even the great medical historian W. H. S. Jones, who correctly translated the passage and knew that only a pessary was specified, nonetheless interpreted its broader meaning to include a prohibition of abortion in any form.[29]

A misunderstanding about what was in the oath concerning abortion began long before our era, however. In the first century A.D. Scribonius Largus, a Roman medical writer, said, "Hippocrates, who founded our profession [*nostrae professionis*], laid the foundation for our discipline by an oath in which it was proscribed not to give to a pregnant woman a kind of medicine [*medicamentum*] that expels the embryo/fetus [*quo conceptum excutitur*]." [30] Two reasons may account for Scribonius' reading the Hippocratic oath incorrectly. Possibly he allowed the Stoic values of his own day to color his reading of the oath. Or Scribonius may have received an incorrect text of the oath, one rewritten to fit the Stoic or some other philosophy. In the latter case, Scribonius would have been guiltless. Placing the statement about the oath in the context of his subsequent statements, however, reveals that Scribonius had a strong pronatal philosophy. In summarizing Hippocrates' belief that medicine was the art of healing, not of doing harm ("scientia enim sanandi, non nocendi est medicina"), he said that Hippocrates protected even the potential for being a person. "How much greater the moral crime [*nefas*]," he asked, "to permit injury to one who is complete than harm the dubious hope for humanity?" [31] By this statement Scribonius plainly reveals that he interpreted the Greek writer to be against abortion (and, possibly, contraception). Also let us not overlook the inference that the expected means of abortions were drugs.

Whatever the reason for his misreading of the oath, Scribonius is but one of many over the centuries who have misunderstood the oath and its statement on abortion. A third-century A.D. papyrus text of the oath justifies the reading of abortive suppositories and therefore stands contrary to Scribonius' earlier reading.[32] Scribonius' misreading has survived in modern times. The error became particularly important in the nineteenth century, when so many states passed antiabortion laws based in part on the misreading of the oath and thus of a doctor's sacred obligations (see chapter 14).

Later the Arabs were under no delusion about the correct Greek text for the oath. An Arabic translation preserved by Ibn Ali Usaybia (d. 1269) reads, "Nor will I contemplate administering any pessary which may cause abortion." [33] Abu al-Hasan al-Tabib advocated abortion in pregnancies if the woman was under fifteen, because of the small uterus and the health risk to the mother. To justify his position he said, "This is the reason Hippocrates demands the use of abortive drugs before childbirth." [34]

Two medieval Latin translations of the oath preserve both traditions; one prohibits abortion completely, and the more literal one restricts the procedure to pessaries.[35] The first, found in a thirteenth-century manuscript, reads, "Neither [will I give] to a pregnant woman a protacted drink [*potio*] for killing a conceived fetus [*conceptum fetum*]." Note that the meaning is unmistakable. The use of the phrase *conceptus fetus* makes clear that there is no intended distinction between a *conceptus* and a *fetus*. Also, in using the word *potio,* meaning "a drink," the translator assumed that the means of receiving an abortion was oral. The second translation, found in a manuscript copied in 1380, is literally translated from the Greek as we know it: "Similarly [will I not give] to a woman an improper pessary [*pessarium corruptivum*]." Although we do not know when these translations were made, the evidence points to a corruption of the text as early as the first century A.D.

Theodorus Priscianus (fl. late fourth century A.D.) began a chapter in his book on gynecology with the statement, "It is not right [*fas*] for anyone to give an abortion." The statement of Hippocrates, he said, made it a matter of honor for a physician not to engage in the practice. Theodorus observed, however, that it is often a matter of life or death that a pregnant woman not bear children, in which case, abortifacients are available (which he proceeded to detail).[36] The point here is that Theodorus thought that the Hippocratic oath prohibited abortion, and thus his reading was similar to Scribonius's interpretation.

It is curious that the Greek and Latin church fathers who spoke against abortion did not invoke Hippocrates to sustain their position. Quite to the contrary, the Latin father Tertullian (c. A.D.160–c. 225) accused Hippocrates of possessing (hence presumably using) one of the brutal surgical instruments designed to dismember the fetus.[37] Scribonius and Theodorus notwithstanding, when combined with the fact that other church fathers fail to mention Hippocrates as being against abortion, Tertullian's accusation suggest that Hippocrates and his followers were indeed associated with abortion procedures.

Soranus (early second century A.D.) had no misunderstanding about the oath on this subject. In his work on gynecology, he is the second writer we know of in antiquity specifically to cite the oath. He understood the text one way but cited it another. Soranus' reading is, "I will give to no one an abortive."[38] Soranus interpreted Hippocrates to be referring to drug-induced abortions because he knew the section in the Hippocratic treatise that prescribed a method to induce an abortion by manipulation. In the treatise *On the Nature of the Child* (attributed to Hippocrates), the author advocated the so-called Lacedaemonian leap, that is "leaping with the heels to the buttocks for the sake of expulsion."[39] The literal meaning of the Hippocratic oath as we presently possess its text is that the one taking the oath swears not to administer an abortive suppository. The implicit meaning is that a physician was free to employ contraceptives, oral abortifacients, and the various surgical and manipulative procedures available.

The citation of Hippocrates might suggest that Soranus was not acquainted with other Hippocratic works that advanced specific abortifacient drugs, but this does not seem to be the case. Even though Soranus said that drug-induced abortions were dangerous, he gave specific recipes for drug abortifacients, some of which were directly or indirectly from various Hippocratic works (discussed in Chapter 8). One of the recipes, a vaginal suppository (details in Chapter 3), he said could be taken to abort "with relatively little danger." [40] Also Soranus recognized that early abortions, those within the first thirty days after conception, were relatively easy. Soranus said that one should merely follow the opposite regimen of procedures, exercises, diet and so forth that he gave to avoid a miscarriage. [41]

Throughout I make frequent reference to ancient, medieval, and modern sources on practical means to induce abortion. Surgical or manipulated abortions were recognized as dangerous. The survival of surgical instruments and surgical texts describing the procedure, however, clearly shows that the Mediterranean and European world, whatever the time, employed abortions to control births, but their presence does not speak to the circumstances. [42] The agreement in the sources about abortion's dangers, notably in late-term abortions, causes modern historians to believe that resort to them was avoided unless the situation was truly desperate. The various medical and social sources present little evidence that abortions were routinely employed for birth control.

Suzanne Dixon enters a caution here, because she observes that all of the negative comments about abortion in antiquity came from "the public male attitude." [43] The principles of ancient law bear out this principle. In the code of Hammurabi (1728–1686 B.C.) a person causing a seigneur's daughter to abort by receiving a blow is fined "ten shekels of silver for her fetus." [44] A later Assyrian law prescribed a penalty of impalement to a woman for procuring her own abortion—and, it added, she shall be buried. [45] In Chapter 10 below I will discuss Roman and Germanic laws, which had as their judicial assumption the rights of family heads to receive children whom they fathered. Neither ancient nor early medieval law protected women, except in some cases against malpractice from a second party (such as a physician or magician).

An extensive report in 1953 by the United Nations concerned the elements determining population trends, this just a couple years before the contraceptive pill was introduced. It concluded that abortion was not an important factor in limiting family size in most countries when compared with the results of contraception. [46]

Infanticide

Infanticide is the explanation for population limitation before A.D. 1750 that commands the greatest attention among scholars. Ancient law protected neither the fetus nor the newborn infant until there was acceptance by the parents, often by some ritualized tribal or community registration.[47] In contrast, during the Middle Ages, religious and sometimes secular law spoke against exposure of infants.

The primary reason for accepting the infanticide theory is that some data from antiquity and the Middle Ages show (or are interpreted as showing) a higher male-female ratio than one would expect in a biologically neutral environment free from interferences. The argument runs: children had to be born before their sex was known; in the premodern period there were more males born than females; biologically, we would expect a male-female ratio closer to 1:1; we know that premoderns practiced some form(s) of birth control; therefore the means of population control practiced was infanticide. During the ancient period, theories vary from denying that the data reflect an infanticide biased against females to believing that a higher male population is natural in certain premodern and modern conditions.[48] One theory argues human intervention; the other, biological normative conditions.

Donald Engels argues that the data and the paucity of evidence in literary texts show that infanticide during antiquity was not extensive. His hypothesis is based in part on the supposition that, if one in five females (20 percent) was exposed, the replacement rate would have had short-term drastic consequences to the socioeconomic fabric, which we know did not happen.[49] As we observed earlier, the birth rate diminished gradually, not dramatically, over centuries. William V. Harris challenges Engels' hypothesis by countering that (1) a female exposure rate of less than 20 percent could be postulated, (2) leading historians, notably P. A. Brunt (*Italian Manpower*) [1971]), accepted the evidence for extensive infanticide, and (3) modern anthropological studies show that in some contemporary traditional societies, where a comparable sex ratio is prevalent, the cause is attributable to infanticide.[50] Mark Golden contends that the exposure of females in classical Athens was higher than 10 percent.[51] Many distinguished historians and classicists have joined sides in refuting Engels' claims, including Sarah B. Pomeroy, Richard Feen, and Ruth Oldenziel.[52] Pomeroy's study *Women in Hellenistic Egypt* (1984), however, observes that the only evidence of exposure in Ptolemaic Egypt is a law prescribing a certain number of days of purification after abortion, childbirth, and child exposure.[53] The papyrus documents from Egypt, to be sure, provide us with by far the most abundant documentation of ancient social life.

Advocates of the infanticide hypothesis always cite an earlier papyrus in which a man writes to his wife, "I urge and entreat you to be careful of the child . . . if it is male, let it be, if it is a female, expose it." [54] The meaning is clear, but the question is how accurate a generalization can be made on the basis of this one, albeit dramatic, piece of evidence.[55]

Whatever the situation in antiquity in regard to infanticide (in particular, of females), the Middle Ages definitely deplored infanticide. Prior to Christianity, Tacitus informs us that the Germans did not practice infanticide.[56] By observing its absence among the Germans, however, Tacitus implied that it was practiced by the Romans. Some infanticide activity by the ancients is acknowledged. The question is the extent of usage and whether it was at a level that affected gross population.

Most historians doubt, however, that there was extensive infanticide during the Middle Ages. Positioned against the conventional opinion is Josiah Russell, a respected medieval demographer, who says that, despite the "apparent strength" of the church, "infanticide must have continued to keep the population from increasing."[57] Agreeing with Russell's position are Yves Brissaud and Barbara Kellum. The former, however, admits that there is only slight evidence for his conclusion. Brissaud's study of letters of remission for crimes in Poitou between 1302 and 1502 shows that only eleven, or less than 1 percent, deal with infanticide.[58] After searching the literary evidence, Kellum asserts, "The rivers and latrines of medieval Europe 'resound with cries of children who have been plunged into them.' "[59]

If there was extensive infanticide during the Middle Ages, one would expect a higher ratio of males to females. Although there is a differential, it is slight, or so says Barbara Hanawalt.[60] Her study of late medieval peasant families acknowledges the lack of evidence for infanticide during the Middle Ages and concludes that the practice was rare.[61] In a prodigious search for evidence, John Boswell argues that an important factor was simply abandonment of children, but even here the evidence is surprisingly slight to maintain such a hypothesis.[62]

The higher ratio of males is evident in data from Florence, London, Berlin, Amsterdam, and twentieth-century United States, as shown by the following.

Place	Period	Males per 100 females
Florence	1451–1470	104.2
	1731–1750	103.7
London	1664–1670	108.1
	1785–1787	106.7
Berlin	1722–1731	105.6
	1787	111.0
Amsterdam	1700–1719	110.6
	1720–1739	106.9[63]
United States (aggregate)	1900	104.4
	1910	106.0
	1920	104.0
	1930	102.5[64]

If there were no interference with the biology of births and survival in early infancy, the expectation is that the ratio should be approximately 1.05, a figure based on twentieth-century global figures and a general consensus among demographers.[65] Because of complex factors, however, small variations within a narrow band are not sufficiently meaningful to draw conclusions. Any figure above 1.10 calls into question the registration of females.[66]

The modern figures above do not take into consideration such factors as migration and war. Given these factors, the above statistics show no pattern of extensive sex bias in raising children. Since in a biologically neutral environment approximately twenty-one males are born for every twenty females, we cannot conclude that a slightly higher ratio of males in antiquity shows significant infanticide practices.

If these and other statistics reflect a practice of sexual bias, there is no necessity to assume infanticide, or (to use the ancients' term) exposure. A recent study in Bangladesh maintains that the data showing more males than females reflects a differential in infant care with a prejudice toward males.[67] Other studies elsewhere sustain this hypothesis. There are indications that relative neglect for a second-born child or for one sex may even be attributable to unconscious parental conduct.[68] Perhaps it is more plausible to accuse ancient and medieval peoples of sexually biased child care than to charge them with murder, as we do in speaking of their practicing infanticide.

Historical data from Germany support the finding that variations in sex ratios do not necessarily point to infanticide. Marriage cohorts among three subpopulations (farmers, smallholders, and landless) were examined in the northwestern German town of Krummhörn between 1689 and 1820. Among farmers, the number of males born per 100 females was 116.2, the highest among the three groups. (These figures are supposedly for live births.) The infant and child mortality rate, however, was higher for males than for females, as the following figures indicate.

Subpopulation	Males surviving to age 15 (%)	Females surviving to age 15 (%)
Farmers	43.5	69.9
Smallholders	46.1	59.6
Landless	50.6	54.5

The authors of this study, Eckart Voland and Eva Siegelkow, believe that social factors led to a bias favoring better care for females.[69]

This brings us back to the question of whether differentials in sex ratios are evidence for extensive infanticide. Both recent evidence from the modern period and the historical records we possess from the distant past suggest they are not.

Paleopathology and Infanticide

Using increasingly sophisticated techniques, the field of paleopathology, with its subfield paleodemography, provides important clues about life and death in bygone days. In the examination of ancient skeletons, especially in graveyards containing a large number of specimens, we can learn about age composition, mortality at different stages of life, longevity of the sexes, ratio of children to adults, average height and probable weight, particular diseases (such as arthritis, certain cancers, and anemia), effects of nutrition, and, as we have already seen, sex ratios. Skeletal evidence is supplemented by microscopic and chemical analysis of other organic artifacts at a habitation site, such as garbage deposits, sewerage remains, and fragmental survivals of soft tissue, even blood, in mummies and peat bogs. J. Lawrence Angel, an American pathologist, and Mirko D. Grmek, a French physician-historian, are major pioneers and contributors to the field in discovering the data by developing techniques for examination and assessing the evidence.[70] Their studies are helpful in informing us about the use of birth control devices, but they are also controversial.

Consider first the evidence that is less controversial. In the eastern Mediterranean, especially among Greek populations (but not restricted to them), the population density increased until about the fifth century B.C., and then, as we have seen, after a few centuries of relative stability, the density decreased. In sharp contrast, the average life span for females was around 31 years from 11,000 B.C. (North African population sample) to 5800 B.C. (Nea Kikomedeia site). Males show an increase in average age from 27 to 30. Comparing females buried at Karatas in 2400 B.C., Lerna in 1750 B.C., and Athens and Corinth in the period 650–350 B.C., we see that the average life span increased from approximately 33 (Karatas) to 37 (Lerna) to 45 (Athens-Corinth), while for males the comparable figures are relatively flat—from 30 to 35 years.[71] Near the first century B.C., a female's life span in the Mediterranean world and in Britain (where comparable figures are available) hits a similar peak of the 45 found at Athens-Corinth and the 36.6 in the Hellenistic-Roman world around 300 B.C. From this relative high, the average female life span in the same regions declined, and it is not until the second half of the nineteenth century that the average of the classical period is surpassed.[72] In all periods, there is a relatively high mortality rate for women during the childbearing years of fifteen to forty in comparison with their male cohorts. Menarche in classical times was between ages thirteen and fourteen.[73]

Therefore, to summarize, at the period when women lived longer and had longer periods of pregnancy liability, the population numbers appear steady and, according to evidence presented above, begin to decline. The data for the average life spans represent only a minuscule number of the people who lived, and as more studies are done, these figures are likely to change. I suspect that they will be revised upward toward a longer life. As we understand them now, however, the long-term trends coincide with other historical data, and probably the trends themselves are acceptable evidence.

This brings us to the controversial evidence. Female skeletons have three features that may indicate the number of full-term pregnancies: (1) dorsal pitting of the pubic plate, (2) scarring of the preauricular groove, and (3) scarring of the groove for the interosseous ligament. When parturition occurs, one or more of these features are produced. Hypothetically, one can study the dorsal pits on a female pubis and determine the number of births she had. From the study of female public bones, J. Lawrence Angel calculates that Middle Bronze Age women around 2000 B.C. averaged 5.0 births; then there is a decline: 4.7 births are osseo-recorded on females alive around 1500 B.C., 4.1 around 1150 B.C., and 3.6 around 300 B.C., and 3.3 around A.D. 120 in imperial Rome.[74] Sarah Bisel's data derived from skeletons at Herculaneum (A.D. 79) show that the mean number of births per menopausal woman was 1.81.[75] Admittedly, these Roman women had died at the same time and included women who, had they not been killed by volcanic eruption, would have lived to have more children. Even so, the birth rate figure is smaller than one would expect.

If the method of determining births by pubic lesions was reliable, we would have hard evidence to show that infanticide was not the significant factor in affecting gross population size because the marks supposedly record births. Considerable doubt, however, has been raised about the precision of this evidence. Researchers have studied the pubic bones of modern American females, comparing the markings with the number of births each is known to have had. According to one study, there is only a weak correlation between the markings and the number of full-term pregnancies.[76] Another study (Kelley 1979) found that the most sensitive indicator of parturition is the preauricular groove, but that all marks can become obliterated in old age. At this time the burden of the evidence supports the conclusion that the markings are reliable indicators in distinguishing females who have had a full-term pregnancy from those who have not, but not as a precise indicator of the number of births, as Angel, Grmek, Bisel, and others claim.[77]

Whether such claims are eventually sustained or not, the alleged facts do correspond with the aggregate data found in the historical sources and in archaeological remains. We can only conclude that classical peoples were somehow regulating their family sizes.

CHAPTER TWO

Evidence for Oral Contraceptives and Abortifacients

No lovemaking of gods can be in vain.

Homer, *Odyssey*, 11.249–250
(Ann Hanson, trans.)

In 1936 Norman Himes published a history of contraceptives. For the classical period he concluded, first, that oral contraceptives ("potions") were not effective and, second, that the knowledge of the few other contraceptive devices that worked (specifically, vaginal suppositories) was "confined largely to the heads of medical encyclopedists, to a few physicians and scholars."[1] In the coming chapters, I suggest that their knowledge was primarily transmitted by a network of women working within the culture of their sex and that only occasionally was some of it learned by medical writers, almost all of whom were male.

P. A. Brunt states clearly that "it must . . . be regarded as doubtful whether any form of contraception was either usual or effective in limiting families in ancient Italy."[2] Norman Himes, J. Knodel, E. van de Walle, and Philippe Ariès agree that existing birth control devices could not have worked sufficiently well to affect historical demography.[3] Marie-Thérèse Fontanille sees a possible "danger démographique" if the drugs had some efficacy because, she suggests, the mortality of women attempting desperate poisonous drugs may account for a "mortalité féminine catastrophique."[4] Her assumption is based on the unsubstantiated belief that any antifertility action by the herbs would be because of their toxicity. Ariès argues for the virtual absence of contraception in medieval Europe before the seventeenth century because of its inconceivability ("l'impensabilité".[5] Supposedly the Christians joined the Stoics in banishing the thought.

In contrast, John Noonan, a Catholic canonist and historian, gives numerous examples in religious, legal, and other sources to the effect that contraception was not only understood but generally strongly discouraged.[6] Keith Hopkins holds out a possibility that contraceptives "might have had some limiting effect upon the fertility of the Romans," but he sees limited effectiveness only in the actions of vaginal suppositories.[7] Danielle Gourevitch dismisses oral contraceptives but advances the possibility that some suppositories may have worked.[8] In respect to oral contraceptives, modern scholars disbelieve what the ancients thought possible. In contrast, Noonan argues that the contraceptives must have had some effect simply on the basis of their persistence in historical records over long periods of time, but he could not cite evidence for their efficacy.

The demographic depression that occurred in western Europe between the 1430s and the 1480s may have been caused by ergotism from a contaminated supply of rye bread, which in turn reduced fertility.[9] Ergot is an alkaloid produced in some kinds of cereals, and one of its effects is fertility suppression. Others are more dramatic, including tremors, spasms, hallucinations, paralysis, and even death.[10] The organism is a fungus (*Claviceps purpurea* Fries) that is especially active on a strain of rye (*Secale cereale* L.), a type of cereal that for periods was especially prevalent in England and Russia. In order to grow, however, the microorganism needs optimum conditions—notably, cold weather in winter and spring and warm summers, conditions prevalent in northern Europe during certain periods. The correlation between birth and fatality rates between 1660 and 1739 is highly significant when compared with temperature and climatic conditions favorable for ergot alkaloid production.[11] In the nineteenth century, European medicine knew about the action of ergotine alkaloids and sometimes used them for abortion.[12] There is no evidence, however, that premodern populations could control the concentration and amount of ergot in order to produce a pharmacological result. While there are periods in history, notably in Russia and England, during which ergot contamination of the bread is suspected of producing low fertility, there is no evidence that the action was the product of a deliberate use of the chemical for birth control. Quite the contrary, lacking the knowledge of microorganisms, premodern people had no means of controlling ergot production and therefore could not depend on it. For a chemical to be a birth control agent, it had to be available and dependable.

The evidence for the concept and existence of contraceptives and abortifacients that were deliberately used is clearly and abundantly in the records. Moreover, classical and medieval peoples believed that they worked. In *Laws,* Plato discussed the measures that could be followed to ensure population stability. "There are many devices available: if too many children are being born, there are measures to check propagation; on the other hand, a high birthrate can be encouraged and stimulated by conferring marks of distinction or disgrace."[13] Although Plato does not specify the measures to be used, he plainly thought that fertility was manageable. In another work, *Theaetetus,* Plato has Socrates say regarding midwives: "And furthermore, the midwives, by means of drugs [φαρμάκια] and incantations, are able to arouse the pangs of labor and, if they wish, to make them milder, and to cause those to bear who have difficulty in bearing; and they cause abortions [ἀμβλίσκουσιν] at an early stage if they think them desirable." To which Theaetetus predictably replies, "True."[14]

Aristotle also considered population control desirable and, in writing about an ideal city, was only a little less vague than Plato was in the *Laws:* "if conception occurs in excess of the limit so fixed, . . . have abortion induced before sense and life have begun in the embryo."[15] Because Aristotle disapproved of abortions after the fetus had formed, implicitly he was calling for either contraceptives or early stage abortifacients (that is, before the middle of the second trimester) as the means of birth control in the wisely led city. Polybius spoke of families in Greece in the second century B.C. limiting children to one or two, and that, he said, was not enough for growth.[16] Musonius Rufus, in an apparent reference to Augustan legislation in 18 B.C. and A.D. 9 that encouraged births (or at least child rearing), said:

> The lawgivers, who had the same task of searching out and finding what was good for the city and what bad, and what helped or harmed it, did not they also consider that it was most beneficial to their cities to fill the houses of the citizens, and most harmful to deplete them? They considered that childlessness, or small families, of citizens was unprofitable, while to have children, and in fact many children, was profitable. Therefore they forbade the women to abort and attached a penalty to those who disobeyed; secondly they forbade them to use contraceptives on themselves and to prevent pregnancy; finally they established honors for both men and women who had many children and made childlessness punishable.[17]

Rufus' curious statement is clearly based on a misunderstanding of the legislation. Whereas the objectives were to encourage fertility and child rearing, no other sources refer to a prohibition of contraceptives.[18] Indeed, had such a provision been there, it would have been unenforceable because the Roman government neither regulated drug trade nor could have done so. In the case of contraceptives and early stage abortifacients, the plants were too common and therefore readily available. The relevant point here is that Musonius viewed contraceptives as a reason for low fertility.

Indeed, Musonius said that contraception was one of the two reasons, the other being abortion. He knew that the intent of the legislation was to increase fertility, and he thought that a reason for the low fertility was the use of contraceptives. Musonius' error supports the point that contraceptives were important in checking population growth.

In a sermon around A.D. 390 John Chrysostom decried those who used contraceptives (ἀτόκια), likening the practice to sowing a field in order to destroy fruit (καρπός) and raising the question whether it was not the same as murder.[19] In order to look pretty, Chrysostom said, women resort to incantations, love potions, and countless other things, and drugs are prepared not against the uterus of a prostitute but against the uterus of an injured wife. Jerome condemned those who "drank sterility [*sterilitas*] and murder those not yet conceived," while others use poison to destroy those yet to be born.[20] Mincius Felix condemned those "women who, by drinking medicaments and drinks, extinguish the source of the future man in their very bowels and thus commit a parricide before they bring forth."[21] Finally, the entire purpose of the elaborate and expensive Alimentary Laws that were enacted in the first century and periodically reintroduced or refinanced was to encourage the begetting, birth, and raising of children. By giving cash incentives to families, the government's presumption was that people could be persuaded to be fertile, something the Roman masses were not willing to do if left to themselves.[22] The historical population studies support the opinion of the people of the time that fertility was being controlled.

Birth Control in Judaica

In Judaic scripture, the Talmud, Tosefta, and Midrash, abortions and "root potions" for sterility are frequently enough mentioned that we can assume the practices must have been widespread and, to some degree, acceptable.[23] What the "root potions" were is left unspecified. The Babylonian Talmud, *Yebamoth*, records: "A man is commanded concerning the duty of propagation but not a woman. R. Johanan b. Beroka, however, said: Concerning both of them it is said, and God blessed them; and God said unto them: 'Be fruitful, and multiply.' Rabbi Ile replied to this statement, "It is the nature of man to *subdue*, but it is not the nature of a woman to subdue."[24]

The rabbinic interpretation is that because men are the sexual aggressors, they may not employ contraceptives. Women, however, who must suffer pregnancy, childbirth, and child rearing, are excused by God from the command to be fruitful. The case is cited under the heading, "A man is commanded concerning the duty of propagation, but not a woman." Judith, the wife of Rabbi Hiyya, came to him after a difficult childbirth ("agonizing pains") and asked, "Is a woman commanded to propagate the race?" When he replied in the negative, she went and drank סַמָא דְּעַקַרְתָּא , *samā d-ʿaqartā* (medicine, potion, or poison that makes one sterile or barren). When Rabbi Hiyya learned of her actions, he lamented that she had not given him one more birthing.[25] Rabbi Aha ben Rabbi Qattina also held that the commandment to be fruitful does not apply to women.[26] This rabbinic ruling is significant because it indicates approval of oral contraceptives. In the phrase *samā' d-ʿaqartā* the root *'qr* has the semantic range of rootlessness, and hence extirpation; to harm by castration, hamstringing, and mutilation, cutting off some vital part; to conceal; to pluck up or harvest (from Eccles. 3:2); to be barren (as of Sarah in Gen. 11:30).[27] The Latin word *sterilis* (adjective) or *sterilitas* (noun) conveys the same meaning as the Hebrew *'qr* and was often employed by Christian writers.

When Is the Soul a Soul?

The Hebrew text for Exodus 21:23 seems to accept abortion implicitly in punishing it (*nefesh taḥat nefesh,* "life is given for life") only if the mother dies because of the procedure. The Septuagint translates the passage as δώσει ψυχὴν ἀντὶ ψυχῆς, which means that the penalty ("life for life") is imposed *after* the conceptus is "formed." The key Hebrew word is *nefesh;* it is sometimes translated "soul" or "self," but it means "soul" in our modern, theological sense only because of Hellenistic influence on rabbinic, speculative theology: "Thou shalt give soul for soul. . . ."[28] It is an example of how the Greek translation supplied a new meaning to the original passage, and from the Greek the interpretation was passed into Latin and modern languages. With the passage of centuries, the Hebrew meaning was lost.

For the most part, the Greek and Latin church fathers accepted the Septuagint/Old Latin interpretation as making a distinction between a formed and an unformed fetus (Exod. 21:22). Using the same vocabulary that was in the Latin translation of Exodus 21:22, Augustine wrote, "If what is brought forth is unformed [*informe*], but at this stage some sort of living, shapeless thing [*informiter*], then the law of homicide would not apply, for it could not be said that there was a living soul in that body, for it lacks all sense, if it be such as is not yet formed [*nondum formata*] and therefore not yet endowed with its senses."[29] Gregory of Nyssa (c. 330–395) expressed the same sentiments when he wrote that the unformed embryo could not be considered a human being.[30]

While Augustine and Gregory expressed what were apparently majority sentiments, Basil (c. 330–379), bishop of Caesarea, called feticide murder at any point of development.

> She who has deliberately destroyed a fetus has to pay the penalty of murder. And there is no exact inquiry among us as to whether the fetus was formed or unformed [ἐκμεμορφωμένου καὶ ἀνεξεικονίστου]. For here it is not only the child to be born that is vindicated, but also the woman herself who made an attempt against her own life, because usually the women die in such attempts. Furthermore, added to this is the destruction of the embryo, another murder, at least according to the intention of those who dare these things. Nevertheless, we should not prolong their penance until death, but should accept a term of ten years, and we should determine the treatment not by time, but by the manner of repentance.[31]

Although Basil here says that feticide is the same as murder, he mitigates the punishment and recommends compassion and a lesser repentance. His sentiments appear to be grounded more in the Stoic value of potentiality to become a human (to be discussed later) than in the Scriptures.

Eventually, Hebrew, Greek, and Roman thought came nearly together on the point that prior to the fetus forming, feticide was not homicide. There was never absolute uniform opinion, however, in Hellenic, Hellenistic, or Roman thought, in pagan philosophy, Judaism, or Christianity.

The question about the soul of the fetus was posed initially by the Greeks, argued by Stoics, and later answered affirmatively by Jews and Christians. Aristotle suggested in one place that the conceptus had a "soul" (ψυχή, meaning "life" or "animation") after forty days from conception if a male, ninety if female (for a similar differentiation , see Lev. 12:1–5); elsewhere, however, he stated that the fetus develops "little by little" and that one cannot make fine judgments.[32]

The Stoics believed that soul (ψυχή) came when the fetus was exposed to cool air, although the potential was present at conception.[33] The idea of cooling air at birth giving rise to the soul was ridiculed by Plutarch, the Greek, and by Tertullian, the Christian. The latter asked what happened to souls in hot climates or warm bedrooms, or whether, since if the air is too cool, the infant dies, anybody could be born north of the Scythians and the Germans.[34]

Aristotle's position that the soul came when the fetus is formed is of critical importance. Augustine of Hippo wrote about Aristotle's position: "If the embryo is still unformed, but yet in some way ensouled while unformed . . . the law does not provide that the act pertains to homicide, because still there cannot be said to be a live soul in a body that lacks sensation, if it is in flesh not yet formed and thus not yet endowed with senses."[35] Jewish rabbinic thought borrows from the same Hellenistic tradition that influenced Augustine. In the Jerusalem Talmud there is the following query and series of answers:

At what point is the presence of the foetus recognized?

Sumkhos says in the name of R. Meir, "In three months, even though there is no clear proof of that proposition, there is at least an indication of it: 'And it came to pass at the end of three months'" (Gen. 38:24).

Said R. Yudan, "And even if she is pregnant only with air: 'We were with child, we writhed, we have as it were brought forth wind'" (Is. 26:18). "'You conceive chaff, you bring forth stubble' (Is. 33:11)."

R. Zeira, R. Ba bar Zutra, R. Haninah in the name of R. Hiyya the Great: "Even if [the fetus is discernible] in the greater part of the first month, and for the greater part of the first month, and for the greater part of the last month [if] the middle [month] is complete, [we deem the three months' rule to apply—that is, after only sixty-two days]."

R. Assis says, "Ninety days, complete."[36]

The Babylonian Talmud has an exchange between Antoninus, a pagan, and a rabbi who admits to having his opinions changed by Antoninus's logic. "Antoninus also said to Rabbi, 'When is the soul placed in man: as soon as it is decreed [that the sperm shall be male or female, etc.] or when [the embryo] is actually formed?' He replied, 'From the moment of formation.' He objected: 'Can a piece of meat be unsalted for three days without becoming putrid? But it must be from the moment that [God] decrees [its destiny].' Rabbi said: 'This thing Antoninus taught me.'"[37] Antoninus is arguing that a person could no more live without a soul from the point of conception than meat could avoid becoming putrified if left unsalted. Stephen Newmyer believes that this passage indicates that rabbinic thought was adopting the Stoic concept of the soul's potential existence from the point of conception.[38] The above exchange is followed by this question: "From what time does the Evil Tempter hold sway over man; from the formation [of the embryo] or from [its] issuing forth [into the light of the world]?" Antoninus replied to the rabbi, "It is from when it issues."[39] In other words, when it takes its first breath of cold air.

Noonan, Himes, and Feen cite the numerous instances in Hebrew, Greek, and Latin sources in which the subjects of abortion and contraception are encountered, and they see no consensus in antiquity about when it was morally wrong to contracept potentially fertile intercourse or to abort once fertilization had occurred. The Stoics had a notion of potentiality at conception but believed that the soul was not present until birth. Aristotle's position was more definite, but still it was not definitive. Marie-Thérèse Fontanille believes that the time interval that at least some of the ancients saw between conception and "animation" ("quickening," it will be called later) was a zone for action without incurring moral or legal wrong. There was an imprecise difference between when the fetus was formed according to Aristotle and when quickening occurred, but the difference was too subjective for precise legal or theological distinc-

tions. Between conception and animation was a window for action by the female. For this reason contraception and early abortions were acceptable.[40] Hebrew religious law allowed for a period of up to thirty days before a fetus was potentially viable. A woman was not to be regarded as pregnant until forty days after conception.[41]

Classical Attitudes

For medical reasons, it was evident to Hippocratic writers, Soranus, Oribasius, Paul of Aegina, and other medical writers that early abortion was preferable to late. Indeed, a woman who took an emmenagogue or abortifacient during the first month of pregnancy would not be able to observe whether there had been fertilization or delayed menstruation. After some months, the fetus's form is observable and the danger of abortion to the mother is greater. The Mishnah says, "If the abortion was a foetus filled with water or filled with blood or filled with variegated matter, she need not take thought for it as for [human] young; but if its [human] parts were fashioned, she must continue [unclean the number of days prescribed] both for a male and for a female." [42] An inscription known as the *Lex cathartica* from Cyrene, dated 331–326 B.C., cites a woman who aborts a fetus whose features are distinct as incurring an impurity, but one who aborted a fetus with indistinct features did not incur pollution.[43]

Clearly Hebrew, Greek, and Roman law did not protect the fetus, but there was a religious distinction made at the point when the fetus had formed recognizable features. Before that point women could either contracept or abort without religious or legal sanction. There were cases where the father had some legal interest in the decision[44] and where a physician or *pharmakos* who gave *pharmakeia* (drugs, poisons) was denounced and, at times, legally punished (or so said the law) for a procedure that resulted in harm to the mother. Neither convention nor the law protected the unborn and the unconceived.[45] According to convention and the law, ancient women could employ contraceptives and early stage abortifacients virtually without consequences. The same was true in medieval Islam and to some degree in Christian society during the Middle Ages. The question is whether they knew the agents to control fertility and how effective these agents were.

Modern explanations have largely ignored chemical means of family planning because, until recent scientific and anthropological findings, we did not believe them to be effective. The writings of the Romans and medieval sources speak often about oral contraceptives. Modern writers, as we noted, have denied the effectiveness of oral contraceptives among the ancients.

Ancient and medieval people often referred to anything as a sterility

poison that intervened between fertile sexual intercourse and the termination of pregnancies.[46] At the same time, the ancients and medieval peoples actually distinguished between contraceptives and abortifacients. One example occurs in an inscription from the first century B.C., from a sanctuary in Philadelphia in the province of Lydia. A devotee named Dionysus described his dream of excluding people who have used "love charms, contraceptives, abortifacients, or others [who] killed infants."[47] Soranus, a writer on gynecology during the time of Trajan (98–117) and Hadrian (117–138), clearly made the distinction. "A contraceptive differs from an abortive [ἀτόκιον δὲ φθορίου διαφέρει], for the first does not let conception [σύλληψιν] take place, while the latter destroys [φθείρει] what has been conceived [σύλληψιν]. Let us therefore call the one 'abortive' [φθόριον] and the other 'contraceptive' [ἀτόκιον] . . . it is safer to prevent conception from taking place than to destroy the fetus."[48]

CHAPTER THREE

Soranus on Antifertility Agents

We've so many sure-fire drugs
for inducing sterility.

Juvenal, *Satire,* 6.595–596

E arly in the second century A.D., Soranus, antiquity's foremost writer on gynecology, clearly distinguished between contraceptives and abortifacients. He included a number of actual prescriptions for birth control, including both vaginal suppositories and oral contraceptives. He began with the suppositories. Although he conceded that contraceptives were preferable to abortifacients, he did not comment on whether suppositories or drugs taken orally were the better of the two. Soranus recommended four oral contraceptives, but warned, "These things not only prevent conception but also destroy any already existing. In our opinion, moreover, the evil from these things is too great, since they damage and upset the stomach, and besides cause congestion of the head and induce sympathetic reactions." [1]

Before analyzing the prescriptions administered orally, let us look first at the suppository recipes, five of which use pomegranate peel or rind (*Punica granatum* L.).[2] Pomegranate is frequently prescribed in classical and medieval medical sources and is recognized as an abortifacient in ancient Indian literature and in modern folk medicine references[3] and, as a contraceptive, in modern science studies.[4] In laboratory experiments using rats, female rats fed pomegranate and paired with males not treated with the plant showed only 72 percent as many pregnancies as the control group; in testing female guinea pigs under the same conditions, none became pregnant. Forty days after drug withdrawal, the fertility of both rats and guinea pigs was restored to normal.[5] Modern testing of pomegranate is incomplete. Different solvents (such as water and alcohol) have not been tested. The parts tested positively come from the fruit skin portion, but certain extracts taken from the seeds, root, and whole plant have shown no antifertility effects.[6] The fruit skin is precisely what Soranus prescribed. The coincidence is too great for this reference not to point to rational usage by rational people. The ancients' pomegranate was, according to their word and ours, an antifertility agent.

Soranus was the first medical writer to prescribe pomegranate for birth control. Similar prescriptions are found in the Hippocratic corpus (to be discussed in Chapter 8), but its use as an antifertility agent appears to have been recognized much earlier than the Hippocratic writers (ca. 430–330 B.C.). The knowledge of the plant's effects went back to the mists of archaic Greek history as preserved in mythology. In the legends, Persephone (Phersephone) was abducted to the underworld by Hades (Pluto), the death god. Her mother (or mother-in-law), Demeter, the goddess who governed the fruits of the earth, asked through Zeus that Persephone be returned so that life might again flourish on earth. Before Hades complied with the wishes of the other gods, he gave Persephone a kernel of pomegranate to eat. This doomed her to the underworld for part of each year. She was obliged to return to the upper world from one-third to one-half of the year. For as many pomegranate kernels as she ate, that many months were given to fall and winter.[7] Curiously, modern scholars have not made the connection that the pomegranate was the substance that kept the virgin goddess Persephone from being fertile.

The other substances in Soranus' suppository recipes will be examined later in the context of works of Aëtius of Amida, in Chapter 4. He said that all the suppository recipes are employed after the termination of menstruation.

Soranus next gave the following four oral prescriptions with the prefatory remarks that "some people" prefer oral contraceptives to the suppositories.

On the other hand to some people it seems advisable once a month to drink Cyrenaic juice [or "sap"; eq *Ferula historica*] in the amount of the size of a chick-pea [= *Cicer arietinum* L.] in two cups of water so as to induce menstruation.

Or, of opopanax [= *Ferula opopanax* Spr.], Cyrenaic juice, and seeds of rue [= *Ruta graveolens* L.] up to two obols [each; 1 obol = 0.8–1.0 g], mold round with wax and give to swallow; then follow with a drink of weak [or diluted] wine or let it be drunk in weak wine.

[Or] the seeds of *leukoion* [= *Matthiola incana* L. and/or *Cheiranthus chieri* L: Cruciferae] and myrtle [*Myrtus communis* L.], three obols each [= ½ drachma]; of myrrh [= *Commiphora myrrha* Engl. + sp.], a drachma [6 obols = 1 drachma = 4.3 g/0.15 oz]; of white pepper [= *Piper nigrum* L., with husks removed], two [seedpods]; give to drink with wine for three days.

[Or] of rocket [= *Eruca sativa* L.] seed, one obol; of cow parsnip [= *Heracleum sphondylium*], one-half obol; drink with oxymel [a vinegar-honey mixture].

However, these things not only prevent conception [συλλήψεως] but also destroy any already existing.[8]

Having listed these recipes, Soranus stated that these were both contraceptives and abortifacients and that they should be avoided because of harmful side effects.[9] In order to evaluate Soranus' prescriptions, we must clarify the definitions of terms. An abortifacient is any agent that terminates pregnancy; the agents that produce this action are called ecbolics, oxytocics, and emmenagogues, in modern medicine. The last is any agent that provokes menstruation, regardless of whether or not a fertilized egg is present and implantation has occurred. The first perceived awareness of pregnancy is an interruption of the menstrual cycle. Amenorrhea—the absence or suppression of menstruation—is commonly caused by a variety of reasons besides pregnancy, including febrile and chronic diseases, malnutrition, and mental depression. A physician, either ancient or modern, or an herbalist would not know the etiology of amenorrhea reported by a patient within, say, the first months of pregnancy unless the physician conducted tests, which were unavailable to ancient and medieval physicians. Idiopathic (genuine) amenorrhea and early pregnancy are difficult to distinguish, especially if a physician did not conduct a careful case history with a patient who was perfectly honest. In classical antiquity, the determination about whether a woman was pregnant came from the woman herself. Helen King, who writes on ancient medicine, remarked that in the Greek culture, where a woman could not even be a witness in a law court, it was commonplace that a woman knew when she had conceived.[10]

For purposes of this paper, I shall use the term "abortifacient" for all forms of pregnancy termination, even those that occur shortly after implantation. Although some religious and ethical doctrines assert that the critical dividing line is the instant that fertilization takes place, the distinction is not the dividing line made in modern medicine; any agent that interferes with the ovary transport, before or after coitus, and prevents or impairs implantation is nonetheless a contraceptive.[11] As we shall see, not until the late nineteenth century did most authorities consider the taking of a menstrual regulator, regardless of whether there is a pregnancy, as an abortifacient. Unless a woman was demonstrably and visibly pregnant, she was not pregnant until she so declared.

In evaluating Soranus' four recipes for oral contraceptives and abortifacients, the first obstacle is determining the meaning of "Cyrenaic juice" in the first two prescriptions. Columella associates Cyrenaic juice with *laser Cyrenaicum* (or *lacer Cyrenaicum* in some texts).[12] References in other classical writers, especially Pliny and Isidore, show that Cyrenaic juice is a species of *Ferula* (English, giant fennel), called by Dioscorides and others σίλφιον or *silphium,* now extinct.[13] Once the plant grew near the Greek city-state of Cyrene in North Africa. In fact, *silphium* made Cyrene famous. Herodotus spoke of the harvesting of the wild plant, and other Greek sources said that attempts to cultivate the plant failed.[14] In 424 B.C. Aristophanes spoke of its high price, and by the first century A.D. Pliny said that it could scarcely be found.[15] For centuries the city's coins had carried the image of the plant, which was its distinctive symbol. One may wonder why a plant would make a city famous. Soranus told us: it was a contraceptive—one of the best in the ancient world. Its popularity, however, drove it to extinction probably soon after Soranus' time.

Closely related to *silphium* is *Ferula assa foetida* L., which the ancients regarded as an inferior substitute for *silphium*. The juice of asafetida's root has an unmistakable—and unforgettable—odor.[16] Dioscorides said that *silphium* was "like ferula" (ἐμφερὴς νάρθηχι [= *Ferula communis* L.]).[17] Asafetida is reported in human tests in 1963 as a contraceptive agent[18] as well as an abortifacient (emmenagogue).[19] Ferujol, the active substance in *Ferula,* has been isolated, and in animal tests it has been nearly 100 percent successful in preventing pregnancy up to three days after coitus at a low dose of 0.6 mg/kg in adult female rats.[20] One species, *Ferula moshchata* Kozo-Polj., is employed in folk medicine in Central Asia as an abortifacient.[21] Because plants of the same family, especially closely associated species, tend to have similar chemistries, we can be reasonably sure that Soranus's Cyrenaic juice was both a contraceptive and an abortifacient. The best of the related plants, the plant found only near Cyrene, was *silphium,* which prevented unwanted pregnancies. It became extinct in part because of its value and restricted habitat.

Besides Cyrenaic juice, the second prescription mentions opopanax, which was once thought to be of the same family and called *Ferula opopanax* Spr. Now the plant is classified as a member of the Pastinaca family, which is closely related to *Ferula*. Its action would be somewhat similar to the other giant fennels.[22] Like asafetida, opopanax was regarded as contraceptive but, again, inferior to *silphium*. In the nineteenth century, opopanax was thought to be an "allied gum-resin" and substitute for *Ferula* resins, with one authority asserting that opopanax was once a species of either *Ferula* or *Opopanax* and that the "botanical source of the genuine opopanax is still unknown."[23] Whatever the plant of antiquity and presumably today, the medical authorities agree that it was kin to the *silphium* or *Ferula* resins.

The third plant in this prescription is rue (*Ruta graveolens* L.), which contains pilocarpine, a substance given to horses to induce abortion.[24] Rue is a traditional abortifacient among the Hispanic people in New Mexico;[25] according to another report, it is used as a tea for abortion purposes throughout Latin America. The same study reports a laboratory study on rats indicating abortifacient activity, but the "clearest effect is a contraceptive one" by preventing implantation.[26] In one animal test, parts of the whole plant were ground up and given to rats, with implantation blocked in 50–60 percent of the animals.[27] Tests in China have identified *yuehchukene* as the active substance in a related species, *Murraya paniculata,* in the same family (*Rutaceae,* or Rue). The substance is 100 percent successful in preventing pregnancies in rats when administered at two mg/kg body weight on pregnancy days 1–6. A single dose at three mg/kg is 100 percent effective on the first day after coitus. It looks promising as a future postcoital interceptor.[28] The prescription would clearly have had an antifertility effect as an abortifacient and a contraceptive.

The third prescription would have been even more effective. It contains *leukoinos,* which is either *Matthiola incana* L. or *Cheiranthus chieri* l., both species being Cruciferae and having a similar chemistry. Both plants are known in modern Indian medicine as abortifacients and emmenagogues.[29] The other plants in the prescription are *Myrtus communis* L.;[30] *Commiphora myrrha* Engl.;[31] and *Piper nigrum* L.[32] Each ingredient in the prescription is known to have the prescribed effect. Myrtle (*Myrtus*) and myrrh (*Commiphora*) will be discussed in greater detail later. Pepper contains piperine as one of its main components, which has sparteine, a known oxytocic (abortifacient). Piperine has been effective in tests on animals in a dose of thirty mg/kg,[33] but for humans heavy doses are required to induce an abortion.[34]

Less certain in its effectiveness is the fourth recipe. Neither rocket nor cow parsnip has been evaluated as a contraceptive, and judgment must therefore be reserved. A plant closely related to cow parsnip, *Heracleum sosnowskyi* Mandenova, is reported in a chemistry study to exhibit estrogenic activity and therefore may be contraceptive.[35]

Of the ten plants Soranus mentioned in these four recipes, modern medical science has judged eight as having an effect as contraceptives and abortifacients/emmenagogues. One of the other two is likely to have an antifertility effect, while the final plant, rocket, has not been studied. In the case of rue, present Chinese, Latin American, and Indian medical authorities recognize its abortifacient quality,[36] with one manual warning that pregnant women should avoid even small amounts of it because of its "emmenagogue properties."[37]

Soranus' prescriptions appear to be early stage abortifacients, although some of the plants (rue and *silphium* or *Ferula*) also interfere with one or more critical ovulatory events. A woman taking these prescriptions will likely either prevent or terminate pregnancy.

Soranus began his discussion of contraception not with drugs but with regime. First, one should avoid intercourse during the most fertile period—thought to be the period when menstruation was "ending and abating." [38] During coitus the woman could draw herself away enough so as to keep the seed from being hurtled deep into the cavity; afterward she was to squat down, induce sneezing, wipe the vagina, and, possibly, drink something cold. Finally, he gave a series of "aids," with the prefatory phrase "It assists the inconception" (συνεργεῖ δὲ τῇ ἀσυλληψίᾳ).

The aids, all ointments to smear on the mouth of the uterus, are:

1. old olive oil, *or*
2. honey, *or*
3. cedar resin, *or*
4. juice of the balsam tree [*Commiphora opobalsamum* Engl.], alone or together with
5. white lead, *or*
6. salve with myrtle oil and white lead, *or*
7. before coitus with moist alum, *or*
8. galbanum [sap from *Ferula galbaniflua* Baiss. and Bushe], *or*
9. a lock of fine wool in the orifice of the uterus, *or*
10. before coitus use vaginal suppositories that have the power to contract and condense.

According to Soranus, "Such of these things are as styptic, clogging, and cooling cause the orifice of the uterus to shut before the time of coitus and do not let the seed pass into its fundus. [Such, however, as are hot] and irritating, not only do not allow the seed of man to remain in the cavity of the uterus, but draw forth as well another fluid from it." [39]

The gums and resins have a mild antiseptic effect and, as such, may act as spermicides. Cedar oil in antiquity came mostly from the juniper tree, whose antifertility qualities are discussed below. White lead, on the other hand, has been employed in modern medicine in dermatological salves, such as for poison ivy; because of its toxicity, however, it has been dropped for the most part from our pharmacy. The myrtle oil and galbanum (from *Ferula* have an antifertility effect. The wool pad and old olive oil are seen as lubricants and devices to block the mouth of the cervix mechanically. It is interesting how Soranus couched this information: these agents are aids, not drugs, and only help prevent conception.

CHAPTER FOUR

Terminology in Dioscorides'
De materia medica

The Chaste Tree destroys generation as well as provokes menstruation.
Dioscorides, *Materials of Medicine*

S oranus said that his oral contraceptive recipes were also abortifacients. In this chapter we consider the works of the foremost authority on ancient pharmacy, Dioscorides, to see whether his distinctions of antifertility agents were sharper. Dioscorides wrote a five-book work called *De materia medica* (Materials of Medicine) in the first century, a little earlier than Soranus. Dioscorides unmistakably recommended oral contraceptives, most of them herbal. Before examining oral contraceptives, however, let us look at usages involving birth control in order to understand his lexical distinctions.

Dioscorides prescribed a number of herbs for birth control, and he used them in various ways. He used the same word as Soranus—ἀτόκιος, meaning "contraceptive." He gave these plants as oral contraceptives: white poplar (*Populus alba* L.),[1] cabbage flowers (*Brassica* sp.),[2] pepper (*Piper* spp.),[3] ivy (*Hedera helix* L.),[4] asplenon (a fern, probably, *Asplenium adiantum nigrum* L. or *Adiantum capillus veneris* L. or both).[5] The chaste tree (*Vitex agnus-castus* L.) "destroys generation [ἐκλύει δὲ καὶ γονήν] as well as provokes menstruation [ἔμμηνα ἄγει]." Here Dioscorides avoided the term for contraceptive but implied the same action in addition to its being an emmenagogue and, presumably, an abortifacient.[6] Dioscorides used the term ἀτόκιος for several plants employed as vaginal suppositories. Juniper berries (*Juniperus communis* L. + sp.), crushed and put on the penis or the vulva before insertion, act as a contraceptive.[7] But cabbage flowers, pepper, and ivy were also vaginal suppositories and acted as a contraceptive and abortifacient in both oral and suppository administrations. What was he saying precisely? Finally, in a similar example, Dioscorides wrote that the leaves of the white willow tree (*Salix alba* L.) cause inconception (ἀσυλληψία).[8]

A larger number of plants are abortifacients and, as will be explained later, early stage abortifacients. The cultivated lupine (*Lupinus angustifolius* L. + sp.), according to Dioscorides, extracts the menses and fetus;[9] rue extracts the menses (without mentioning the embryo/fetus);[10] similarly he said that *silphium* (Soranus' Cyrenaic juice), drunk with pepper and myrrh, moves the menstrua;[11] birthwort (*Aristolochia clementitis* L. + sp.), drunk with pepper and myrrh, expels the menstrua and embryo/fetus (ἐν προσθέτῳ ἐμμήνων ἀγωγὸς καὶ ἐμβρύων), and it does the same as a suppository.[12] Another fern, *thelupteris* (*Pteris aquilina* L.), causes inconception (ἀσυλλημψία) and, if the woman is pregnant, a miscarriage (ἐκτιτρώσκει, using a verb);[13] and the root of the alpine plant called barrenwort (*Epimedium alpinum* L.; the English name itself suggests birth control usage) causes contraception (ἀτόκιος), and "its leaves, beaten and drunk in the amount of five drachmas [approx. 20.5 g/0.7 oz.] in wine after the menstrual period for five days preserve inconception [ἀσύλληπτος]."[14] Great arum (*Arum dracunculus* L.) aborts a newly conceived fetus.[15]

Of the plants that Soranus recommended as oral contraceptives and abortifacients, Dioscorides prescribed only *silphium* (*Ferula historica*) and pepper as oral contraceptives, but he identified opopanax as "expelling the menstrua and killing the fetus [ἔμμηνά τε ἄγει καὶ ἔμβρυα φθείρει]";[16] myrrh expels the menstrua and fetus when administered with wormwood (*Artemisia absinthium* L.), lupin, and rue;[17] *leukoion* (wallflower or stock) is an emmenagogue-abortifacient;[18] myrtle is good for menstrual problems as a sitz bath but not specifically as an emmenagogue.[19] Dioscorides gave no birth control usages for rocket, parsnip, and pomegranate, although rocket was declared to stimulate sexual desire.[20] Inexplicably, Dioscorides listed no specific birth control usages for rue in his chapter devoted to it (book 3, chapter 45), but he called it an emmenagogue. In his chapter on myrrh, he stated that rue was part of the prescription for an abortifacient.

Sex Hormones and Plants

The oral contraceptives that Dioscorides recommended have a basis in fact according to modern medical knowledge. The strictly oral contraceptives that Dioscorides added to Soranus' list are white willow, white poplar, cabbage leaves, ivy, and barrenwort. The use of plant contraceptives is complex and requires an introduction. In recent years, the physiology of reproduction has undergone careful scrutiny by medical research to show that the onset of female ovulation is controlled by hormones secreted in the hypothalamus and pituitary. The processes of releasing the follicle-stimulating hormone and the luteinizing hormone take place in mammals and were thought to belong only to the animal kingdom, not to plants. In 1933, two studies were produced that eventually changed these understandings. Boleslaw Skarzynski reported that he obtained from the willow a substance that resembled a human female hormone (trihydrooxyoestrin).[21] In the same year, Adolf Butenandt and H. Jacobi reported that the date palm and pomegranate produced female sex hormones.[22] These reports were at first received skeptically because plant substances were not thought of as functioning as human hormones; furthermore, scientists could not duplicate Butenandt and Jacobi's laboratory results.[23]

In recent decades, however, many studies and reports indicate that plants do have antifertility effects on animals, including humans. These discoveries emerged when researchers in animal science observed that grazing animals reacted to certain plants by miscarriages (abortions), ovulation failures, and other forms of infertility. Some plants have the means of disrupting and/or desynchronizing one or another of the preovulatory and preimplantational events; they exert their antifertility effects through chemical classes known as estrogenic sterols, coumestrols, and isoflavones and through uterine contractors. Some plants, such as those containing estrogenic steroids, act on the hypothalamus (and perhaps on the pituitary, as well). Certain plants can stimulate the production of prostaglandins that can have a variety of antifertility effects such as causing the endometrium of the uterus to resist implantation and inhibit transport of the sperm.[24] A delicate hormonal balance is necessary in order to ensure the postovulatory events necessary for reproduction.

Dioscorides and Oral Contraceptives

Dioscorides' use of the white willow and the white poplar bark has probable verification in modern science and in medical studies. Skarzynski reported that estriol is found in the willow.[25] In a rough screening test, willow bark was found in one experiment to interfere with ovulation.[26] In another test a crude drug from the plant of a related species, *Salix babylonica* L., was 50 percent effective in preventing implantation.[27]

Although I have found no modern testing of white poplar, willow (*Salix alba* L.) and poplar (*Populus alba* L.) are both members of the willow family (Salicaceae); as a rule, phytochemistries are similar, but not exactly the same, among species of the same family. Furthermore, one is intrigued by the other ingredient associated with white poplar, which is given with the kidney of a mule for contraception.[28] There may be some connection between this recipe and modern contraceptives. The "pill," as we refer to the most commonly used antifertility agent today, is a combination of estrogen and progestin. A major source for conjugated estrogens (estriol) is taken from the urine of pregnant mares[29] and has been isolated from human placenta (not surprising, since it is produced there).[30] Estrogen would be present in a pregnant horse's kidney tissue as well as in its urine. But the prescription says the kidney of a mule, not of a pregnant mare. Assuming Dioscorides truly meant mule, not horse, another theory is more plausible. The mule is sterile; according to the ancient principle of "like causing like," eating a mule's kidney could be thought to cause sterility, on the same principle that a man would eat a bull's testicles for virility. If this is the interpretation of Dioscorides' ingredient, it is an anachronism infrequently seen in the rational medicine of Dioscorides' time and even less in Dioscorides' work.

The case of barrenwort makes it difficult to determine what action Dioscorides intended. He said that the root produces *atokios,* a word whose context in various writings, including Soranus and Dioscorides, suggests temporary lack of conception ("sterility," "unfruitfulness," or "barrenness")—that is to say, a contraceptive effect. As we shall see, barrenwort in classical and medieval medical writings and in folklore usage is traditionally said to cause sterility. In Jean Ruel's Latin translation of Dioscorides, published in 1516, *atokios* is translated as *sterilitas,* thus supplying some evidence that a "sterility maker" was the same as a contraceptive.[31] The question arises whether the drugs that Dioscorides identified as *atokioi* are the same as Jerome's *sterilitas* ("sterility drug") or the Talmud's "root poisons" that were discussed in Chapter 1? Even though there is no direct evidence, likely the authors of these various texts had much the same formulas in mind. A contraceptive was a temporary sterility agent, and some of the more effective ones were roots. A number of other root antifertility agents will be discussed later.

Dioscorides noted that a solution of five drachmas of barrenwort's perforated leaves in wine, drunk for five days after the termination of menstruation, causes "inconception" (ἀσύλληπτος). Both the context and pharmacological actions suggest that the activity envisioned was a temporary period perhaps as long as a month, or the menstrual cycle. Barrenwort's folklore use as a sterilizer is reported in the journal *Science* (1954);[32] I could find no laboratory reports to support its alleged fertility effects. A closely related plant, *Epimedium sempervirens* Nakai, is reported by Japanese investigators to be a uterine stimulant, thus interfering with fertility.[33] My postulate is that neither the intent nor the effect was permanent sterility but that, in a carefully regulated way, it would produce temporary contraception, reversed by deprivation of the drug. This premise is based on the hormonal action of many of the substances and the modern pharmaceutical knowledge that interference or chemical disfunction of sexual hormones results in no permanent change and is reversed by drug cessation. In effect the plants are causing the same anti-fertility process that the body instigates with pregnancy.

Dioscorides' statement that cabbage flowers and seeds were used in a suppository as a postcoital contraceptive (*atokios*) is another example where understanding language is important in interpreting the intent. Modern studies attest that drugs from cabbage seeds have abortifacient properties, but also two species of *Brassica* have reported estrogenic properties. Thus, they may be contraceptive as well.[34] And we shall en-counter instances in later medical writers that point to oral administra-tion of cabbage.

Ivy is a contraceptive (*atokios*), Dioscorides said.[35] The uppermost part is pulverized and given as a vaginal suppository to provoke menstruation, and "being drunk in the amount of one drachma after the cleansing pe-riod [of a woman] it is a contraceptive." Pepper, Dioscorides stated, is applied as a vaginal suppository "after coitus [*meta sunousian*] as a con-traceptive [*atokios*]."[36] On cabbage, ivy, and pepper Dioscorides appears to be confused about the difference between contraceptives and abortifa-cients. At first glance, Dioscorides seems not to have Soranus' verbal pre-cision. This is not necessarily the case, however. Aristotle asserted that the seed could live (in the uterus) for a maximum of seven days without conception occurring.[37] There is agreement on this point between ancient and modern thought: modern medical usage knows of postcoital contra-ceptives.[38] Dioscorides did make precise distinctions; he also said that pepper "dries out" a fetus/embryo (ἔμβρυον), thus implicitly distinguish-ing two actions—one a postcoital contraceptive and another an aborti-facient. The modern recognition of pepper's antifertility effects has al-ready been discussed. Pepper, cabbage seeds, and ivy were recommended throughout the medieval period. Finally, modern medical references re-port ivy's usage as a contraceptive and as an abortifacient.[39] The plants that Dioscorides called contraceptives (*atokoi*) have been shown to be exactly that.

The last two examples of Dioscorides' oral contraceptives are the fern *Pteris aquilina* (he called it also an abortifacient) and the chaste tree. I find no modern evaluative scientific studies of this particular fern, but studies of related ferns reported below show a common substance that causes abortion and has a limited estrogenic activity. The chaste tree, Dioscorides said, "destroys generation." One study shows that it has no contraceptive effect,[40] but several other studies indicate that it has abor-tifacient qualities.[41] One study in a modern Indian journal says that 200 mg/kg of the whole plant were given to rabbits, with ovulation and hence pregnancy prevented in at least 60 percent of the test animals.[42] We can see that the modern English name associates sexuality with the plant; the chaste tree could keep someone, if not chaste, at least nonpregnant. Even so, its strength was apparently not sufficient for this plant to be considered among the more important antifertility drugs.

Vaginal Suppository Contraceptives

In a study reported in 1986, researchers orally administered 200 mg of an extract of juniper root (*Juniperus communis* L.) to laboratory rats, with the result that implantation was blocked in 60 percent of the cases.[43] But these tests were as oral contraceptives (which is how I refer to anti-implantation agents, following medical convention), whereas Dioscorides' prescriptive was as a vaginal insertion. In this form, too, it may have some proven effectiveness. Juniper berries were a part of our pharmacopoeia until the last century as a uterine stimulant.[44] Juniper seeds in animal tests block implantation 60–70 percent of the cases.[45] Juniper berries act as an emmenagogue affecting the menstrual cycle; oils from the leaves are uterine stimulants as shown by in vitro and in vivo tests in animals and in experiments on the isolated human uterus and Fallopian tubes; the oils cause relaxation and inhibition of movement to the extent that could lead to an abortion. In fact, there are medically reported cases of abortion induced by juniper toxins.[46]

Whether a substance is more effective if used as a suppository or if taken orally is not always clear—either in modern medicine or in its ancient counterpart. There is some evidence that hormonal drugs, specifically estrogen and progesterone, are more effective if introduced directly into the uterus than if taken by mouth. Dioscorides said that the Mediterranean mezereon (*Daphne gnidium* L., Thymelaeaceae fam.) "on a pad expels the fetus/embryo [προστεθεὶς δὲ ἔμβρυα κτείνει]."[47] Four diterpenoid orthoesters have been isolated in a related species, *D. genkwa* Sieb. and Zucc. In human and monkey tests, when administered either intraamniotically or extraamniotically in monkeys, there were induced trimester abortions.[48] Fetal death occurs before the abortion, but there is an interval between administration and abortion of from 69 to 142 hours. Dioscorides named another species of the same plant the *mezereon,* which is either or both *D. mezereon* L. or *D. laureola* L. (or laurel spurge), but this plant, he said, causes menstruation or, in his expression, "puts in motion the menstrua [κινεῖ . . . ἔμμηνα]" in a context suggestive of oral application.[49]

In modern tests of extracts from *Daphne* there have been uterine irritation and some damage when used as a suppository. This reaction may have been what Soranus meant when he said that suppositories cause more damage than do oral drugs (see Chapter 3). In tests on nine monkeys four to five months pregnant, extracts from *Daphne genkwa* Sieb. & Zucc. were injected intraamniotically. Six aborted in 1.6 ± 0.2 days, but the other three showed adverse side effects. One aborted on the third day with a dead fetus, while the other two did not abort but lost body weight and had adverse reactions. The active substances in the plant had two actions revealed in autopsy. The level of progesterone was decreased, and there was inflammation, degeneration, and necrosis of the decidua (the endometrium, or mucous membrane that forms when conception occurs and that envelopes the impregnated ovum).[50] It is interesting that in the case of *Daphne,* its use as an abortifacient occurs in the second trimester and not in an early stage, as do most of the others encountered in this study. Dioscorides did not indicate, however, when during the pregnancy *Daphne* was taken.

Another suppository was the lily, the first plant that Dioscorides discussed in his work. He said that a drug made from the root "is applied as a pessary with honey to draw down the embryo [προστεθεῖσαι δὲ ὡς κολλύριον μετὰ μέλιτος ἔμβρυα κατασπῶσι]."[51] A substance called Pallasone A (irisquinone A) has been isolated from the seed coat of a related iris (*Iris pallasii* or *I. lactea*) and given to pregnant mice at a dose of 6.7–10.0 mg per animal with the result that implantation was blocked in 85 percent of the cases. A dose of 10 mg similarly administered was 97 percent effective. In human clinical trials, however, sixteen women were given the substance, with a resulting abortion rate of only 62.5 percent.[52]

Dioscorides recommended that the root be drunk with wine in order to remove the menses. As we have learned, this expression could mean to abort a pregnancy.[53] On the basis of limited evidence, iris appears to be a plant whose use could result in abortions, perhaps more effectively when employed as a suppository, but whose effectiveness was limited. If we may judge from its infrequent mention in works similar to Dioscorides' *Materials of Medicine,* iris was not widely used in early medicine as an antifertility drug.

Likely the action that occurred in some vaginal suppositories was not hormonal but spermicidal. Garlic (*Allium sativa* L. and/or *A. prassum* L.) was given as a suppository to "bring down the menses," by which we can infer it was an abortifacient, according to Dioscorides.[54] Tests conducted in China and reported in 1986 show that allitridum, the active principal in garlic, was highly spermicidal in both animal and human tests. In vitro tests with human spermatozoa show complete immobilization at a dose level of 7.5 mg/ml.[55] Dioscorides' action, however, was for abortion, not contraception. In tests garlic is demonstrated to have estrogenic activity.[56] The use of garlic is reported in Indian folk medicine as an abortifacient; thus the matter must rest with less than conclusive evidence about its efficacy.[57] On the basis of modern reports, Dioscorides' garlic was likely effective as an abortive suppository, but it might have contraceptive action as well.

If garlic is a contraceptive or abortifacient, one might wonder why there is any population in the Mediterranean at all. In answer, we should note that garlic is often an ingredient in compound prescriptions and does not appear a drug of preference. That is to say, like pepper, its use does not appear extensive. Second, as an abortifacient garlic was administered topically, not orally. Furthermore, in the modern world we are conditioned to think of an "effective" drug as one that is 100 percent effective, whereas in natural-product drugs such is seldom the case.

"Root" Medicines and Abortifacients: Sequence #1

Dioscorides organized his pharmaceutical work on the basis of arranging plant, animal, and mineral drugs first by categories (e.g., pot herbs, roots, trees, aromatics) and then, within these groups, by drug affinities.[58] By affinity, he meant the sum total of all its actions. An example of the importance of sequence is afforded by spurge (plants of the *Euphoria* genus). Dioscorides lumped various species together in one chapter under the term *euphorbion*. The plants in this chapter are not specifically given as antifertility agents or as regulators of menstruation. Dioscorides, however, mentioned that spurge is put in a *collyrium*, a type of medicine usually translated as "salve" but, in Dioscorides' usage, sometimes as "suppository." The location of the chapter tells us more. Chapter 82 in book 3, devoted to spurge, is in a sequence of chapters on drugs made from tree roots. The sequence of surrounding chapters is as follows:

Chapter	Greek term	Modern ID
80	*silphion*	*Ferula historica*
81	*sagapēnon*	*Ferula persica*
82	*euphorbion*	*Euphoria* sp.
83	*chalbanē*	*Ferula galbaniflua* Boiss. and Buhse
84	*ammōniakon*	*Ferula orientalis* or *F. tingitana*

Earlier we learned that all species of the giant fennel, or *Ferula,* are contraceptive. Even with different names, Dioscorides appears to have made a botanical classification system but for the interruption of spurge, which is an entirely different genus. The system is not botanical, however. It is a pharmacological arrangement by drug affinity. In recent human clinical trials a 50 percent ethanol extract of the root of *Euphorbia kansui* was intraamniotically injected, with the result being abortion. The experiment showed that the substance acted to stimulate prostaglandin synthesis and had few side effects.[59] Even though Dioscorides said nothing about its antifertility effect, he nonetheless related that the root could be substituted for silphium and other known contraceptive and abortifacients, whose usage he had explicitly discussed. Failure to know Dioscorides' system results in the information not being transmitted to the reader. Perhaps it is for this reason that spurge is not often mentioned as an antifertility drug in most later medical works.

In the beginning of book 3 of *Materials of Medicine,* Dioscorides discusses root herbs in chapters 1–7. Here one might expect some indication of the "root poisons" mentioned by the Talmud and Jerome. (See table 1.)

Book 3 begins with *agaricon,* prescribed for a number of ailments and afflictions, mostly having to do with the digestive tract, spleen, liver, and urogenital system. It was given as an emmenagogue—that is to say, an abortifacient for practical results. The identification of *agaricon* is problematic. Likely it is a fern of the Polyporaceae family, the same family as the other two ferns that we encountered already in this study. Scholars have identified it as *Fomes officinalis* Bredasola, *Polyporus sulphureus* Bull., or *Polyporus officinalis* Fries.[60] I have found no laboratory studies of these three possible ferns, but in a folk medicine report, *Fomes auberianus* is used in New Guinea both as a contraceptive and an abortifacient.[61]

Chapter 2 discusses rhubarb, a familiar laxative to us, which Dioscorides recommended for a similar battery of problems with the digestive tract, kidney and bladder, spleen, and liver, but no antifertility or menstruation problems—unless it is the nonspecific "suffering in the womb."[62] One modern manual, however, says that rhubarb is toxic to pregnant women.[63]

The third chapter begins the sequence of abortifacients that are explicitly so labeled. As an example, the phrase describing gentian is ἐκβάλλει δὲ ἔμβρυα.[64] One modern manual lists gentian as an emmenagogue; a pharmacognosy textbook called it an ecbolic (abortifacient) in its 1966 edition but then dropped reference to its antifertility use in the 1978 edition.[65] Dioscorides' application was as a poultice.

In chapter 4, birthwort was prescribed by Dioscorides both as an oral abortifacient (together with pepper and myrrh) and as a vaginal suppository for abortion.[66] Birthwort is known in modern science studies to prevent conception in humans[67] and to cause an abortion in humans.[68] Aristolochic acid (or its methyl ester or p-coumaric acid) is a uterine stimulant; it is 100 percent effective in blocking pregnancy in mice after a single oral dose (100 mg/kg) on the sixth or seventh day after coitus.[69] A dose of 20–90 mg/kg was sufficient to block implantation, and a dose of 30 mg/kg interrupted midterm pregnancy.[70] This action of aristolochic acid is unusual because most of the plant substances are effective only for the early stages of pregnancy.

Table 1.   Root Medicines in Book 3, Chapter 1–7

Chapter	Greek name	Modern ID	Family	Birth control use in Dioscorides
1	*agaricon*	a fern, perhaps *Formes officinales* Bredasola, *Polyporus sulphures* Bull., or *P. officinalis* Fries	Polyporaceae	provokes menstruation (abortifacient)
2	*ra*	*Rheum rhaponticum* L. (rhubarb) *R. officinales* Baill.	Polygonaceae	none, but helps "suffering in the womb"
3	*gentianē*	*Gentiana lutea* L.	Gentianaceae	abortifacient
4	*aristolocheia*	*Aristolochia pallida* L. (birthwort)	Aristolochiaceae	abortifacient
	stroggylē makra	*A. rotunda* L. *A. sempervirens* L.		
	klementitis	*A. clementitis* L.		
5	*glykyrriza*	*Glycyrrhiza glabra* L. (licorice)	Leguminosae	none
6	*kentaureion makron*	*Centaurea centaurium* L. (giant century plant), or *C. thapontica* L.	Compositae	abortifacient
7	*k. mikron*	*Centaurium umbellatum* Gilib. (feverwort) = old, *Erythrae centaurium* L.	Gentianaceae	abortifacient

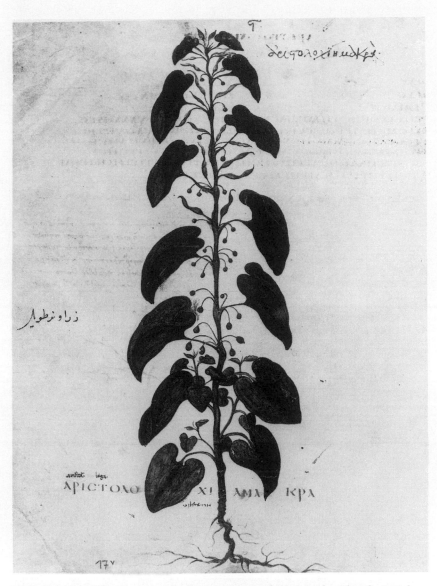

Birthwort, from the Constantinople manuscript of Dioscorides (dated around A.D. 512), which arranged herbs in alphabetical order. The artist has accurately depicted the flowers, budding, stems, and veins in the leaves of the plant. (Vienna, Nationalbibliothek, MS gr. 1, fol. 17v)

The fifth chapter discusses another familiar plant, licorice, but Dioscorides' description causes a problem: in the sequence of chapters four through seven, licorice is the only one not called an abortifacient. Actually licorice is estrogenic, containing active principals of β-Sitosterol, estriol, and estrone,[71] which puts it more in the contraceptive category. A laboratory test screening an extract of licorice found that implantation was prevented in only 33.3 percent of the albino rats fed the substance.[72] Dioscorides failed to include it, however, since he placed it between birthwort and two abortifacients. He indicated that, if either birthwort or the great century plant was not available, licorice could be substituted. Doubtless the dosage of licorice would have to be greatly increased if it was a substitute for birthwort, but unfortunately such information is not in the documents. That knowledge came from the experience or inexperience of the physician, midwife, or herbalist.

The last two chapters are on plants that Dioscorides called the large *kentaureion* and the small *kentaureion*. We know that these two plants belong to two families, the great century plant (*Centaurea centaurium* L., possibly also *C. rhapontica* L., or giant knapweed) of the Composita family; and feverwort, or common century (*Centaurium umbellatum* Gilib., formerly *Erythraea centaurium* L.), of the Gentianaceae. Despite being different plants physically, Dioscorides saw them as similar pharmaceutically. Both were abortifacients, the latter used as a suppository, the former as a poultice, and possibly taken orally.[73] The great century plant and feverwort are known as abortifacients today.[74]

Herb Roots: Sequence #2

There is another sequence, this one also involving root drugs. Because the drugs can come from either the upper plant parts or from the roots, Dioscorides placed them in the category of herb roots. (See table 2.)

Barrenwort's antifertility qualities were attested to above. While the bur reed and stinking iris were not specified as being emmenagogues/abortifacients, their position in the arrangement indicates that, if one did not have a gladiolus plant, one could substitute bur reed. Similarly, one could substitute stinking iris for alkanet. Of these six plants, I can find modern evaluations of only two—barrenwort and the mallow-leaved bindweed—and the latter is reported as an abortifacient. Nonetheless, stinking iris and gladiolus contain isoflavonids (irigen and tectorigenin), which can have a contraceptive effect and, possibly, an abortifacient one as well.[75]

Of the plants whose active antifertility effects come from their roots, two appear to be strong abortifacient substances: birthwort and barrenwort. Although because of his classification scheme Dioscorides did not

Table 2. Herb Roots in Book 4, Chapters 18–23

Chapter	Greek name	English name	Modern ID	Family	Action	Route
18	*mēdion*	mallow-leaved bind weed	*Convolvulus althae-coides* L.	Convolvula-ceae	emmenagogue	oral
19	*epimēdion*	barrenwort	*Epimedium alpinum* L.	Berberidaceae	contraceptive	oral
20	*xiphion*	common gladiola	*Gladiolus communis* L.	Iridaceae	emmenagogue	vaginal suppository
21	*sparganion*	burreed	*Sparganium simplex* Hud.	Sparganiaceae	unspecified	oral: expels poisons
22	*xyris*	stinking iris	*Iris foetissima* L.	Iridaceae	unspecified	oral: fertility not specified
23	*anchousa*	alkanet	*Anchusa tinctoria* L. *A. officinalis* L.	Boraginaceae	abortifacient	vaginal suppository

Table 3. Sharp Herbs in Book 2, Chapters 159–166

Chapter	English name	Modern ID	Family	Antifertility use
159	pepper	*Piper nigrum* L.	Piperaceae	orally for abortion; suppository to hinder conception after coitus
160	ginger	*Zingiber officinale* Roscoe	Zingiberales	none—regarded as pepper substitute
161	water pepper	*Polygonum hydropiper* L.	Polygonaceae	none
162	sneezewort	*Achillea ptermica* L.	Compositae	none
163	soapwort	*Saponaria officinalis* L.	Caryophyllaceae	dries out menses and kills embryo
164	Greek cyclamen	*Cyclamen graecum* Link	Primulaceae	as applicant, causes an abortion; mixed with other medicines for abortions
165	cyclamen	*Cyclamen hederifolium* Aiton	Primulaceae	purges afterbirth
166	edderwort lords-and-ladies	*Arum dracunculus* L. *A. maculatem* L. *A. italicum* Lam.	Araceae	aborts newly conceived

place them as drug affinities, these two plants appear likely as ingredients in the "root poisons" in the Talmud and Jerome and later in medieval sources. Their actions were abortifacient, although their pharmacological action is due not to toxicity but to hormonal action. As is true with all these plant drugs, the exact details concerning preparation, amounts, and frequencies are crucial.

Sharp Herbs as Abortifacients: Sequence 3

The sharp herbs provide a group of abortifacients and contraceptives in sequence near the end of Dioscorides' book 2. (See table 3.)

Pepper's antifertility properties have already been discussed. The following two plants, ginger and water pepper, were ascribed no antifertility properties, even though modern studies attribute abortifacient qualities to ginger and strong contraceptive qualities to water pepper.[76] Sneezewort, or milfoil, is cited in medical reports as an abortifacient,[77] but one test on animals yielded no significant antifertility effects.[78] Soapwort is reported as an abortifacient.[79] The two cyclamens, of the same or related species, are known as abortifacients.[80] The greatest difficulty comes with the interpretation of the usages for the two arums (edderwort and lord-and-ladies). Edderwort, sometimes called the great arum (*Arum dracunculus* L.), aborts a developing [or "early stage"?] fetus. Wellmann's text of Dioscorides says that a "smell" is enough, but other textual readings add that thirty seeds in a drink will have the same results.[81] *Arum maculatum* L. is reported as an abortifacient, and a related species of the Araceae family was tested experimentally in humans as an oral contraceptive. In male and female mice, it produced temporary sterility; five of its species are employed as antifertility agents in folklore reports.[82] Finally, there is another member of the Araceae family, *Acorus calamus* L., which Dioscorides called an emmenagogue both for oral and suppository application, whose properties will be discussed later.[83]

CHAPTER FIVE

Early Stage Abortifacients in Dioscorides and Soranus

An abortive vaginal suppository . . . causes too great a sympathetic reaction and heat.

Soranus, *Gynaecology*, 1.65

S oranus began a section on abortion by telling a woman who wanted to destroy a fetus in the first thirty days to do just the opposite of the regime he had earlier prescribed to prevent miscarriages. First, there were the "aerobic" exercises: walking energetically, horseback riding, jumping, and carrying heavy loads. She should take diuretic concoctions to bring on menstruation. Likely, these would be in the category known to us as dietary diuretics, such as asparagus, but Soranus did not specify the precise agents. Laxatives are helpful, he added, as well as pungent clysters. He recommended daily baths with a warm, not hot, soaking for a long time, with a little wine beforehand and a diet of pungent food. If the exercises do not work, then a sitz bath is in order, consisting of a decoction (that is, a boiling until concentrated) of linseed (*Linum usitatissimum* L.), fenugreek (*Trigonella foenumgraecum* L.), marshmallow (*Althaea officinalis* L.), and artemisia (*Artemisia* sp.).[1] Following the bath she must apply a plaster composed of the same substances together with (1) old olive oil, alone or with rue juice, or (2) honey, or (3) iris oil, or (4) wormwood together with honey, or (5) opopanax fennel by itself or with rue and honey and the Syrian unguent, a formula that is not known. If these poultices or plasters do not work, then she must go to a stronger one made of lupine meal together with ox bile and wormwood.

All these plants, except linseed, were suggested as oral contraceptives as well, either in Soranus, Dioscorides, or later writers.[2] Their use in sitz baths and poultices was clearly seen as the milder, first step to terminate in the first month of pregnancy. If a woman's condition remains unchanged or if she decides to abort after the first month, there is a regimen to follow, plus harsher abortion drugs.

If the pregnancy should persist, she must move to different treatments. For two or three days, she should take protracted baths, eat little food, use softening vaginal suppositories (unspecified), and drink no wine. She is then to be bled; according to Soranus (and to Hippocrates earlier), "A pregnant woman if bled, miscarries." [3] Following the bleeding she can be shaken by riding draught animals (e.g., horses) and can use softening vaginal suppositories. If these procedures, including reapplication of poultices, are ineffective, she must take an "abortive vaginal suppository [πεσσὸν φθόριον]. Of the latter one should choose those which are not too pungent, that they may not cause too great a sympathetic reaction and heat." [4] Soranus related several of the "more gentle ones":

1. myrtle, wallflower (or stock), bitter lupines (*Lupines pilosus* L.) in equal quantities; mix with water and mold into pills the size of a bean.
2. 3 drachmas of rue leaves, 2 drachmas of myrtle, and 2 drachmas of laurel (*Laurus nobilis* L.); mix with wine and give her a drink.
3. "Another vaginal suppository which produces an abortion with relatively little danger: wallflower [or stock seed?], cardamom, sulfur [or brimstone θερῖον], wormwood, myrrh, equal quantities, mold with water." [5]

Myrtle and wallflower (stock) in the first recipe are known antifertility agents. Lupine, on the other hand, appears here and in Dioscorides.[6] Lupine is a type of bean that is poisonous unless properly prepared. As mentioned above, Dioscorides indicated that it would abort a fetus. Again, his report is correct. Lupanine and possible other constituents of lupine (*Lupinus* sp.) produce contractions of isolated pig uteri.[7] In tests in vivo, the resulting uterine contractions were "very effective" in the interruption of the second half of pregnancy in guinea pigs.[8]

The second recipe is somewhat anomalous in that it is given as a drink under the heading "vaginal suppositories." Such a labeling, however, must be an editing error, because the description of the compounding and molding into a pill points to oral administration. In any case, the recipe appears effective. Rue and myrrh are antifertility drugs, as shown above, and laurel is employed in Indian medicine as an abortifacient and in a Western manual as an emmenagogue.[9] Dioscorides was more direct about laurel: he said that it aborts the fetus (*embrya kteinei*), without mentioning provoking the menses, as he so frequently did.[10] Modern Lebanese mountaineers use the raw berries to induce abortion, but Dioscorides said to use the juice of the roots.[11] In situations of this kind where different parts of the plant are employed, the operative difference is apt to be the amounts of concentration. Likely, the same substances appear in both the berries and roots. The time of the year that the substance is extracted and how it is extracted is of critical importance. Unfortunately, such information is seldom found in the sources. In general, however, Dioscorides said that any drug taken from a root should best be made when the plant begins to lose its leaves.[12]

The third recipe, the one he said was a suppository with little danger, mentions wallflower (or stock), myrrh, and three substances not previously discussed: sulfur, wormwood, and cardamom. Sulfur was prescribed by Dioscorides as a fumigant to expel the fetus.[13] Wormwood (*Artemisia absinthium* L., *A. sp.*), along with myrrh, is mentioned as an ingredient by Dioscorides, who said that it expelled the menstrua.[14] Wormwood is known today as a poisonous plant that causes abortions.[15] It is also a contraceptive, since it delays the production of estrus and ovulation and prevents implantation.[16] Cardamom is a seed from *Elettaria cardamomum* Maton and has used been continuously from antiquity to today as part of people's pharmacies and pharmacopoeias. Today it is used as a vehicle and flavoring agent and as an adjunct to other aromatic drugs. Dioscorides recommended it as an abortifacient, and it is employed in Indian medicine for the same effect.[17] Likely, however, because of its widespread and intensive use, the amount of cardamom given by Soranus would within itself not have a primary active quality.

Soranus concluded his discussion of abortifacients with this significant advice: "In addition, many different things have been mentioned by others; one must, however, beware of things that are too powerful and of separating the embryo by means of something sharp-edged, for danger arises that some of the adjacent parts be wounded. After the abortion one must treat as for inflammation."[18] Here, Soranus' omissions are also important. Relating only what he thought to be safe, effective abortifacients, he did not name some of the important drugs in Dioscorides, such as barrenwort and birthwort. He approved of drug abortifacients early in the term, but he disapproved of surgical procedures. He was doubtless familiar with the second part of the Hippocratic aphorism on bleeding a pregnant woman: "The larger the embryo, the greater the risk."[19]

Dioscorides, for all his genius with drugs and medicine, did not state drug preference. He would list drugs and their qualities but did not compare them. Seldom would he say that a given preparation was the mildest drug for, say, an abortion, or that another one was good but strong and dangerous. Such comparisons are rare in the other medical works in classical antiquity, as we shall see later. Soranus, in contrast, informed us of

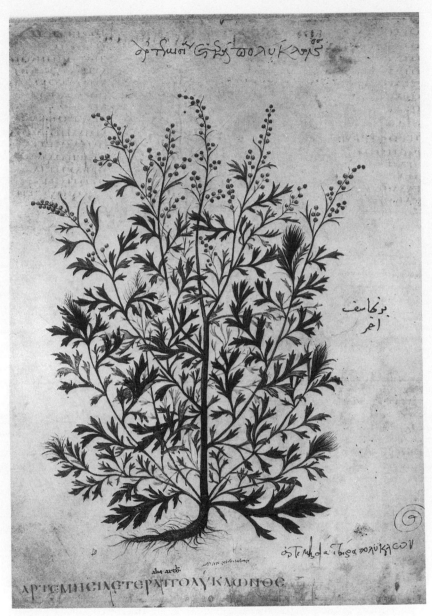

Artemisia (*Artemisia vulgaris* L.), the plant named after the Greek goddess associated with fertility and childbirth, as depicted in the Constantinople manuscript of Dioscorides (Vienna, Nationalbibliothek, MS gr. 1, fol. 20v)

the various regimes that went with pregnancy prevention and termination.

Other Abortifacients in Dioscorides

Ploughman's spikenard (*Inula conyza* DC + sp.) "carries away the menses and aborts the embryo fetus [πρὸς καταμηνίων ἀγωγὴν καὶ ἐκβολὴν ἐμβρύων]," and dittany (*Origanum dictamnus* L.) "shakes out a dead embryo [τὰ τεθνηκότα ἔμβρυα ἐκτινάσσει]."[20] Spikenard is an abortifacient frequently encountered in a variety of folk usages. In a rough screening laboratory study, it was found to have an antiovulatory activity.[21] If pregnancy had taken place, the presumption is that spikenard, if taken in sufficient amounts, would have aborted the fetus. Dittany is reported in a modern medical guide (1963) as an abortifacient.[22] In tests on rats, an extract of dittany's root was administered orally up to ten days after coitus, with the results of decreased fertility.[23]

The statement about expelling a dead fetus was sometimes used by Dioscorides and other writers, especially Pliny, but quite likely there is an unresolvable ambiguity as to whether the words describe an action or a desired effect.[24] Because the results are the same (even if the conditions might not have been), the agents to expel a "dead fetus" are the same as an abortifacient, especially since various authors appear to interchange the terms.[25] The only writer whom I could find who was explicit about the matter is a thirteenth-century Muslim medical authority, Ibn al-Baitar (1197[?]–1248), who said of juniper that more than any other drug it is for "menstruation, causing bloody urine, killing the living embryo, and expelling a dead one."[26] The assumption is that the terms for "fetus" and "embryo" were interchangeable and not given technical meanings as they are today. The "dead" or "unhealthy" fetus could be a mask for rationalizing a simple abortion, as possibly when Galen spoke of the expulsion of the "weak" or "unhealthy" fetus (ἀδύνατον τὸ ἔμβρυον).[27]

A member of the same birthwort family as *Aristolochia* is *Asarum europaeum* L., which Dioscorides recommended as an emmenagogue but not specifically to abort a fetus.[28] He did the same thing with rue, as previously stated. Evidently, Dioscorides intended an emmenagogic action to be interchangeable with an abortifacient action. Reports in scientific studies disclose that Canadian asarum (*A. canadense*) allegedly prevents conception, according to North American folklore reports. The roots are boiled down slowly over a long period and drunk.[29]

In some instances, Dioscorides said only that a plant was an emmenagogue, such as he did for cyperus (*Cyperus rotundus* L.),[30] but the presumption is that they were known and used as abortifacients. In the case of cyperus, the plant has an estrogenic compound and thus presumably has an antifertility effect.[31] Paraguayan Indians take a closely related species, *C. redolens,* in a juice made from macerated stalks and roots as a drink every five days.[32] The evidence of the plants' actions (see those called only emmenagogues) justifies the presumption that they were also abortives, especially since it is impossible to determine the action if very early in the pregnancy.

Folklore Reports

On rare occasion, Dioscorides included information that he had received through reports but had not personally verified. For two plants he gave birth control information with this indirect approach. Annual scorpion-vetch (*Coronilla scorpioides* L. + sp.) "is thought to act as a contraceptive," which is Dioscorides' way of reporting folklore without his endorsement that it is factual.[33] I have found no modern medical studies about the possible antifertility effects for the annual scorpion-vetch. The plant had a historical gynecological connection: the scientific name of one of its species is named *Coronilla vaginalis* Lam.

The hawthorn (*Crataegus oxycantha* L.) was another of Dioscorides' plants about which he had either heard or read. "It is told that the property of its roots is such that it causes abortions [ἐκτρωσμοὺς ἐργάζεσθαι] if [the root is] hit three times on the abdomen or anointed thereon." [34] In reports published in 1952 and 1953, hawthorn was found to possess therapeutic properties through the action of crategolic acid and a mixture of sapogenins, sometimes called crategus lactone. The plant depresses respiration, affects the heart, relaxes the uterus and intestines, and constricts the bronchi and coronary artery. Drugs from this source currently are used to treat elderly patients with heart disease and patients with mitral stenosis.[35] With such a marked effect on the body, it seems possible that the plant could cause an abortion.[36] Regulated dosages of the root are administered in modern China for menstrual pain and postpartum lower abdominal distension and pain.[37] Dioscorides, though, was certainly justified in his skepticism—at least the part about striking it on the abdomen. In the section where he related therapeutic qualities, he said that hawthorn stopped menstrual bleeding.[38]

Modern Studies

Estrogenic Plants

A textbook authority (Harborne 1977) has named five plants that have female steroids (i.e., those that are either estrogenic or prostogenic): date palm seeds and pollen (*Phoenix dactylifera* L.), pomegranate seeds, willow flowers, apple seeds (*Malus pumila* Mill.), and scotch pine (*Pinus*

sylvestris L.).[39] Between them, Dioscorides and Soranus knew the actions
of willow and pomegranate, and Dioscorides is probably correct in adding willow's close relative, poplar. In Soranus' work and, obliquely, in
Dioscorides's, pomegranate was given as a vaginal suppository. Estrogen
may be administered by implantation or by iniunction for systemic activity at an efficiency level greater than if given orally.[40]

In other words, of the five plants having true oral contraceptive activity
listed by Harborne, Soranus and Dioscorides identified three and added
another; pine, Dioscorides said, was an abortifacient (ἔμβρυά τε καὶ δε-
ύερα [ὑστέρα] ὑποθυμιαθεὶς ἐκβάλλει),[41] and the gum of the doom
palm cast out the fetus.[42] The date palm helps regulate menstruation.[43]
Later, Galen prescribed date palm as an emmenagogue.[44] Earlier in the
Hippocratic treatise *On Women's Diseases,* pine resin is prescribed as an
abortive suppository; later in the sixth century, Aëtius of Amida recommended pine bark as a contraceptive suppository.[45] Only the apple seed's
gynecological applications were not noted by Dioscorides, Soranus, or
other early medical writers. With allowances for the imprecise correlation of ancient and modern medical expressions, the coincidence of four
out of five birth control agents is too great to attribute to chance. The
reasonable interpretation is that the ancients discovered and employed
birth control means present in plants. Modern scientists want to know
the details of harvesting, preparation, and concentration of active substances, as well as the amounts and frequencies of administration, before
they can be sure that the recipes were effective. Such information is not
found in the sources. The proof of the efficacy of drugs must rest with a
reasonable case probability.

Comparing the ancients' knowledge of birth control substances with
Harborne's list of estrogenic plants, we see clearly that the plants listed
were known as birth control agents long before their rediscovery in recent
years. To complete our understanding of what premodern peoples knew
about contraceptives and early stage abortifacients for the control of fertility, let us examine more extensively Dioscorides' and Soranus' knowledge of antifertility substances.

Menses-Inducing Plants

In 1974 Wolfgang Jöchle surveyed the plant-derived drugs mentioned in
Dioscorides that induced the menses, killed the fetus, or delivered or expelled the fetus (dead or alive), all of which were abortifacients when
pregnancy is indicated. He encountered 161. In comparing them with
two modern pharmacognosy guides, he found 90 (or 56 percent) listed
for emmenagogic or abortifacient activity.[46] Because Jöchle used the
flawed seventeenth-century Goodyer and the nineteenth-century Berendes translations, he relied on some incorrect plant identifications,

missed several important plants altogether, and could have extended the pharmacognosy reports to a broader base. The correlation percentage is thus too low. But even with the figure of 56 percent, his study establishes that Greek medicine as seen in Soranus and Dioscorides was capable of distinguishing abortifacient-emmenagogic agents.

In a symposium held in Beijing in September 1980, Norman R. Farnsworth and others presented a summary of their findings on antifertility plant agents. They surveyed more than eight hundred scientific articles that report on one or more plant extracts for various pharmacological activity in affecting fertility. In the category of anti-implantation agents alone, some seventy-five plant species are listed.[47] In these publications, however, the same plants are consistently identified as those having the greatest degree of activity. Those plants are almost always the same ones that were historically used in folk or premodern medicine. In large measure, modern science has rediscovered the past without benefiting from the past by knowing where to look.

As stated above, the first scientific report on plant sex hormones came in 1933 by Skarzynski, who found them in the willow, and, in the same year, by Butenandt and Jacobi, who identified the date palm and pomegranate. Perhaps it was not sheer coincidence that these modern scientists randomly selected for the testing the same plants that are prominent in ancient medicine.[48] It is clear that, on the basis of what we know today, what there is to be discovered had been discovered long before modern science. Unfortunately, scientific and historical studies often proceed on unconnected tracks.

Before looking at the picture of antifertility agents more generally, let us look at the mint plant family, for surely the ancients saw common relationships between plants (after all their lives were more closely dependant on them than are ours). These characteristics of plants gave them clues as to where to test for new drugs.

Mints

There are a number of other plants designated in antiquity as emmenagogic and abortifacient, on the properties of which modern studies are mixed. In addition to dittany, already discussed, Dioscorides recommended five other members of the mint family (Labiatae): hulwort (*Teucrium polium* L.), thyme (*Thymus vulgaris* L.), sage (*Salvia* sp.), betony or woundwort (*Stachys officinalis* L.), and marjoram (*Origanum vulgare* L.).[49] Thyme, sage, and marjoram are antigonadotrophic and thereby interfere with fertilization in laboratory tests on animals. Sage is estrogenic.[50] Hulwort and betony are said to be abortifacients in folklore reports.[51]

Another mint, pennyroyal (*Mentha pulegium* L.), is an attested abortifacient according to Dioscorides and modern science.[52] Pennyroyal is used in Europe as an emmenagogue. In 1978, three women in Colorado, believing themselves pregnant, read that pennyroyal induced an abortion and took its oil, which was marketed as an insect repellent and herbal fragrance. One became ill and, after a hospitalized recovery, was persuaded to receive a legally induced abortion; the second woman was examined and discharged, but no follow-up was made. The third died as a result of taking the pennyroyal oil.[53] Pennyroyal oil is very concentrated; the amount of oil was the equivalent of fifty gallons of pennyroyal tea.[54] The plant cannot be legally sold as a drug in the United States, but it is employed in modern folk medicine both as an abortifacient and an emmenagogue.[55] Finally, the great century plant has antifertility properties.[56]

Abortion Wine

Resembling patent medicines among the ancients are "medicinal wines." Dioscorides was reluctant to include a section of his work on them because he knew them to be compounds of a number of drugs and therefore simply the composite of the parts. Nonetheless, since these wines were popular, Dioscorides said that he felt it necessary to include them, lest his poorly educated readers think him incomplete. Among the wines was a so-called abortion wine (φθόριος ἐμβρύων οἶνος). It consisted of:

> hellebore, either white hellebore (*Veratrum album* L.) or black hellebore (*Helleborus niger* L.)
> squirting cucumber (*Ecballium elaterium* L.
> scammony (*Convulvulus scammonia* L./Convol. fam.)
> Give the wine mixed with water to a woman who has fasted and vomited, in the amount of eight cups [*kyathou*].

While this recipe appears straightforward, Dioscorides did not give the details on how to prepare the recipe. He said only that the plants, when growing among grape vines, cause wine made from those grapes to assume the property (*dynamis*) of the plants. This appears farfetched. It is as if Dioscorides had fallen for a medicine-show artist who would not tell exactly how he made the formula. The squirting cucumber is highly active as an antifertility device, although modern testing confirms a contraceptive, not abortifacient, activity. When mice were given daily doses of between 20 and 100 mg/kg of extracts derived from both the whole plant and the flower alone, they failed to ovulate.[57]

Which one of the hellebores Dioscorides intended is somewhat irrelevant (except to a botanist) because he regarded both as abortifacients.[58] Sheep grazing on *Veratrum californicum* (Durand.) have prolonged gestation associated with cycloptic fetuses, and the same study revealed that it had estrogenic activity.[59] An active principal in *Veratrum* plants is veratrine, which is said to cause miscarriages in humans and, not as strange as it may appear, used for hypertensive toxemia during pregnancy because of its quality of lowering the heart rate.[60] Black hellebore contains two active glucosides (helleborin and helleborein) that are emmenagogic and, according to Indian medical authorities, abortifacient.[61] Hellebore affects the heart in the manner of digitalis drugs and similarly to veratrine alkaloids from white hellebore or *Veratrum*. Whereas black hellebore is seldom used in modern pharmacy because of its harmful side effects, the effective dosage is two to three grains (or 120–200 mg). The dosage for an abortion is three to five grains (200–300 mg).[62] In view of the pharmacological similarities, Dioscorides was probably not careless in naming just "hellebore," because either of the two plants from unrelated species would have done the job. Finally, there is scammony, which is known as a drastic purgative, an action that both hellebores also have. A modern report on scammony focuses attention on the ergot alkaloids which grow on it and speculates that the historical use of scammony as an abortifacient could come from the action of this known abortifacient.[63]

In review, the abortion wine of the ancients would have worked, provided the proper mixture. Still we are faced with a problem. Dioscorides (at least according to his text as we have it) did not say that abortion wine is a compound but that it is made from grapes growing in proximity to these plants. Rationally this strikes us as unlikely, but, at the same time, it is unlikely that a wine composed of these three (or four) plants is a hoax. If it was a ruse, why would those plants out of hundreds of thousands have been selected? A plausible explanation is that the abortion wine was sold by vendors who gave out the story and therefore were protecting the secret of their mixture. The surprise comes in believing that Dioscorides in this instance accepted the tale, since he was so ready to challenge other equally absurd stories.

A Male Contraceptive

There is one drug from the plant called *periklymenon*,[64] possibly honeysuckle (*Lonicera periclymenum* L.),[65] which Dioscorides said makes men barren (ἄγονος) if drunk for thirty-seven days. The description of the plant, however, leaves considerable doubt as to its identity, although probably Linnaeus thought Dioscorides' plant was honeysuckle. Most likely the plant was identified as honeysuckle during the Middle Ages. The plant is taken by women, Dioscorides reported, to hasten birth, but after the seventh day of taking it, blood appears in the urine.

Summary

Dioscorides named fourteen of the fifteen drugs specified by Soranus as emmenagogues/abortifacients: artemisia (*Artemisia* sp.), cardamom, fenugreek, iris, laurel, lupine, myrrh, opopanax (*Ferula*), pepper, rocket rue, *silphium,* wallflower/stock (*Matthiola incana* and/or *Cheiranthus cheiri*),[66] and wormwood. The one exception is myrtle, which Dioscorides did not list as this type of agent.[67] And sulfur appears in Soranus' compounded prescription, but Dioscorides listed it as a fumigant. Since we know that Soranus did not borrow from Dioscorides, we may conclude that the ancients by the first two centuries of the modern era had reached a consensus about what were the contraceptive plants and the abortifacient drugs. There was some degree of overlap, as the modern understanding of their pharmacological actions makes clear. The fact that Dioscorides related more information than Soranus is due to two factors: first, the nature of Dioscorides' work was to examine the whole of materia medica, or pharmacy; second, Soranus deliberately excluded the dangerous abortifacients.

For the most part, the method of analysis has been to compare Soranus' and Dioscorides' antifertility drugs with modern lists. Another, perhaps more instructive means is to produce a modern list and to compare it with the knowledge of these two ancients. The latest and probably the best modern reference about medicinal plants is James A. Duke's *Handbook of Medicinal Herbs* (1985). Duke reports on twenty-seven contraceptive plants, but of these only eight are in Dioscorides. Of the eight, Dioscorides reported two as contraceptives (ivy and pepper) and another two, fenugreek (*Trigonella foenumgraecum* l.) and henbane (*Hyoscyamus* sp.), as being used to regulate menstruation and, in the case of henbane, to assist in childbirth.[68] Moreover, Dioscorides included white willow and poplar, which Duke did not list. Other scientific evidence, however, indicates that they act as oral contraceptives. When the statistical likelihood is taken into consideration of any overlap at all between ancient and modern lists, along with the statistical evidence generated by Wolfgang Jöchle, the presumption must be that Soranus and Dioscorides knew effective drugs.[69] Especially this is true when one considers that there are around 750,000 plant species. The evidence is very strong that Soranus and Dioscorides recorded folk usages we now know to have had an antifertility effect as contraceptives and early stage abortifacients.

CHAPTER SIX

Ancient Society and Birth Control Agents

A very lovely land,
Well cropped, and trimmed, and spruced with pennyroyal.

Aristophanes, *Lysistrata*, 88–89.

There should be an only son to feed his father's house, for so wealth will increase in the house.

Hesiod, *Works and Days*, 375

Soranus and Dioscorides showed us that the ancients differentiated between contraceptives and abortifacients, and most of the agents they identified were likely effective. The question becomes: how widespread were contraceptives and early stage abortifacients in the ancient world? Already we observed that even before Soranus pointed to the pomegranate as an antifertility remedy or before the advent of classical medical writings in the Hippocratic corpus, there were strong indications that pomegranate was associated with antifertility: its seeds caused Persephone to be sterile. There are other similar indications.

Myrrha

From the dawn of ancient Greece and West Asia comes the story about Myrrha. The fragrant substance myrrh was not only named by Soranus and Dioscorides as an antifertility drug, but it was also listed as an ingredient in a number of recipes for the same purpose. In mythology, Myrrha was the daughter of Theias (or Cinyras), legendary king of Assyria. Myrrha was doomed to an incestuous relationship with her father, who ravaged her because Aphrodite, goddess of vegetation, was angered by

Theias' refusal to worship her. Myrrha bore a son from the union, Adonis, but when her father continued to ravage her in drunken advances, she fled with the assistance of other gods, who transformed her into a plant known by her name Myrrha, and by us as *Commiphora myrrha*. As told by Ovid, "Even the tears have fame, and that which distills from the tree trunk keeps the name of its mistress and will be remembered through all the ages."[1] Thus, the plant became a rescuer of daughters caught in the distress of incest.

Queen Anne's Lace and Folklore

Behind the dormitories and surrounding the tennis courts at Meredith College in Raleigh, North Carolina, Queen Anne's lace grows profusely. Because there is a sharply sloping bank, the campus gardeners leave it untouched. The carrotlike plant will grow where grass will not. It has a reddish, slender, strongly aromatic root and stems about two feet high; leaves and stems are covered with coarse hair. In the autumn, its whitish flower withers into many small seeds that fall for the next year's growth.

Not too many miles from the gently rolling Piedmont landscape of this women's campus, a small number of women in Watauga County in the Appalachian Mountains gather some of the seeds of Queen Anne's lace. Each time these women have sexual intercourse, those who wish not to be with child put a teaspoonful of the seeds, saved from the autumn harvest, in a glass of water and drink it. They are confident that they will not conceive.[2] The question arises why on a sophisticated college campus there seems to be no knowledge about the uses of Queen Anne's lace, but in a rural, backwoods mountain region a few women continue to know what was common knowledge to women two thousand years ago.

Dioscorides knew about Queen Anne's lace, or wild carrot (*Daucus carota* L.). He said that it brought forth the menses and aborted an embryo. To do this, he said, take its seed.[3] Scribonius Largus (fl. A.D. 47) is the earliest medical writer who discussed the wild carrot in connection with fertility. Scribonius placed the plant in a recipe for abortion.[4] Queen Anne's lace inhibits implantation. An extract of its seeds has estrogenic activity, meaning that it is also a contraceptive.[5]

Rural populations in Rajasthan, India, chew dry seeds of Queen Anne's lace to reduce fertility. In order to test what might be the reasons for the Indian practice, an experiment was conducted using mice. Varying dosages from 80 mg to 120 mg, given between the fourth and sixth day of pregnancy, reduced implantation by 100 percent.[6] In another experiment, Queen Anne's lace seeds were found to inhibit "implantation, ovarian growth . . . [and to disrupt the] estrous cycle."[7] A Chinese laboratory test of *Daucus carota* showed clearly that the seed terpenoids block progesterone synthesis in pregnant animals.[8] The drug is viewed as a promising substance in the development of a postcoital antifertility agent.[9]

Women in modern China, India, and the mountains of North Carolina are connected to antiquity through the knowledge about Queen Anne's lace. How did they learn what they know? Surely not through books. Why do so few now know what so many once did?

Pennyroyal

Aristophanes' play *Peace* was produced in Athens in 421 B.C., during a period that was anything but peaceful. For over ten years, despite a truce, Athens and Sparta were engaged in a long struggle known as the Peloponnesian War. In the play, Hermes speaks with Trigaius, who is in need of a female consort.

> Then on these terms I'll give you Harvesthome
> To be your bride and partner in your fields.
> Take her to wife, and propagate young vines.

Trigaius replies:

> O Harvesthome! come here and let me kiss you.
> But, Hermes, won't it hurt me if I make too free
> With fruits of Harvesthome at first?

Hermes:

> Not if you add a dose of pennyroyal
> (βληχώνιαν = *Mentha pulegium* L.).[10]

A Byzantine scholiast explained that pennyroyal was used in a medicinal draught that counteracted the effects of eating too much fruit.[11] Pennyroyal, however, was in fact both a contraceptive and an abortifacient, as Aristophanes' audience knew. Otherwise, the humorous point of Hermes' final line above is lost.

Pennyroyal made its way into another of Aristophanes' plays, *Lysistrata*. In the plot, the women of Athens could bring about peace by withholding their bodies from the bellicose men, who, once the female strike occurred, clearly wanted their women. An Athenian woman named Calonice, seen by the audience as clearly pregnant, is being persuaded to hold off sexual advances from her husband. A woman from Boeotia, who is not pregnant, is described as "A very lovely land, / Well cropped, and trimmed, and spruced with pennyroyal."[12] The line is interpreted by scholars to be a pun. The Greek word for "land," πεδίῳ, also means the female genitalia.[13] Actually Aristophanes was doubly clever: the playwright's audience must have caught the pun on the word for land and associated women's fertility with the plant.

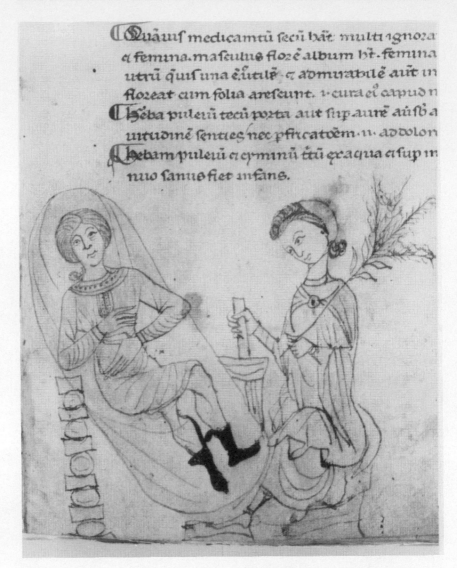

Pennyroyal being used as an abortifacient. This drawing accompanying a thirteenth-century manuscript of Pseudo-Apuleius' herbal shows a person holding a sprig of pennyroyal and preparing the drug with a mortar and pestle, while the patient waits with her legs demurely crossed. (Vienna, Nationalbibliothek, MS lat. 93, fol. 93)

The Chaste Tree

Athenian women celebrated the festival of the Thesmophoria during the month that corresponds to our October. To honor Demeter they remained chaste during the celebrations and strewed boughs of the chaste tree beneath the pallets of their beds.[14] In Greek it is called the ἄγνος, which, by folk etymology, was associated with the word ἁγνός, meaning "chaste" or "pure."

The plant is not a tree. A member of the vervain family, it is a small aromatic shrub no bigger than three meters high, with leaves somewhat like those of a willow and with lilac flowers on spikes. In *The Golden Bough*, Sir James George Frazer reports the behavior of the Athenian women during the Thesmophoria, but he misunderstood its meaning entirely. He thought that the chaste tree was an aphrodisiac and as such was a ritual that went back to the primitive rites of maintaining women's important duty of perpetuating the purity of the seed.[15] It is unlikely to have been as Frazer thought. Pliny, in contrast, said that the chaste tree suppressed sexual desire.[16] For this reason Pliny said it was given as an antidote in a liniment for bites of spiders whose venom excited sexual desire. Whether this is true or not, the Athenian women had at least an additional motive to place it beneath their beds while they sought chastity. It contracepted. Not only was it given orally for this purpose (see Chapter 3), but the chaste tree seeds were also put in vaginal suppositories and fumigants. Drunk with pennyroyal, it cleaned the uterus and cleared away headaches.[17] It would appear that women celebrated this shrub because it enabled them, if not to be chaste, to be nonpregnant as long as they knew how to use it. The ritual dated from the earliest Greek culture, long before the medical writings. It indicates that knowledge of chemical birth control predated the learned recognition that Dioscorides and Pliny gave to the small shrub with the sweet lilac flowers.

Contraceptive in the Talmud

What was the herbal, oral contraceptive that we encountered in the Talmud passage and mentioned in Chapter 1? This was in reference to Judith's question to Rabbi Hiyya about whether the biblical injunction to propagate the race applied to women. When she learned that it did not, she "went and drank *samā' d-'aqartā*." One surmises that, were she already pregnant, the question would not have been phrased in this manner. The likelihood is that the herb was a contraceptive. Since by now in our study we have learned that the use of these plants has a rational basis, we seek to learn more about the herb that Judith took.

Samā' d-'aqartā is identified in the modern Hebrew-English dictionary as heteranthelium, which is *Heteranthelium piliferum* in the binomial system and a member of the genus *Triticeae* of the Gramineae family.[18] As best I can determine, the name does not appear in the Bible.[19] A few species of this genus and more from the family have estrogen, various isoflavonoids, and coumestrols.[20] The plant has not been tested for antifertility activity and does not appear elsewhere in such a context.[21] It is possible that the plant possesses antifertility qualities and possible also that the plant is misidentified, inasmuch as it is not common in the Palestine area.

Attention, however, shifts to the plant name that has as a root *'qr*, which means "rootless" or "barren." [22] In effect the plant in Hebrew has the same root as the English term barrenwort for *Epimedium alpium* L.—that is to say, the plant's use is its name. Whatever the plant's identity, it surely is associated with fertility, and at least one Jewish woman took it. By reasonable inference, however, we know that when she was given permission to use a contraceptive, she had to have known from someone what to take. The knowledge was part of her culture.

Ancient Law and the Fetus

By and large, ancient law—Greek, Roman, or Hebrew—did not protect the fetus, as we saw briefly in Chapter 1. There was some recognition, however, of rights of the father in a marriage, and a survey of those laws indicates the use of chemical birth control. As we saw in Chapter 1, ancient law did not protect the newborn until the legal acknowledgment of the child by the father and the registration of the child in the tribe, community, or polis. In such a case, legal restrictions on abortion appear incongruous.

In Greek law, a single exception is encountered in Thebes, but the law (undated) is late and probably in the Hellenistic era. Aelian recorded:

> No Theban man should be allowed to expose a child . . . But if the father of the child should be extremely poverty stricken, the law orders that he immediately after the child's birth (be it male or female) carry it to the magistrate together with its swaddling clothes, and they shall sell the child received to the person giving a low price for it . . . that he should bring up the child in good faith . . . and receive his service as payment for the upbringing.[23]

In the nature of Greek law, we do not have extensive records available nor are those we have consistent enough to allow many generalizations. Normally a Greek jury of a given city-state did not feel bound by precedents of similar cases; a clever lawyer dare not inform a jury that they were compelled to reach the decision for which he argued. Greek juries were apparently governed less by statutes than by their sense of generally acceptable norms of behavior. It should come as no surprise that there is some evidence that the Greeks afforded to the father some rights as a father; he, after all, was the one responsible for deciding the life or death of the newborn.

Sopater, a Greek parodist who lived in Alexandria, Egypt, shortly after its founding in the late fourth century B.C., referred once to an Athenian trial involving abortion. The lawyer Lysias is quoted by Sopater in his oration "On Abortion" (Περὶ τοῦ ἀμβλωθριδίου)"[24] as referring to a trial "in which Antigene accuses his own wife of homicide, the woman having voluntarily aborted, and he says that she had, by aborting, impeded his being called the father of a son."[25] How extensive a father's rights were to protect a fetus is unknown, according to what we know of Greek law. Clearly, as Richard Feen concluded, the crime of abortion was not the killing of a fetus or embryo but the depriving the father of his right to an heir.[26]

Roman law is much more orderly and precise. The earliest known case on abortion rights is cited by Cicero, who refers to a Milesian woman who received bribes from "alternative heirs" to secure on herself an "abortion through drugs [*partum sibi ipsa medicamentis abegisset*]," an offense for which she was sentenced to death.[27] This case was cited in the *Digest* once by the great jurist Ulpian (d. A.D. 228) and by Tryphonius (*Disputations,* bk. 10), who invoked the precedent but added that if a pregnant woman after a divorce should commit "a violent act upon her insides [*visceribus*] . . . [because] she wanted an abortion [*partum abigeret*] so as not to give a son to her husband who is now hateful to her, she ought to be punished by temporary exile as was stated by our most excellent Emperors in a Rescript."[28] Tryphonius is likely citing the ruling of Septimius Severus (A.D. 193–211) that "a woman who procured an abortion for herself should be sent into temporary exile by the governor; for it would appear shameful that she could with impunity deprive her husband of children."[29] By these examples Roman law is seen changing in the early second century, but nowhere is there a clear statement that the embryo/fetus was being protected, only the rights of the living.

Another legal principle invoked in late Roman law is the defense against magic. Those who gave *maleficia* ("evil deeds") were held legally responsible for malpractice, should harm to life or property be incurred.[30] Paulus, the celebrated jurist alive at the same time as Ulpian and Emperor Septimius Severus, wrote in his *Sentences:*

Those who administer a beverage for the purpose of producing abortion, or of causing affection, although they may not do so with malicious intent, still, because their act offers a bad example, shall, if of humble rank, be sent to the mines; or, if higher in degree, shall be relegated to an island, with the loss of a portion of their property. If a man or a woman should lose his or her life through such an act, the guilty party shall undergo the extreme penalty.[31]

The civil code is making a point about malpractice of a magician or someone who is using "poisonous drinks," as Jerome called them, to secure an abortion or to increase sexual activity. Malicious intent need not be proven, because the act "offers a bad example." Reading between the lines, one might interpret Paulus' opinion as a culmination of policies of the Roman government to encourage child raising and to restrict magical practices, mostly by charlatans, even though he said that malicious intent need not be a factor. The law also punished those who gave drugs that promoted conception and resulted in harm. In the latter case, clearly the intent was benevolent, but the malpractice was the crime.

Left unstated or only alluded to is an example where ancient law accepted the Stoic principle that an unborn fetus was potentially a human and therefore should be protected for its own sake. The inference in Paulus is that the fetus is not the object of protection. Instead, the object of protection is society because of its rights to unrestricted childbirth. Plainly this was a principle of legal jurisprudence without statutory force or implementation.

Finally, specific mention of the means of abortion referred invariably to chemical means—namely, a drink. For the sake of comparison, note that the first English criminal abortion law (1803) mentioned explicitly only one kind of abortion—chemical (see Chapter 15). One could reasonably conclude that drug abortions were the normal means and, on the basis of our study, so were mostly early stage abortifacients. A woman who had not previously divulged her pregnancy would almost certainly not be proven guilty of abortion because, during the first months, pregnancy would be nearly impossible to prove in a court to satisfy legal requirements of evidence. The Romans, at least, were noted for strict definitions of evidence. Also, no legal statements were made against a successful abortion administered by the woman and unassisted by another person, including, we might suppose, by advice. From the Hammurabi Code through Roman law, even though the details are sketchy, a second party could be held legally liable for harm to the mother. This observation underscores the point that abortion per se was not criminal; it was the right of the family, perhaps too of the state, to have children. From what we know about the Roman Empire, however, most abortions were not the subject of litigation.

Roman Literary References to Birth Control

Enzo Nardi, John Noonan, and Marie-Thérèse Fontanille have collected the classical references in literature to birth control.[32] The corpus of references is substantial. The evidence is compelling that abortion and contraception were a part of the everyday world of classical antiquity.

In *Truculentus,* a play by Plautus (c. 251–184 B.C.) about three young men who seek to divert the attention of the women of a house by amourous advances on the household's matron, the young men come, a clever maid observes, not with "barren hands" (*steriles*) but with intent to steal. The maid discloses that the matron is pregnant. "She hid it [pregnancy] from you, fearing you'd urge her to have an abortion [*abortioni*], and be the death of her baby boy." [33]

Juvenal satirized even the most intimate details of Roman life.

> Yet these at least endure the dangers of child birth, all
> Those nursing chores which poverty lays upon them:
> How often do gilded-beds witness a lying-in
> When we've so many sure-fire drugs [*medicamina*] for inducing
>   sterility [*steriles facit*]
> Or killing an embryo child [*homines in ventre necandos*]? Our
>   skilled abortionists
> Know all the answers. So cheer up, my poor friend,
> And given her a dose yourself.
> Things might be worse—just suppose
> She chose to stay pregnant. [34]

Besides Plautus and Juvenal, Ovid,[35] Philo,[36] Lucretius,[37] and Seneca[38] discussed or alluded to contraceptives and/or abortifacients, generally disapprovingly. So did early Christian writers, including Clement of Alexander, John Chrysostom, Lactantius, Ambrose, and Jerome.[39] The number of such references clearly indicates a widespread early knowledge of birth control agents.

CHAPTER SEVEN

Egyptian Papyrus Sources

You should [make] for her a prescription to loosen semen.

Berlin Papyrus, c. 1300 B.C.

The notion that women could regulate their fertility through chemical means is as old as medical records. In practical terms, it means that the idea is older than the record. The earliest medical writing from Egypt, the Kahun Medical (or Obstetrical or Gynecological) Papyrus, dating from around 1850 B.C., has three fragmentary prescriptions for preventing conception, all involving vaginal suppositories.

Recipe 1 (Kahun. No. 21 [3,6]):
Not to become pregnant,[1] that . . .
Feces of crocodile, smash up with fermented dough [or paste];
    soak . . .[2]

Recipe 2 (Kahun 22 [3,7]):
Another Recipe.
6/7 Pint of honey; sprinkle in her vagina.
This is done with [ḥr sḥm] of soda/saltpeter.[3]
Another Recipe.
[. . . mashed up] with fermented dough/paste, sprinkle in her
    vagina . . .[4]

The first recipe calls for crocodile feces. No classical medical writings call for the use of crocodile feces as a vaginal birth control suppository; in Arabic medicine, however, elephant feces are frequently recommended as a suppository.[5] Al-Razi (A.D. 865–925, in the *Kitaba l-Hawi*) prescribed elephant feces either by itself or mixed with henbane.[6] From the

Kahun Papyrus to al-Razi is a separation of almost three thousand years, definitely too long for a possible link in literary transmission when there is no direct evidence. Folk continuity is possible, but again the hypothesis is too frail and tenuous.

A suggestion is made that feces may have actual birth control properties, as an agent that either blocks mechanically the seminal fluid at the os of the cervix or changes the pH level.[7] In the absence of more and better evidence, this hypothesis represents too great a modern effort to impose scientific rationality. A simple explanation—probably incorrect—is that inserting feces into a woman's vagina would be an excellent contraceptive merely by decreasing the libido of a squeamish male. More inferential evidence assists our understanding even if it does not lead to a definitive conclusion. The crocodile is associated with the Egyptian god Seth, the deity who sought to injure Isis in her difficult pregnancy.[8] Ancient Egyptian uterine amulets often have Seth on them. The amulets were employed both for "opening" the womb, thus assisting menstruation, conception, and birth, or for "closing" the womb, thus causing hemorrhaging, miscarriage, or abortion. Robert Ritner observes that Thoueris, the Egyptian goddess who protected pregnancy and childbirth, rarely appears on the uterine amulets, but Seth is often represented.[9] At least one statue of Thoueris, however, portrays the goddess with the body of an obviously pregnant hippopotamus and a head of a crocodile.[10] Thus, the crocodile was associated with abortion, the hippopotamus with pregnancy, but the two animals are mixed on the statue. It is curious that in nature the principal enemy of baby hippos is the crocodile.

The second and third recipes give us some clues. Soda or saltpeter (perhaps in various forms, such as bicarbonate of soda) will be employed from time to time in medieval recipes for the same purpose.[11] Again, modern speculation revolves around the possible relevance of the pH level of the vaginal chemistry or spermicidal action. The fermented dough or paste may have been only a vehicle for the active substances, or it may have been productive through ancillary effects of its own through the microorganisms causing the fermentation.

A magical papyrus from the third century A.D., written partly in hieratic and partly in demotic, has a lengthy formula for a male who wants to seduce a woman. He must take various scented oils (some details of which are lost in the text), store them for a month, and then place in the vessel a black *kesh* fish, nine fingers long and with variegated eyes. The fish is kept in the oil for two days, during which time incantations are recited before exiting the house and speaking to any other man. A ripened grapevine shoot is taken in the left hand, transferred to the right hand, and allowed to grow seven fingers long. The fish is extracted from the oil and hung head down until its oils drip down onto a new brick for three

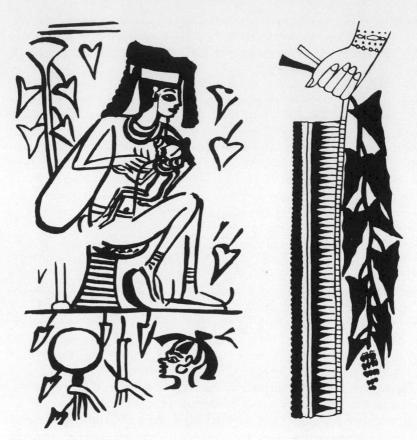

The scene on the left, from a vase found in the Egyptian city of Thebes, shows a woman nursing a baby with *Aristolochia,* or birthwort, in the background. (B.M. 8506) The drawing on the right, from a tomb in Thebes, also shows birthwort. The plant assisted with childbirth, but caused an abortion taken early in pregnancy. (Drawing from Theban tomb no. 217, courtesy of Dr. Lise Manniche)

days. This liquid is put with myrrh and soda/saltpeter and hidden in the bedroom for two more days. Then, for seven days recitations are delivered to the mixture and finally it is rubbed on the penis. A woman will be attracted to lie with the man who does all this and who says the proper prayer.[12] Certainly, a man who went to that much trouble would have heightened expectations, but surely there is more to be understood about the magic than that. The rubbing of myrrh and soda may have had a contraceptive effect, as previously seen with the myrrh. The rituals and formulas are combined with what we call magic, but to our understanding it may have had some physical effects as well. The soda/saltpeter ingredient in the Kahun Papyrus, unlike the crocodile feces, appears frequently throughout history, as in the example of the Leyden Papyrus. Whether the woman in the Leyden Papyrus allows herself to be seduced because of the knowledge that fertility is unlikely is open to our imagination.

Our analysis of these contraceptive formulas may be too involved for the meager evidence here. Still, the Kahun Papyrus is the earliest document that we have that mentions a birth control measure, albeit a suppository, and for that reason alone merits as full an understanding as is possible. The fact that the Kahun is not an original but a copy from an even more ancient archetype adds to the intrigue.[13]

Ramesseum Papyrus

Another papyrus, the Ramesseum Papyrus IV, dated 1784–1662 B.C., contains the same contraceptive formula using crocodile feces and fermented dough as was found in the Kahun Papyrus.[14] Although we do not know whether these substances may have assisted in birth control, the importance of these documents lies in the fact that these earliest of medical records show that the concept of contraception was present and that the means used was vaginal suppositories. The preservation of the prescriptions are in two unrelated texts; both reflect earlier archetypes. The belief that people could control conception through substance use is, therefore, older than the extant records themselves.

Ebers Medical Papyrus

The Ebers Medical Papyrus is dated between 1550 and 1500 B.C. Like the other two texts, it contains a contraceptive, a vaginal suppository, but the recipe is entirely herbal. It reads:

> [Ebers 783] The Beginning of Recipes that are made for women to cause a woman to stop pregnancy in the first, second or third period [trimester][15]
> Unripe fruit(?)[16] of acacia
> Colocynth [d 3 r.t]
> Dates
> Triturate with a 6/7 pint of honey; moisten a pessary of plant fiber (ftt)[17] and place in vagina.[18]

Likely, the acacia (literally "thorn") is one or more species of Acacia, probably *Acacia nilotica* Del.[19] The colocynth in Egyptian is identified as colocynth (*Citrullus coloquinthus* [L.] Schrad).[20] This is the same plant that Dioscorides recommended also as a vaginal suppository.[21] Two researchers have studied this prescription, noting that, if it is compounded and fermentation occurs, lactic acid anhydride is produced. Dissolved in water, lactic acid is liberated. Lactic acid is employed in contraceptive jellies in the United States and United Kingdom. In laboratories it is rubbed over cervical rubber vaginal diaphragms to prevent spermatozoa from passing the diaphragm's edges.[22]

Even if fermentation was not assumed, there is evidence that each of the plants may have had antifertility effects. *Acacia koa*'s leaf was fed to mice twice daily for five days with 88–100 percent reduction in the number of litters, and its seed reduced pregnancy by 100 percent.[23] *Acacia nilotica* Del. is reported as an emmenagogue (abortifacient) when its leaves are eaten.[24] A traditional contraceptive pill used in modern, rural Bangladesh consists of mixing the exudations of *Acacia catechu,* the powdered stem bark of *Acacia arabica,* and the seed powder of *Tragia involucerta*. The prescription was administered to rats with the result that fertility was inhibited in 87.5 percent of the cases, but the tests showed no interruption of the estrus cycle, thereby leading to speculation that the action may be anti-implantation.[25] While it is impossible to disentangle all the plants in classical antiquity known as *Acacia,* especially by species and in early Egyptian documents (when examples of usage are so few and when descriptions are not given), nonetheless the evidence is sufficient to conclude that plants of the *Acacia* genus do have antifertility effects.

The second plant in the prescription, colocynth, is a known and attested abortifacient, but at least part of its action may be attributed to its toxicity.[26] Modern Arabic women take it for abortions. (One woman who took 120 grains in a powder to induce abortion died fifty hours later.)[27] In animal tests a leaf extract of colocynth was found to be 60–70 percent effective in preventing implantation.[28] Colocynth is in the same family as *Ecballium elaterium,* and both have a very active substance known as α-glucosidase elaterase.[29] The combination of acacia and colocynth is not unambiguously anticontraceptive insofar as the Egyptian recipe is topically administered, but the scientific testing was for oral administration.

The Ebers Papyrus contains a number of prescriptions for abortions, if, as seems most likely, the sign for "loosening" (sf*h*) or "stripping off" means abortion. The verb also is used to mean "discard; set aside";[30] many of the substances are abortifacients, which seems to make much less likely a translation as an aid to childbirth. The first recipe in the series is for a fumigant consisting of lower Egyptian salt, emmer seeds, and a plant called *sw.thm.t*. The recipes that follow are either taken orally or applied topically.

[Ebers 801] Another [for loosening a child in the belly of a woman]. One part fresh beans and one part honey are pressed together and drunk for one day.

[Ebers 802] Another. [An unknown plant called] *bsbs* one part, terebinth resin [from *Pistacia terebinthus*] one part, one part onion [*Allium* sp.], *3sr.t* beer, fresh beans one part, bird dung one part: made
into a suppository and placed in her vagina.

[Ebers 803] Another. Terebinth resin one part, oil/fat one part: made
into a salve for abdomen.

[Ebers 804] Another. [An unknown plant called] *nj3j3* one part, *ksntj*
[unknown] one part, wine one part: these are mixed together and
drunk for four days.

[Ebers 805] Another. Fruit of *išd* one part, *dsr.t* beer; these are poured
into her genital [*iwf*].

[Ebers 806] Another. Fruit of juniper [*wᶜn*] one part, [unknown plant
called] *nj3j3* one part, pine resin one part; these are made into a
suppository and placed in her genital [*iwf*].

[Ebers 807] Another. *njs*—part of a turtle, *ḥkwn*—beetle one part,
pine oil one part, *3sr.t* beer one part, oil/fat one part: these are
mixed together in a pill and thereby becoming united.[31]

The use of onions (*Allium* sp.), juniper, and pine products, as we
learned from Dioscorides, indicates that at least some of the recipes were
abortifacients as labeled. The unknown part of the beetle may be the indication of an early discovery of cantharides, or Spanish fly. Because
some of the plants are not identified, we cannot judge these prescriptions
with certainty. If, however, the beans are kidney beans (*Phaseolus vulgaris* L.) or closely related, this fact would be significant, since this bean
plant has four estrogenlike substances that are found in the flowering
beans, with amounts of estrogen varying from 8.5 µg equivalents in the
leaves to about 3 in the stems.[32]

In the same papyrus two other series of prescriptions probably pertain
to abortions, as follows:

[Ebers 797] Another [recipe] for inducing that a woman gives forth to
the ground. *nj3j3* [the same unknown plant as in Ebers 804]. This is
brought about by a woman, who is stripped and sits over it.

[Ebers 798] Another [recipe] for inducing that everything which is in a
woman's abdomen is expelled. Potsherd of a new earthern pot; it is
ground in oil/fat, it is warmed, and it is placed in her genital [*iwf*].

[Ebers 799] Another [recipe]. Date-palm juice in the *mšš* condition;[33]
upper Egyptian salt; oil/fat; these are cooked and drunk lukewarm.

[Ebers 828] Recipe for the extraction of a woman's blood. Onions one
part, wine one part; these are mixed together and placed in the genital [*iwf*].

[Ebers 829] Another [recipe for menstruation]. Acacia leaves one part,
oil of ben, drying (?) oil [*mrḥ.t*] one part, the plant *p3ḫ-srj.t* one

part, fruit (?) of the pea [*tḥwj*] one part, honey one part; these are placed in the genital [*iwf*].

[Ebers 830] Another [recipe for menstruation]. *bsbs* [unknown plant] ⅛; honey ⅛; *mhw.t* 2½ *ro;* sweet beer 5 *ro;* these are placed in her genital [*iwf*] for four days.[34]

While enough about these recipes is known for an evaluation, the use of acacia and date palm is particularly noteworthy, since they provide antifertility substances. In contrast, Ebers 798, where potsherds are mixed with oil in a suppository, would appear nothing more than an extreme irritant and abrasive. If all of the prescriptions cited here are abortifacients, as we surmise, one might ask why there are different rubrics. Why distinguish, for instance, between recipes to cause abortion and those that "induce a woman to drop forth to the ground" or "to expel what is in her abdomen" or "to extract [menstrual] blood"? First, there may be some distinction because a recipe for menstruation would be taken only during the earliest stages of pregnancy. Second, in the nature of complications of the Ebers type, the scribe is merely making lists of recipes and engages in little editing from the variety of sources.

Berlin Papyrus

The earliest mention of an oral contraceptive is found in the Berlin Medical Papyrus, dating from the Nineteenth Dynasty (c. 1300 B.C.). As in all the medical papyri, there are linguistic indications of archetypes. Although fragmentary, the translation reads:

> [...] emissions of semen[35] [...] a woman without becoming pregnant. You should fumigate her vagina with emmer seeds [*Triticum dicoccum* Schrank.] to prevent her receiving the semen. Then you should [make] for her a prescription to loosen [or release] semen: oil [or fat] 5 parts [*ro*], celery [*Apium graveolens* L.] 5 parts [*ro*], sweet beer 5 [*ro*]; heat and drink for four mornings.[36]

Assuming that the oil or fat and sweet beer are vehicles, the attention turns to celery. Emmer seeds were mentioned in the Eber Papyrus as a fumigant and elsewhere in the same papyrus as a (magical) indicator of a fetus's gender.[37] In fact, celery seeds are conspicuously found in the Indian Ayurvedic, Unani, and traditional medical systems, including African,[38] but the scientific laboratory reports are mixed. On the negative side is the report that extracts of celery seeds were taken separately with ethanol, petroleum, and water, and the amount of 100 mg/kg was administered to rats on days 1–7 with no inhibition of implantation.[39] Different results were reported in 1983. Here a higher dose of 250 mg/kg of extracts taken from the whole plant was administered to six rats for days 1–7 with the result of pregnancy termination in two, or 33.3 percent.[40] But these tests were conducted on pregnant rats. I have found no report of laboratory testing for contraceptive effects. All the implications for the use of celery are not clear, but other classical sources do not mention celery as an antifertility agent as did the Indian sources.[41] Not until the eleventh century is celery found in a medical work, one by Constantine the African, who reports that it is a strong abortifacient.[42]

On the basis of current information, sketchy though it is, there are indications that the first mention in medical literature of an oral conceptive may indeed have been to some degree effective. Certainly, the prescription for the abortifacient containing acacia and colocynth was effective, possibly with some danger to the woman unless care was exercised in the amount taken. In contrast, vaginal suppositories appear in the oldest of Egyptian medical records and continue to appear in later papyri; all appear to draw on an archetype, or traditional formula, whose activity may have some basis for action. Given the uncertainties about texts, translations, and identifications, however, and given the lack of definitive pronouncements in modern science studies, one cannot draw conclusions. The importance of the Egyptian material is the presence of the concept that certain agents can prevent conception and cause an abortion. The idea of a chemical means of birth control is thus as old as the surviving medical records. As for abortifacients, some were likely effective. Less confidence can be placed in the contraceptives, but here too there are grounds to postulate a rational use of drugs.

CHAPTER EIGHT

Greek and Roman Medicine from Hippocrates to Galen

When a woman has intercourse, if she is not going to conceive, then it is her practice to expel the sperm from both partners whenever she wishes to do so.

Hippocrates, *Nature of the Child*, 5.1

Writings Attributed to Hippocrates

The earliest explicit statement in Greek about an oral contraceptive occurs in two Hippocratic treatises. The work *On the Nature of Women* says, "If a woman does not wish to become pregnant, give to her in a drink of water moistened [or diluted] copper ore [*misy*] in the amount of a *vicia* bean, and she will not become pregnant for a year."[1] In *Diseases of Women* much the same appears: "Contraceptive [*atokion*]. If a woman does not want to be pregnant, moistened [or diluted] copper ore, as much as a *vicia* bean, in water, and have her drink it. For a year, thereabouts [*hōs epos eipein*], she does not get pregnant."[2] The different text, although related, differs only in what appears to be some kind of qualification about the time period that copper ore is supposed to have worked.

Being the earliest, specific contraceptive in Greek and, moreover, being found in works allegedly by Hippocrates, the reference to *misy* is cause for attention. If it was a true contraceptive, it would be noteworthy. The Egyptian papyri indicated that the ancients may have been able to control their reproduction without dangerous side effects, but the evidence was too scant for definitive conclusions. Since the measure of evidence is greater in ancient Greek medicine, our chances are therefore better of knowing how early such birth control was known. As we learned from Soranus and Dioscorides, the knowledge was acquired by the first century.

Misy is a copper compound, probably an ore, such as a copper sulphate. Dioscorides said that it came from Cyprus, but he gave no antifertility uses for it.[3] Neither did Galen, who also spoke of its use in salves.[4] Curiously in his work on metals, ores, and stones, Theophrastus did not mention it, although he did discuss copper.[5] Even more curious is why there are no other references in classical medicine for a copper compound as a contraceptive. Even Galen, who was well acquainted with writings attributed to Hippocrates, did not repeat the formula. According to the available documents, it is not until the sixth century A.D. that *misy* is recommended again as a contraceptive, this time by Aëtius of Amida (see Chapter 9 below).

While I can find no modern scientific studies on ingested copper compounds (which is what *misy* is), studies reveal that copper intrauterine devices (IUDs) are the most effective material allegedly because trace amounts of copper separate and cause chemical changes harmful to sperm and the conception event.[6] In an experiment performed at Zhejiang Medical College, Hangzhou, China, and reported in 1980, copper wire inserted in utero corroded in the first month of insertion 6 mg, or 0.2 mg daily, and for up to eighty months thereafter 0.014 mg daily.[7] In experiments with rabbits, after insertion of copper wire in utero, the copper did not prevent fertilization, even though there was some spermicidal action. The copper salts inhibited the lysis of the semen coagulum.[8] The action appears to be in the endometrium, that is, where implantation occurs, because the tissue there absorbs copper ions. Urine tests of women wearing the copper IUD show that about one half of the copper corroded from the IUD was excreted, and thus the remainder stayed in the body in some way. Copper salts in very small amounts (about 25 μg per kilogram) applied directly to the hypothalamus in rabbits caused ovulation and pseudopregnancy.

The work of two scientists, Gerald Oster and Miklos Salgo, has led to their hypothesis that copper metal inhibits enzyme activity "at very low concentration," possibly through prostaglandin synthesis. Copper causes increased prostaglandin production, and prostaglandins increase inflammation in the endometrium, especially affecting the mucus that causes the fertilized egg, the blastocyst, to attach.[9] Oster and Salgo's hypothesis has been countered by Warren Levinson, who believes that the possible mechanism is that copper sulfate is absorbed by three proteins in human fibroblasts and that it is this action with the function of proteins necessary for early cellular growth that is the cause.[10] Whatever the mechanism of its action, copper as a material for IUDs is actually a "pharmacologic agent."[11]

The reference in the Hippocratic work is to copper being orally taken and not directly induced as the modern studies have researched it. Could

copper possibly be effective as an oral contraceptive? The answer is unclear because there has not been experimentation. There is no reason a
priori to suppose that copper would have a systemic action other than
some toxic affects. Copper ingested, however, would be excreted via
urine and feces. Since only trace amounts of copper are responsible for
the pharmacological action, it is quite possible that ingested copper
would contaminate the vagina and continue to do so until there was a
cleansing action, such as would occur with menstruation.[12] Hence, the
recommendation by Aëtius of Amida that copper as a contraceptive was
effective for only one month, not a year according to the Hippocratic
treatise, is more believable. Too much should not be made of this puzzling
passage, because of the uncertainty about its effectiveness and the paucity
of references to copper compounds in subsequent medical documents.[13]
There is sufficient evidence, however, to merit the hypothesis that the first
contraceptive mentioned in Greek medicine is based on rational observations by women who were seeking to control their fertility through contraception.

In the same Hippocratic treatise, *Diseases of Women,* there are a number of abortifacients, most of which are vaginal suppositories.

An efficacious pessary [προσθετὸν δυνάμενον], which expels the afterbirth
[χόριον] and draws down the menstrua [ἐπιμήνια κατασπάσαι] and the
crippled embryo/fetus [ἔμβρυον ἀπόπληκτον]. Remove wings, legs and
head from five cantharine beetles; next, bruise the leaves and roots of the
small caltrop [*Tribulus terestris* L.], a shell amount of the crushed hard outer
part of *boanthemon* [*Chrysanthemum coronarium?*],[14] a shell amount of celery seed [*Apium graveolens* L.], fifteen cuttle fish eggs, mix in sweet wine
and insert.[15]

Virtually the same recipe is repeated in the same treatise, but with a
slightly different wording for the crucial passage referring to an abortion;
rather than "crippled embryo/fetus," this time the phrase is "it releases
the half-completed embryo/fetus [ἔμβρυον ἡμίεργον ἕλκει]." The Hippocratic medical writers generally expressed a pronatal policy. Perhaps
that spirit caused the authors to refer to a "crippled" fetus, but who can
be certain, especially in light of the repeated formula as an incomplete
fetus?

Commonly called Spanish fly, cantharine is a drug from a beetle.[16] The
cantharine beetle was mentioned, so we interpreted, in the Ebers Papyrus,
and the celery seed appeared in the Berlin Papyrus. The two plants, one
possibly the small caltrop and the other one known as *boanthemon,* are
not identified with certainty. The Egyptian formulas also contained references to unidentified plants. The similarities between the Hippocratic
prescriptions and the earlier Egyptian material are to great for there not
to have been a connection, albeit undocumented.

Following the recipes for disguised abortifacients, there followed a recipe clearly labeled ἐκβόλιον ὑστέρων, for "uterine abortive." In a context that suggests a suppository, the author cites the squirting cucumber (see Chapter 5) as a good abortive for the uterus—an author adds, "there is nothing that is better." [17] (I say "an author," even though the treatise is thought to be a composite of three separate works by different authors.)[18] We have in this statement something rarely encountered in ancient medicine. Here the unknown author (attributed to Hippocrates) tells us the preferred drug for abortion—namely, the squirting cucumber. This plant, *Ecballium elaterium* L., looks somewhat similar to the familiar garden cucumber, but it has no tendrils. A perennial, it grows in waste places, waysides, and cultivated areas. Its leaves are heart shaped and rough, and the fruit is ovoid-cylindrical (4–5 cm). The English term derives from the fact that, when its fruit dries, it squirts out its seeds. As we saw above in Chapter 5, the anonymous author's judgment is not contradicted by the evidence that we know of its antifertility effects.

Next in *Diseases of Women* are nine recipes, the first beginning with the ambiguous word πειρητήριον, which Emile Littré thought meant "agent to test for fertility" (*moyen explorateur de la fécondité*).[19] The meaning is perhaps simply "agent for testing." What follow are agents for abortion. Other than the term πειρητήριον, the recipes either have no labels regarding their use or have the rubric "Another." The recipes are, as follows:

1. a head of boiled garlic as suppository
2. scorpion of the sea on wool pad
3. cantharine beetle/Spanish fly
4. bulb [βόλβιον = Narcissus?]
5. lees of white wine
6. galbanum [= *Ferula galbaniflua* Boiss. and Buhse.], soda [*natron*], copper ore [*misy*] with myrtle rose, applied on a linen pad
7. elaterium [squirting cucumber] in double amounts, honey and wine on linen pad
8. butter and alum on coarse flax
9. scammony juice, animal fat, barley meal, and wine applied on a linen pad.[20]

References to Spanish fly, natron (soda/saltpeter), and alum were encountered in the Egyptian papyrus. Most of the other active ingredients are found in either Soranus or Dioscorides.

In the same Hippocratic treatise, there are a number of early stage abortifacients, but these are clearly labeled ἕτερον ἐκβόλιον (sometimes, ὑστέρων) or "other abortives" (or "uterine abortatives"). The administration is oral, and most specify that they are taken with wine or water.

1. *Another abortifacient* [ἐκβόλιον]: shake her under the armpits and give her to a drink the petals of the chaste tree in wine, or grind an obol of Cretan dittany [*Origanum dictamnus* L. or *Amaracus dictamnus* Benth.], or a handful of spikenard [*Inula* sp.] in leek juice with a large shell of oil of bitter almonds.[21]

2. *Another.* Take a decoction of pine in sweet wine and add three obols galbanum and myrtle [preparation instructions follow].

3. *Or another.* A decoction of leek juice, myrtle, and sweet wine mixed together.

4. *Or,* grind down purslane [*Portulaca oleracea* L.] given with a double amount of white wine.

5. *Or,* nine seeds of black poplar from Crete, ground, boiled in wine.

6. *Or,* buttercup [*Ranunculus* sp.] leaves and flowers, ground, boiled with an Aeginetan drachma of sweet wine.[22]

The prescriptions generally appear to be effective. We have already learned the effects of the chaste tree, dittany, spikenard, leek, pine, galbanum (*Ferula*), myrtle, and poplar. Two plants here are heretofore unencountered: purslane and buttercup. Although Dioscorides knew of their medicinal qualities, he did not mention any antifertility properties.[23] Buttercup, however, is encountered in folk medicine in India as an abortifacient.[24] Purslane is reported in one scientific study as having an abortive or antifertility effect on rat uteri in vitro.[25] The absence of these plants in later writings and the scarcity of notices in the scientific studies, however, point to plants that may have an antifertility effect but not a pronounced one. Once we disregard the prescription items that are unknown or not found in scientific studies, we find that these recipes indeed have antifertility effects as described.

The list of recipes continues under the several different headings.

1. *Potent uterine abortifacient* [ὕστερον δύναιται ἐκβάλλειν], the roots of sweet earth-almond [*Cyperus esculentus*], that is like a bulb, small like an olive, and let her drink it. If small, two are needed; if not, one will do. Mix together some seeds of Ethiopian cumin [*Carum copticum* B. & H.?),[26] Massilian hartwort [*Seseli tortuosum* L.], dried Lybian leaves [*silphion* or *Ferula historica?*] with three cotyls [approx. 0.7 l] of wine; boil down to a half and let her drink this.[27]

Almost certainly the Lybian leaves are *silphion* because of the fame of the plant and the association with Lybia, its only habitat. The Ethiopian cumin is uncertain, but *Cyperus* has recently been found to have estrogenic activity.[28] Dioscorides said that a species of hartwort (*Tortylium officinale* L.) was a menstrual regulator or emmengagogue. The next plant is *sisōn*, likely a closely related plant; Dioscorides said that it also has the same property.[29] Interestingly, Pliny said that *seselis,* probably the same plant, is eaten by pregnant deer in order to purge themselves and cause an easier delivery.[30] Other recipes follow under this rubric:

2. *Another.* Fruit of the chaste tree [λύγος], hartwort likeness, myrtle, ground and given as a drink in water.
3. *Abortifacient* [ἐβόλια]. Fresh white chaste tree [ἄγνος], well-boiled and given as a drink in a saucer in white wine.[31]

Note that in recipe 2 the word for chaste tree is λύγος, but in the next recipe the word for the same plant is ἄγνος. This evidence suggests that the writer(s) of the treatise was functioning more as compiler than author.

4. *A different kind.* Castoreum [from a beaver] and an obol of *saga-pēnon* [*Ferula persica*], a drachma [4.3 g/0.15 oz.] of *asphaltion* [*Alhagi maurorum?* or possibly the fern *asplēnon?*], two of soda/saltpeter, boiled down in sweet wine and with a half koros [3.2 ml] and drunk with warm water.
5. *Another somewhat similar.* Sea urchin [*Echinus* sp.] boiled in sweet wine and given as a drink.
6. *Another.* A small handful of mint [*minthe*], rue, coriander [*Coriander sativum* L.], juniper or cyperus chips [*Cyperus rotundus* L. + sp.], boiled down in sweet wine and drunk . . .
7. *Another similar one.* Anise [*Pimpinella anisum* L.], juniper, celery seed, Ethiopian cumin, hartwort, . . . [preparation instructions].[32]

Neither Soranus nor Dioscorides listed antifertility purposes for coriander, but Dioscorides said that coriander generated seed, whether in males or females is unspecified.[33] In animal tests reported in 1987, an extract of coriander seeds was administered orally to female rats at doses of 250 and 500 mg/kg. The rats showed significant, although not complete, blocking of implantation on days 5, 12, and 20 of pregnancy. Treatments that began later in pregnancy caused no reduction in the number of pregnancies. Importantly, there were no abnormalities or any significant changes in the weight and length of the fetuses.[34]

The identification of "mint" is unclear as to the exact plant, but if it is pennyroyal (*Mentha pulegium* L.), it is a noted antifertility drug, as mentioned above.[35] If it is corn mint (*Mentha arvensis* L.), a recent laboratory animal test using its leaves shows that a dose of 100 mg/kg resulted in antiovulatory activity in 40–60 percent of the cases.[36] Another rat experiment with corn mint significantly reduced pregnancy from day 1 to day 10 after coitus, and was especially pronounced during the post implantation period. A daily administration of 10 mg/kg from day 7 through day 10 resulted in 90–100 percent loss.[37] Again, the uncertainty about the exact plant should not be too troubling to the historian because of shared phytochemical characteristics of plants of the same genus. Anise has been reported as having abortifacient qualities by blocking progesterone production.[38] The identification of *asphaltion* is not known, and the actions of the sea urchin and castoreum are not known as fertility regulators.

The recipes continue:

> 8. *Another similar one.* A handful of dittany, two drachmas of Queen Anne's lace seeds, black cumin [*Nigella sativa* L.], ground and given as a drink in white wine; afterwards the woman should bathe in warm water.[39]

Here is the first recorded use of Queen Anne's lace for abortion, but, as we saw, it is also contraceptive in that it interferes with implantation. The actions of black cumin are not known.

> 9. *Another.* Galbanum [*Ferula galbaniflua*] ground with oil in juniper, applied, its destroys and aborts a sluggish one [τοῦτο δύναται διαφθείρειν καὶ ἐκβάλλειν τὸ νωχελές].[40]

Much the same recipe is repeated later in the same treatise but this time with the heading Διεκβόλιον, ἢ ἀποθάνῃ τὸ ἔμβρυον, which I interpret to mean, "Somemore expulsives (abortives) to remove a dead embryo/fetus." [41] There follow eight recipes of a similar nature with the heading "Other" (ἕτερον or ἄλλο). These recipes contain much the same ingredients as those that have been previously encountered: silphium (*Ferula historica*), juniper, galbanum (*Ferula galbaniflua*), spikenard, cantharine, plus one that will be encountered later in this study: sweet flag (*Acorus calamus* L.). The series ends with the ninth recipe, "An expulsive to reject an embryo/fetus that is dead in the interior," that is a mixture of squirting cucumber and *batrachion* (*Artemisia absinthium* L.?).[42]

After recipe 9 above, there follow another twelve abortifacients, one of which is a fumigant made by burning willow leaves, but most have diverse headings. The first two have the following headings, with the principal ingredients in brackets: (1) "An abortifacient infusion for the uterus: whenever it suppurates, chilled by cold, whenever the wind is cold" [saffron and goose grease];[43] (2) "A drink mixture for the same thing" [spikenard, meal, pine resin];[44] (3) "Another abortifacient suppository when the child and insides are bad" [copper or bronze: χαλκός];[45] (4) "Another similar drink if it is dead" [pottery and goose grease].[46]

These are followed by six recipes, similar to those above, and introduced by the heading "Another." In one of these there is a plant not encountered heretofore: to expel a fetus that has been battered, *helxinē* (probably *Convolvulus arvensis* L., or field bindweed) is taken in wine.[47]

The next recipe is unusual in both its heading and its contents: "It expels [φθεῖραι] an embryo/fetus that is not moving and works to abort [ἐκβαλεῖν] it." It is a drink composed of black hellebore with myrrh, spikenard, pine resin, and soda/saltpeter.⁴⁸ Black hellebore (*Helleborus niger* L.) and field bindweed were not employed by Soranus, while Dioscorides recommended black hellebore only as a suppository.⁴⁹ Black hellebore is recognized as an abortifacient and emmenagogue today,⁵⁰ whereas bindweed is not known for these effects, although it contains coumarin (an abortifacient). Bindweed is poisonous to livestock in South Africa.⁵¹ Finally, there is a recipe to abort (ἐκβαλεῖν = ἐκβολεύς) a fetus/embryo that is not moving; this consists of one drachma of cleaved alum and three obols of black hellebore blended and mixed with wine and added acorns.⁵² Cattle who eat large quantities of acorns have miscarriages.

If we are somewhat confused by all this information, the reason is that the data were poorly presented by the author(s) of *On the Diseases of Women*. Recipes pile on top of one another with little or no editing. For instance, in one recipe above there was one Greek word for chaste tree (*lugos*), followed in the next recipe with another word (*agnos*) for the same plant. Similarly, two different words were used for copper, *misy* and *kalkos*. What are we to make of the different headings about the status of the embryo/fetus—it is variously described as weak, not moving, healthy, livid,⁵³ palsied,⁵⁴ and crippled within?⁵⁵ Evidently the author or authors simply copied or listed recipes as they encountered them, without attempting to understand the material themselves. Even though the immediate author may have employed one or more written source(s), the variety of headings points to oral transmission. Also, the indications are that the author(s) did not know well the content of what was being listed.

Modern scholars regard the Hippocratic authors as all being male. But were not Soranus and Dioscorides also males, and was not their understanding of the information impressive? Women's matters were women's matters, despite the presence of this new line of physicians who traced their inspiration to Hippocrates. The authors of these work(s) probably did not understand the data and merely recorded it without assimilating and reformulating the material. Later readers may not have understood that this treatise gave information about how to have a safe abortion. Since the work was not translated into Latin until the Renaissance period, it was unavailable to the Western Middle Ages. It was, however, used by the Arabic medical authorities, who made more sense of the material.

The Hippocratic author(s) knew most of the plant, mineral, and animal substances that there were to know. Later writers added substances to the list, but fewer than one might expect. It is clear that the Hippocratic writers drew upon a body of information that was very old indeed. The substances (as best we know them) that were found in the Egyptian papyri are present in Hippocratic works. Consider, for instance, this Hippocratic abortifacient: "Ecbolic (abortive) suppository: Egyptian salt, mouse dung, wild colocynth; pour in a fourth-part honey, boiled to a half; take a drachma of resin and put into the honey and mouse dung, grind all together well. Make suppositories, insert in the uterus, until the proper time."[56] Here, and elsewhere above, the Egyptian use of dung, pottery, colocynth, Egyptian salts, resin, juniper, leeks, and celery seed, most of which are mentioned in the Ebers Papyrus in the same way, produces a connection too similar to disregard. The Hippocratic writers related time-tested abortifacients much older than their own times.

Pliny the Elder

Pliny the Elder (A.D. 23–79) was a learned, eclectic Roman, who authored a large encyclopedia called the *Natural History*. In his writings, Pliny allowed his personality and personal values to intrude. Stoic that he was, he said that he was reluctant to transmit birth control information. Pliny could not resist informing us, however.

For the white poplar and willow, Pliny gave no contraceptive information, but willow is, he said, a sexual depressant.[57] In discussing a spider known as a phalangium used as an amulet, Pliny remarked that the phalangium "is the only one of all contraceptives [*ex omni atocio*]. This only would be right [*fas*] for me to mention, to help those women who are so prolific that they stand in need of such respite."[58] Pliny was not restricted by consistency. About juniper, he said, "Gossip records a miracle: that to rub it all over the male part before coitus prevents conception."[59] About rue, "Pregnant women must take care to exclude rue from their diet, for I find that the fetus is killed by it."[60] Unlike Soranus and Dioscorides, who prescribed rue as an abortifacient, Pliny pointed to this quality as an item to avoid in diet—but the information is related just the same.

Inexplicably for any writer other than Pliny, he showed no reluctance to give herbal prescriptions inducing sterility: parsley (*Petroselinum sativum* Nym.; *P. crispum* Miller) as *sterilesco* and two ferns of uncertain species identification, known as *asplenon* and *felix* (var. *filix*), as *sterilitatem facit* ("it causes sterility" = "it is a contraceptive").[61] Dioscorides said that *asplenon* was a contraceptive. *Asplenium* is probably the fern known to us as *Asplenium adiantum-nigrum* L., and *felix* is likely the fern known to us as the male fern *Dryopteris filix-mas* (L) Schott (var. *Polypodium filix* or *P. vulgare* L.). This fern is taken in Hungary as a contraceptive.[62] One possible identification for this fern is *Adiantum capillus* L., which was shown in recent tests on rats to be an active inhibitor of postcoital implantation.[63] All these ferns contain filicic acid, which is probably the pharmaceutically active substance. Filicic acid from the root of *Dryopteris crassirhizoma* was administered subcutaneously to rats (dose of 2–3 mg/rat on pregnancy days 7–9), and it terminated 100 percent of the pregnancies.[64] The activity here suggests that it is most effective during early pregnancy.

In summary, Pliny failed to give complete information about contraceptives and sterilizers. Although he disfavored such things, he found grounds for doing so in at least one instance to save poor mothers who were having too many children. Despite his moral reluctance to advocate birth control, Pliny not only related information about abortifacients but also extended the information known in the sources. Generally, his method was to relate that a plant was an emmenagogue and add that it also expelled a dead fetus. For example, for cabbage stalks he observed, "purgationem feminis . . . emortuos pellit"; for rue, "feminarum etiam purgationes secundasque etiam emortuos partus." In such expressions he related this information about these plants already discussed: cabbage, rue, mint, pennyroyal, hulwort, thyme, *silphium* (ferula), sage, *galbanum* (from *Ferula galbaniflua* Boiss. and Buhse.), lesser century plant, dittany, birthwort, mandrake, artemisia, wormwood (*absinthium*), Queen Anne's lace, myrrh, pepper, scammony, and opopanax.[65] Most were for oral administration, although a few were used as suppositories. Scammony was taken both ways. A modern report on scammony focuses attention on the ergot alkaloids that grow on it and speculates that the historical use of scammony as an abortifacient could come from the action of this known abortifacient.[66] Scammony's use was not widespread, judging from the paucity of its listing in early medicine. Pliny named the important plants in more frequent usage. For instance, he said that rue was "among our chief medicinal plants," but, of all emmenagogic drugs, dittany had "greatest efficacy [*vis est*]." Dittany is so powerful that it should not be in the same room with a pregnant woman.

Water mint (*Mentha aquatica* L.), Pliny said, "should not be eaten by pregnant women unless the fetus be dead, since even one application of it produces abortion."[67] Pliny named thirteen plants that were emmenagogues or expelled a dead fetus but that had not appeared in earlier sources, including chicory (*Cichorium intybus* L.), chamomile (*Anthemis rosea* Sibth.), ground pine (*Ajuga chia* Schreb. or *A. chamaepitys* Schreb.), and false dittany (*Ballota acetabulosa* L.).[68] Each of these plants is known in folklore as an antifertility agent, but except for mallow and false dittany, they are not reported in scientific studies.[69] A species of mallow (*Malva* [*viscus*] *conzattii* Greenm) was given orally to rats with the result of 71 percent inhibition of fertility.[70] Interestingly, in a recent laboratory finding, an extract of mallow's flower was found to inhibit spermatogenesis and therefore is promising as a male contraceptive drug.[71] Mallow's antifertility effect is high when the drug is extracted from the flower in the winter but relatively weak when taken during the summer.[72]

Like Dioscorides, Pliny related information about betony (or wound-wort).[73] Finally, despite his reluctance to give explicit details about abortions in some of his passages, just the same, for three plants—rue, wild mint (*Mentha silvestris* L.), and pennycress (*Thlaspia avense* L.)—Pliny said that ingestion "kills the fetus [*partus necat*]."[74] A number of plants he labeled as outright abortifacients (*abortum facit* or *infert; abortivum est*): squirting cucumber, mallow (*Malva* spp.), cyperus, hulwort, ground pine, arum (*Arum dracunculus* L.), and the fern *filix*.

Pliny's medical knowledge was limited. He passed on the information he had, however; in doing so, he extended and transmitted fertility information. Some of the plants he mentioned had marginal value, if any. The fact remains, however, that for the principal plants, such as rue, dittany, and squirting cucumber, his encyclopedic *Natural History* was a repository for birth control information.

Scribonius Largus

A near contemporary of Pliny and Dioscorides, Scribonius Largus (fl. A.D. 47) prescribed in his medical work one recipe for the aftereffects of an abortion (*ex partu abortuve*), which consists of valerian (*spica nardus = Valeriana celticia* L.), saussurea (*Saussurea lappa* Clarke), white pepper, black pepper, long pepper, myrrh, opium, mandrake root, cinnamon, *asarum* (*Asarum European* L.), *acorus* (*Iris pseudacorus* L. or *Acorus calamus* L.), lavender, frankincense, cabbage seeds, castoreum, opopanax, French lavender (*Lavandula staechas* L.), Queen Anne's lace, *ammi* (*Ammi copiticum* L.), and *seselis Creticum* (*Bulpeurum fruiticorum* L.).[75] This concoction would indeed be a strong drug. We have already encountered pepper (various species and preparations), myrrh, cabbage seeds, Queen Anne's lace, and opopanax as abortifacients. The opium and mandrake have strong, toxic alkaloids. The atropine in mandrake blocks the ovulatory surge of luteinizing hormones in animals.[76]

Scribonius gave the amounts for each ingredient in this prescription, which would have a predictable effect on fertility and pregnancy. His recipe, however, was for *after* an abortion. Likely, it would be so strong as to be dangerous as well. It is difficult to know the problem it was expected to cure. The recipe does not make medical sense for postabortive therapeutic care, but the ingredients are an awesome compound of strong antifertility agents. In Chapter 1, we observed Scribonius' opposition to abortion. A possible explanation for the inclusion of the recipe is that Scribonius simply did not know what he was recording inasmuch as the recipe appears a strong, possibly fatal, abortifacient and he recorded it as postoperative care.

Opposed as he was to abortion, Scribonius doubtless did not know that he delivered practical information about the procedure when he discussed emmenagogues. The menses that are difficult to purge, he said, can be stimulated by such herbs as artemisia and dittany.[77] Other herbs that can be taken include those on the familiar list: colocynth, opopanax and other *Ferula* plants, parsley, birthwort (*malum terrae*), white pepper, nard, myrrh, and saffron.[78]

Galen

Galen was the foremost physician in classical antiquity, as far as number of surviving works and historical influence are concerned. He described a number of abortifacient prescriptions, most of them vaginal suppositories. He named only three oral contraceptives (ἀτόκιος): one is unidentified,[79] and the other two are barrenwort (ἀναμέμικται γὰρ αὐτῷ τις ἀλλόκοτος ποιότης)[80] and juniper, the latter which he said was both a contraceptive (ἀτόκιον ἐστι φάρμακον) and an abortifacient (verb: ἐκβάλλω, meaning "abort" or "expel").[81] Galen named the following abortifacients that Dioscorides also identified: lupine,[82] death carrot,[83] two juniper species,[84] wallflower or stock,[85] great century (*Centaurium erythraea* Rafn. + sp.),[86] cyclamen (*Cyclamen hederifolium* Aiton),[87] golden drop (*Onosma* sp.),[88] squirting cucumber (*Ecballium elaterium* L.),[89] myrrh,[90] woundwort (*Stachys* sp.),[91] pepper,[92] opopanax,[93] and the fern known as *pteris*.[94] The latter fern, Dioscorides said, was both a contraceptive and an abortifacient. Both Dioscorides' and Galen's prescriptions for squirting cucumber as an abortifacient are paralleled in recent animal tests as an abortifacient.[95] Linnaeus gave the plant the name "Ecballium," a scientific name from the Greek meaning "abortion" (the ancient Greek name is *sikus agrios*).

Galen and Dioscorides both cited calamint (*Calamintha* sp.) as an abortifacient, but Galen said it was for oral administration, while Dioscorides stipulated suppository.[96] Galen listed pennyroyal only as an emmenagogue.[97] In the treatise "On Simple Drugs according to Temperaments and Faculties," which contains the citations, Galen did not specifically say that willow had antifertility properties,[98] but in the work "On Compound Medicines according to Site," Galen gave two prescriptions for emmenagogues. The first has willow and rue, and the other contains willow, rue, ginger, and date palm.[99] As observed earlier in this study, willow and date palm are regarded by modern science as contraceptive. Concerning white poplar (Dioscorides' contraceptive), Galen related other medicinal usages but not for contraception.[100] On *silphion*, or

Cyrenaic juice (ferula), he gave no fertility usages.[101] In one place, Galen said that rue dries out the semen and in another that it represses sexual urges, but he did not explicitly say that it is a contraceptive, abortifacient, or emmenagogue.[102] In other treatises, however, Galen related a number of compound prescriptions for abortions that contain familiar plants previously discussed, including pepper, parsley, rue, juniper, artemisia, aloe, opopanax, and mandrake.[103] One recipe containing twenty-four ingredients was taken "to expel a fetus/embryo without pain [ἀλύπως ἔμβϱωα ἔκκϱίνει]."[104] In an oral-route prescription for abortion named after Orbanos, Galen included pepper, birthwort, and rue.[105] In nonpharmaceutical medical treatises, Galen discussed the harm to the mother that is done by taking abortifacient/emmenagogic preparations,[106] especially after the beginning of the second trimester.[107]

CHAPTER NINE

The Late Roman Empire and Early Middle Ages

It is not right for anyone to give an abortion.

Theodorus Priscianus, *Euporiston*, 3.6.

By itself [rue] does not bring these results; they are due to the people who employ it without considering its strength, its dosage, or the circumstances.

Gargilius Martialis, *Medicines from Oils and Fruits*

Clearly the ancients discovered what we only recently rediscovered. How did the ancients learn this information, and how much of what they learned was known during the Middle Ages? Why was this knowledge seemingly lost, only to be rediscovered? And why, in the rediscovery, did we believe it to be new?

Neither period of time had controlled laboratory and scientific methodology. They learned through observation of what worked on them and, to some degree, on animals. The Hippocratic physicians, Soranus, Dioscorides, Galen, and the hundreds of writers from whom Pliny copied information had themselves not made many, or perhaps any, of the discoveries. One way in which medicine differs from pure science is that its principles are constantly being tested empirically. When Norman Himes said that knowledge of effective abortifacients and contraceptives was confined to a few medical encyclopedists, physicians, and scholars, he failed to ask how this elite would know in the first place what to give for what, if not through intelligent, critical observation of folk practice. Drug usage was discovered in much the same way that nutritious plants were separated from those that were not, namely, by countless experiments, mostly long before the written word.[1]

How modern medicine made the rediscoveries that plants have antifertility effects is informative in understanding ancient medicine and folk practice. When in the 1930s Skarzynski, Butenandt, and Jacobi published their studies of the production of female sex hormones in willow, date palm, and pomegranate, the findings appear to have had little impact or acceptance. The field of animal science is the principal area where research on antifertility effects of plants in mammals produced results now accepted as valid.[2] In the 1940s, Australian sheep, grazing on a type of clover (*Trifolium subterraneum*), had sharply reduced fertility. The reason was found to be isoflavonoids in the clover, which induced estrogenic activity in mammals.[3] In following up on reports that Burmese and Thai women take orally an extract of the root *Pueraris mirificia* (kin to kudzu) to induce abortion, Bounds and Pope, in 1960, isolated a compound called miroestrol that has a medicinally higher activity than estrone.[4]

But how did the ancients learn that plants affected fertility? First, they would observe the connection between what people ate for nourishment or took for medicines and the resulting activity the foods or substances may have had. In the case of miscarriage, they would observe that certain things caused them. This knowledge would be useful to those who wanted pregnancy and to those who did not.

Another way would be to observe the behavior of animals. The death carrot (*thapsi* al. *Thlapsi*), mentioned above as an abortifacient, was described by Theophrastus (died c. 287 B.C.), who gave us this insight: "The cattle of the country [Attica] do not touch it, but imported cattle feed on it and perish of diarrhea."[5] While not specifically pointing to an antifertility effect, some people observing the behavior of cattle were probably induced to experimentation. Whether it was during Theophrastus' time, later, or long before, the historian can probably never know. All that can be said is that by the first century A.D., death carrot was being prescribed as an antifertility agent, and this information was not the product of any research laboratory or a known, learned physician. It was the learned physicians, however, who recognized the effectiveness of this plant and recorded this information. The question now becomes how much, if any, of this information was conveyed to the Middle Ages.

Gargilius Martialis, a retired soldier in North Africa in the third century A.D., wrote about the medical knowledge that an estate leader should have.[6] As such, he gave scant attention to female problems, making only one mention of contraceptives and abortifacients. He praised the powers of rue but ended with a message urging wise practice.

> Some very foolishly declare the damage rue causes: that it inhibits libido, debilitates the generative seed, and kills embryos in the womb. By itself it does not bring these results; they are due to the people who employ it without considering its strength, its dosage, or the circumstances. Therefore a

man of judgment employs it in moderation so that it may not become a poison, rather than a remedy.[7]

Oribasius, Learned Physician

The noted physician Oribasius (fl. under Julian, 359–361) gave a recipe of fern root and willow leaves to be drunk after coitus.[8] In the section devoted to simple drugs Oribasius identified wallflower (or stock: φθό-ριόν ἐστι φάρμακον) and squirting cucumber as emmenagogues and abortifacients.[9] Birthwort and germander he called menstrual regulators but said that juniper was both a contraceptive and an abortifacient, and plowman's spikenard, germander, and myrrh were abortifacients.[10] The plant called κυκλάμινος, possibly honeysuckle, which Dioscorides called a male contraceptive, Oribasius said was a menstrual regulator.[11]

In his *Synopsis,* Oribasius discussed the remedies effective for stimulating menstruation, which were common juniper, savin juniper, iris, pennyroyal, calamint, spignel, rue, horned poppy, dittany, asarum, costus, cassia, and birthwort, as plant drugs, and oils made from cyperus, storax, wormwood, artemisia, and black hellebore.[12] Of these plants, this is the first usage encountered for horned poppy (*glaukion* = *Glaucium* sp.).[13] Costus (*Saussurea lappa* Clarke) was also employed by Dioscorides as an emmenagogue.[14] Juniper was named also as a contraceptive (ἀτόκίον ἐστι φάρμακον) in addition to causing an abortion (ἐκβάλλει).[15] As vaginal suppositories, Oribasius recommended artemisia, dittany, cabbage juice, peony (*Paeonia officinalis* L. and *P. corallina*), leek or garlic (*Allium prassium* L. or *A. sativa* L.), rue, and scammony.[16]

Oribasius named another contraceptive: axe-weed (*Securigera coronilla* DC.) juice is rubbed on the penis prior to insertion to prevent conception. Repeating Dioscorides in part, he said that willow leaves drunk with wine causes barrenness (*asyllēpsia*), and cabbage flowers do the same.[17] This is the same plant that Dioscorides had recommended as an abortifacient. From the Hippocratic corpus through Galen, medical writers provided information about contraceptives and abortifacients, but no work is a copy of another. While there is a strong consistency in the principal plants employed as antifertility agents, no prescription is simply a copy of another. Many works add new plant drugs. Clearly, even with Pliny, who certainly culled his information from many sources without personal knowledge of all of them, there is a sense of vitality in the information as new experiences are gained with plants. Some drugs that were considered less effective drop out or seldom appear, such as pomegranate and *misy* (the copper compound in the Hippocratic work) while almost all works have as antifertility agents plants such as rue, birthwort, wormwood, and dittany. Even with the familiar plants, however, the information appears not to be static, as these plants are used in medical prescriptions with varying formulas.

Another way to see changes is in the Latin translations of Greek medical works, most of them being done around the fifth and sixth centuries. During this period, Dioscorides' *Materials of Medicine* was translated anonymously by someone probably in the Ravenna area of Italy. The translator exhibited no inhibition in dealing with birth control and, by his choice of words, revealed that he understood the subject matter. For example, where Dioscorides used the word *atokios,* meaning "contraceptive," as a use for white poplar, the unknown Latin translator wrote, "Its leaves drunk after a menstrual cleaning in a similar way interfere with conception in a lesser way [than with the bark]." [18] Elsewhere in the same work, where the Greek text reported that pepper "drives out the embryo; if applied as a suppository after intercourse, it prevents conception," [19] the Latin translation reads, "It is thought after coitus that it kills by poisoning; let it be applied after intercourse into the genital." [20] The translation was certainly not a literal rendering of words but an interpretation. It was not that the translator did not know the languages; Dioscorides's comment on death carrot—"*embrya phtheirei* [it aborts an embryo]"—became "abortum facit [it makes an abortion]." [21] In the Latin translation of Oribasius' work, there is a discussion about abortions (*ekballonta embrya*),[22] where many of the same plants (rue, dittany, birthwort, myrrh, pennyroyal, juniper, cyperus, asarus, artemisia, and iris) are referred to, but rather than abortifacients they are called emmenagogues (e.g., "purgat menstruam").[23]

Not always, however, do the Latin texts of the early Middle Ages (when the Latin translation of Oribasius was done) reflect a reluctance to specify about abortions. A near consensus about the drugs is seen in the Latin *Synopsis* of Oribasius. In the discussion of menstrual regulators and emmenagogues, a number of agents are mentioned as follows: "beaten wormwood, pennyroyal, century plant, thyme, rue and others which have those qualities." [24] Clearly, the author assumed that the reader would know what the remaining plants were.

Marcellus Empiricus

Marcellus Empiricus, a late Roman-early medieval writer (fl. 385), recorded the now-familiar herbs to induce menstruation (artemisia, dittany, opopanax, pepper, saffron, giant fennel, myrrh, colocynth, etc.), but he mentioned no contraceptives as such.[25] Marcellus' pharmacy includes many ingredients in single prescriptions that have multiple purposes. For example, the following recipe is cooked and given for inflation of the stomach, indigestion, acrid belching, stomachaches, difficulty in urinating, internal dislocations, and all ruptures and stiffness. Also it moves the menstrua of women, if there is difficulty in purging, and it pulls downs (or expels) if after childbirth or abortion internal corruptions are substituted (*si ex partu et aborsu intrinsecus nociua substiterint*).

> 7 denarii parsley, 4 den. phu [= *Valeriana phu* L.],[26] 19 den. white pepper, 5 den. ploughman's spikenard [*inula* = *Inula conyza* DC], 6 den. walnuts, 12 den. pine nuts, 8 den. false bishops' weed [*ami* = *Ammi maius* L.?], 12 den. lovage [*ligusticum* = *Levisticum officinale* Koch], 8 den. ginger, 12 den. sedge (*careus* = *Carex* sp.), 12 den. celery seeds, 8 den. anise, 8 den. cardamom, 6 den. sweet flag [*acorus*, either *Iris pseudacorus* L. or *Acorus calamus* L.], 8 den. wild carrot seeds [Queen Anne's lace], 12 den. coriander seed [*olisandri?*], [and] 6 den. fenugreek seed.[27]

(A denarius is weight of a Roman coin and, according a treatise on weights and measures attached to Marcellus' works, the same as an Attic drachma [= approx. 4.3 gr/0.15 oz].)[28]What can we make of this prescription? Most of the ingredients are abortifacients, but the combination of so much in one prescription causes one to wonder at what its effect must have been. Unstated, of course, is the means of administration and how much was to be taken at a single time. Marcellus often gave recipes without a good grasp of medicine. For example, he had one recipe with two giant fennels (*Ferula*: *galbanum* and *silphium*), opopanax, rue, artemisia, Queen Anne's lace, asarum, and juniper, but he said that it was for various aches and pains of the belly region, among them retention of the urine.[29] Whatever this recipe would do, a pregnant woman should not take it. Marcellus recorded an immense lore about drugs, but he does not appear expertly knowledgeable about medicine in general, or women and fertility in particular.

Quintus Serenus

Another late Roman writer, Quintus Serenus (d. A.D. 212), was much more open about birth control than was Marcellus. Quintus Serenus said that, when the pregnancy was less than eight months and the fetus was weak, one should "rush into the bedroom" and give to the woman pennyroyal in tepid water.[30] A mixture of egg, rue, and dill in a vaginal suppository is a good expulsive, or abortifacient. Also as an aid to pregnancy, Serenus prescribed dittany, and either the smell of vulture's dung or a recipe of egg, rue, and dill for childbirth.[31]

One wonders whether Serenus understood clearly his sources, whether written or oral. The working knowledge of fertility plants was likely held by women and transmitted orally. Men, who wrote on the subject, were dependent on women as well as on their written sources. Just so, most medical writers of the late Roman and early Byzantine period not only faithfully transmitted the agents for contraceptives and abortifacients but also contributed new formulas, seldom just copying their sources.[32] Familiar plants dominate the formulas: pepper, birthwort, dittany, rue, wormwood, iris, myrrh, lupine, and opopanax.

Theodorus Priscianus

Living in the late fourth century A.D., Theodorus Priscianus exemplifies the contradictions under which late Roman physicians labored. The third book of his major medical work in Latin was devoted to gynecology. The book was separated in manuscripts during the Middle Ages, when it was copied and cited as a distinct work. In the book a long chapter 6 deals with abortions. Ominously he began by asserting that it was not right (*fas*) for any one to give an abortion.[33] The word *fas* means that which is religiously right to do, not right in the sense of law (*lex*). *Fas* is the same word that Pliny had used. The reason for this, he noted, were the words of Hippocrates (*Hippocratis attestatur oratio*). In what appears an allusion to the oath, Theodorus implied that the matter of abortion was not within the realm of conscientious medical practice. But there are times, he countered, when the opening to the womb is too small or the age of the woman is too young, in which case a full-term pregnancy could lead to death. The situation is the same as when the health of a tree depends on pruning branches or when a ship is too heavily laden in a storm and must lighten its weight to be saved.[34] When action is required, there are means to save the woman from a potentially fatal pregnancy, which means he related in detail. The means were chemical.

Theodorus gave some nine prescriptions, plasters, pessaries, and, mostly, oral compounds to produce an abortion. The ingredients are familiar. One oral prescription was myrrh, artemisia, and violet seeds, pulverized, and drunk in water with mint, to be followed by a bath. A lozenge consisted of a decoction of artemisia and dittany; another, of opopanax roots, myrrh, and aloe taken with mint water.[35] The importance of this chapter is that the work circulated throughout the Middle Ages.[36] Not only was information available about how to have an abortion, but, accompanying it, was a moral justification: to save lives.

Aëtius of Amida

In his medical work *Biblia iatrika ekkaideka*, Aëtius of Amida (fl. c. 502–525) displayed a knowledge of contraceptives and abortifacients greater than anyone else in antiquity, except Soranus and Dioscorides. In fact, it would appear that he knew Soranus' work because he opened the discussion with the same sentences: "Contraception differs from abortion. The first prevents conception, the second destroys the product of conception and drives it out of the uterus."[37] He began the discussion by giving a reason why it was sometimes proper for a person to avoid pregnancy and childbirth: when a woman's uterine neck or the uterus itself is too small, or a lump or "something similar" blocks the neck of the uterus. With any of these conditions, women are endangered by pregnancy.

On the means to avoid the condition, he began with contraceptive vaginal suppositories. His borrowed words relate to Soranus' text either as a direct source or, more likely, indirectly through the works of Philumenos (whom Aëtius acknowledged, although not specifically in this context).[38] The information contains some important alterations with obvious similarities in the prescriptions' ingredients.

Aëtius:

1. Πίτυος φλοιοῦ, ῥοὸς βυρσοδεψικοῦ ἑκάστου ἴσον τρίβε μετ' οἴνου στεμφυλίτου καὶ προστίθει μετ' ἐρίου πρὸ τῆς συνουσίας, καὶ μετὰ ὥρας β. ἀφαιροῦσα ἡ γυνὴ συνουσιαζέτω.

1. Pine bark and tannin in equal amounts, soaked in grape wine and made into a pad with wool. Insert in vagina and leave it for two hours and withdraw it before coitus.

2. *Another.* Fresh pomegranate flowers mixed with water and ground in and inserted [into the vagina].

3. *Another.* Two parts pomegranate and one part oak galls, pulverize by grinding, shape into a small suppository and administer at point of cessation of menstruation.

Soranus:

1. πίτυος φλοιόν, ῥοῦν βυρσοδεψικόν, ἑκάστου ἴσον, τρίβε μετὰ οἴνου καὶ προστίθει μετρίως πρὸ τῆς συνουσίας περιειληθεντος ἐρίου, καὶ μετὰ ὥρας δύο ἢ τρεῖς ἀφαιροῦσα συνουσιαζέτω.

1. Pine bark and tannin in equal amounts, soaked in grape wine and made into pad with wool. Insert in vagina and leave in for two or three hours and withdraw it before coitus.

2. *Another.* Cimolian earth [gypsum and/or lime],[39] root of opopanax [*panax*][40] in equal quantities and when stricky apply in like manner [to recipe no. 1].

3. *Another.* Fresh pomegranate flowers mixed with water and ground in and inserted [into the vagina].

4. *Another.* Two parts pomegranate and one part oak galls, pulverize by grinding, shape into a small suppository and administer at point of cessation of menstruation.

5. Moist alum, the inside of pomegranate rind, mix with water, and apply with wool.

4. *Another.* Three drachmas unripe oak galls, two drachmas myrrh fashioned with wine the size of a bitter vetch [pea] [*orobos* = *Vicia orobus* DC], dried in the shade and applied as suppository after intercourse.

5. *Another.* Mixture of dried figs and almonds with soda and applied [as suppository].

6. *Another.* Two drachmas flower of pomegranate, two drachmas oak galls, one drachma wormwood [*Artemisia absinthium* L.]; pulverize by grinding, make up with cedar [oil and] make barley size and apply [as a suppository] immediately after the cessation of menstruation for two days. One should remain calm for a day and thus if so resolved she may have intercourse but not before. It is infallible because of many trials [in testing it].[42]

6. Of unripe oak galls, of the inside of pomegranate peel, of ginger, of each 2 drachmas, mold it with wine to size of bitter vetch [peas] [= *Vicia orobus* DC] and dried in the shade and give applied as a vaginal suppository after intercourse.

7. *Another.* Mixture of dried figs and almonds with soda and applied [as suppository].

8. Apply pomegranate peel and an equal amount of oil of roses.[41]

Aëtius' recipes 1, 2, 3, and 5 are taken virtually word for word (again, probably indirectly) from Soranus' recipes 1, 3, 4, and 7. Aëtius' recipe 4 took most of the wording from Soranus, but the text substituted myrrh for Soranus' pomegranate peel and ginger. Interestingly, he kept Soranus' unit of comparative size for the pill—a vetch pea.

For the most part, Aëtius' recipes appear vaguely familiar; no recipe (except those from Soranus) is a copy from another source for which we have a record, and there are a few innovations. This is the first mention of pine bark we have encountered. A recent study showed that pine needles exert a "very significant effect on implantation and early stages of pregnancy in rats."[43] The use of soda, of course, dates back to the ancient Egyptian papyri. Figs and almonds appear to be employed as vehicles or flavoring agents for the soda in that suppository.

Oak galls (var. nutgalls) are obtained from the excrescence of young twigs of the oak *Quercus infectoria* Olivier, plus other species, which have been infected with insect larvae and attacked by nematodes and fungi. In modern medicine, oak galls are used as a powerful astringent, and so had Dioscorides recommended it as a suppository to staunch bleeding.[44] Tannin is prepared from galls, usually from oak, myrobalan, or sumac, by exposing them with moisture to the air for a month or more, during which time a fermentation takes place resulting in tannin. Medically, oak galls are employed as a mild astringent but do not cause blood to coagulate and are not considered for regular topical application. Aëtius' and Soranus' use of tannin appears in no other recorded sources prior to their time. It is interesting to note that acorns are abortifacient in large quantities to cattle. During the 1988 drought in the southeastern United States, oak trees produced a larger crop than normal, with the result that farmers had to fence off oak trees to protect the cattle.

The last recipe, with pomegranate, tannin, and wormwood, Aëtius said was infallible. Aside from the activity of the drug itself, the time of its administration (two days after menstruation) would lead one to expect a low fertility rate. Given the known actions of pomegranate and wormwood, plus the instructions, conception would be highly unlikely.

Aëtius introduced a number of oral contraceptives by referring to them as "strong potions that hinder conception [*syllēpsin*]."

1. Cyrenaic juice [*silphium* or *Ferula historica*] the size of a vetch [pea] with two cups of water and wine mixed, take twice a month. It starts menstruation.
2. *Another.* Cyrenaic juice, opopanax, rue leaves in equal amounts shaped up and mixed with juice and take in an amount of the size of a bean and swallow with wine mixed in. It starts menstruation.
3. *Another.* One drachma of aloes [*Aloes* sp.], three obols of wallflower [or stock] seeds, two drachmas of pepper, and two drachmas of saffron [*Crocus sativus*]. Give in wine divided into three equal portions and administer immediately after the cessation of menstruation.

The giant fennel (Cyrenaic juice), opopanax fennel, rue, and the wallflower (or stock) are in Soranus' and Dioscorides' antifertility drugs, but the recipes are different. Saffron appears in Dioscorides' work as an ingredient in both vaginal and rectal suppositories but without any specific medicinal action attributed to it.[45] Likely, Aëtius' inclusion of saffron here was not as an active substance but for coloring and aroma. Aëtius' text is the first to cite aloe as an antifertility agent. Tests on guinea pigs reported in 1961 showed that *Aloe barbadensis* L., in small amounts, has some oxytocic (abortifacient) properties.[46] But the prescription called also for stock and pepper, so there is no doubt about its possible efficacy.

Aëtius continued with the oral contraceptives.

4. A contraceptive [*atokion*] is taking both copper water in which a hot iron has been extinguished, drunk vigorously, and continuously after the cessation of menstruation in this order: one drachma of poplar tree root taken in a small cup of water once a month for six months.

Poplar has been discussed. The use of copper was in the Hippocratic corpus, but the term used there was *misy;* Aëtius used the term *chalkos,* an approximate synonym.[47] This is more evidence that he was not directly copying sources, at least not those known to us. The copper compound prescription found in the Hippocratic treatise *On the Diseases of Women* is to be taken monthly as an contraceptive, not annually as is the case in this Hippocratic work. In any case, the familiar drugs are cited, and the important distinctions are made between contraceptives, abortifacients, and those that have both actions. The instructions call variously for administration orally and in suppositories.

Following the copper water prescription, Aëtius related three contraceptive prescriptions for what we would call magical, superstitious, and, more charitably, psychological effects. The amulets are a cat liver in a tube worn on the left foot, the testicles of a cat in a tube around the umbilicus, and the uterus of a lioness in an ivory tube. The latter, he said, was very effective.

Next, Aëtius listed vaginal suppositories. This time he used the term ἀσύλληπτον, or "inconceivers" or "sterilizers."

5. White lead with oil in a suppository before intercourse [*mixeus*] takes place.
6. And, even stronger, the flower and peel of pomegranate, nut gall, the juice of unripe grapes, each two drachmas, one drachma wormwood; mix cedar [juniper?] oil and form into a barley-size [pill] and administer in the vagina two days before intercourse.
7. *Another contraceptive* [*allo atokion*]. As long as she desires barrenness [*asyllēpton*] to last, she should take black ivy berries in a moderate wine mixed with water and drink after the menses are over.

White lead was listed by Dioscorides but not as a suppository or as an antifertility agent. Galen used it in a uterine poultice but not specifically against fertility.[48] The sixth prescription is composed of previously discussed agents except for the juice of unripe grapes, which is probably the vehicle for the active substances. The seventh recipe contains black ivy berries. The white ivy (*Hedera helix* L.) we have discussed. Ivy has berries that are black to deep purple; it is not known whether Aëtius was referring to another ivy species or just to the black berries. Following the seventh contraceptive recipe, Aëtius related another amulet consisting of ass's milk, myrtle, black ivy berry, or flowers (corymb) to be worn wrapped in a rabbit, mule, or stag skin and never allowed to touch the ground.

Next, Aëtius gave two more oral contraceptives, these being both familiar and, for at least one of the two, rational.

8. Or give to the woman who is fasting a cold drink of copper [water] in generous amounts.

9. *Another.* Decoction of willow bark with honey to temper its bitterness. To be drunk continually.[49]

Ending the section on women's contraceptives, Aëtius closed with an amulet of henbane seed washed in a mare's milk nourishing a mule and carried on the left arm. Then, he said,

10. And give the wormwood seed in a drink; these [recipes] guard against conception for a year.[50]

Note that the amulet is taken in conjunction with the oral prescription. Aëtius appeared to have copied no particular source, because, even compared with those of Soranus (the closest account), each prescription differed in important details. In respect to the amounts, none appears at a hazardously toxic level, with the possible exception of the lead compound. The very fact that, from the earliest mention of a contraceptive in the Hippocratic work to Aëtius of Amida, the prescriptions are being refined and improved points to continuous folk usage rather than to a sterile literary transmission of medical texts. Illustrative of this folk refinement is the prescription for willow bark that says it must be concentrated and drunk continually for effectiveness and tempered with honey. The concentration of tannins alone would produce a very bitter taste without the honey.

Aëtius also gave male contraceptives, which, as materials applied to the penis, are complements of the vaginal suppositories. A man should rub astringents on his penis, such as alum or pomegranate or oak galls with vinegar, and then he will not fertilize. One oral contraceptive is given for men: the burned testicles of castrated mules drunk with a decoction of willow.[51]

Aspasia on Abortions

Following the same sequence as Soranus, Aëtius followed his discussion on contraceptives with a discourse about abortion methods, and he related that he took this section of his work from Aspasia, who wrote about gynecology in the second century A.D. Aspasia is likely a pseudonym; although the name is feminine, there is no reason to assume that the author was female.

The section taken from Aspasia begins by telling a woman who wishes to destroy an embryo in the first thirty days to do just the opposite of the regime prescribed earlier. If the exercises do not work, then a sitz bath is in order, consisting of a decoction of fenugreek (*Trigonella foeum gaecum*

L.), marshmallow (*Althaea officinalis* L.), and artemisia (*Artemisia* sp.).[52] Following the bath, she should rub herself with the juice of rue or honey. All these plants are used as oral contraceptives as well, as certified by either Dioscorides or by later writers.[53]

If the pregnancy should persist, she should take five drachmas each of wormwood, Cnidian seed (*kokkos* = pomegranate?), eight drachmas of soda, five of squirting cucumber, ten of opopanax (*Ferula opopanax*), one drachma of lupine, *chelidona* root (*Chelidonium maius* L.?), wallflower (or stock) seed, all mixed with Cyprian oil for a plaster to apply on the abdomen. Following this, one can put dried figs with soda in the vagina or, with oil, rubbed on. A simple but good remedy, Aspasia observed, is the boiled leaves of cyperus applied after the bath to remain overnight on the abdomen. Of value is a suppository of opopanax salve and a fumigation of burned garlic and female hair.[54] Aëtius warned: "If all these [first month] measures do not induce an abortion, it will be necessary to proceed with stronger remedies, but these must not be done haphazardly. For all efforts to destroy a fetus are dangerous, particularly if the woman has a strong constitution and possesses a robust and sturdy uterus. For that reason it is necessary to exercise judgment and to avoid interference at the second and particularly the fourth month."[55]

Aspasia explained that the time for an abortion is not the second or the fourth month, but the third month, if the first month has passed. For the third-month period, he gives elaborate regime and drug procedures. First, there is bleeding This procedure he said comes from Hippocrates (as indeed it does).[56] The woman should vomit after meals and then on an empty stomach eat a boiled broth of female annual mercury (*Mercurialis annua* L.),[57] prepared with *garum*, an oily fish sauce, or "she should drink honeyed *agaric* [either a tree fungus or a fern],[58] or a drachma of wall flower (or stock) seeds, or a drachma each of the seeds of artemisia [*Artemisia* sp.], or dittany, or gentian, or castoreum [from the beaver], or ammoniacum [from *Ferula tingitana* L.] or myrrh, or laurel [*Lauris nobilis* L.] with honey water. Or she may drink one drachma of ivy flowers (or berries) or a cooled [congealed?] bull's gall with a large amount of peeled fruit with scented wine."[59]

These ingredients occur in the border area between diet and drug therapy. Many of the items are drugs that are strong laxatives, and strong laxatives are a means of producing an abortion, according to Hippocrates.[60] Aspasia through Aëtius said that, if these measures do not work, one must move to the next level, which involves a suppository that "destroys the embryo/fetus [*embryōn ekballei*]." The text does not make it clear, however, whether the recipes derive from Aspasia or from Aëtius' composition. The suppositories consist of the following:

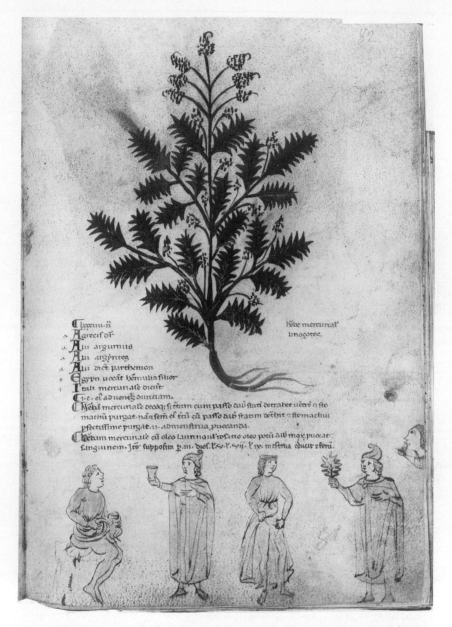

An emmenagogue (menstruation-producing herb): the mercury plant, as shown in a thirteenth-century copy of Pseudo-Apuleius' herbal. At the lower right, a man holds up the herb while the woman facing him shows that she is not menstruating. (Vienna, Nationalbibliothek, MS lat. 93, fol. 82)

Recipe 1:
1 drachma iris [*Iris germanica* L. and/or *Iris florentina* L.]
1 drachma Cnidian grain [pomegranate flowers?]
1 drachma galbanum [*chalbanēs* = *Ferula galbaniflua* Boiss. et Buhse)
1 drachma turpentine
Mixed in equal parts with lily oil, Cyrian oil (consisting of omphacine
    oil [Lesbian wine], sweet flag, myrrh, *aspalathus* [*Alhagi maurorum*
    L. or *Astragalus* sp.]), cardamom, and flowers of Cyperus [*Cyperus
    rotundus* L.] Rose oil . . .
Insert into the vagina before a bath and retain it for a night. In the
    morning let her take a sitz bath with fenugreek and artemisia. If this
    does not produce an abortion, let her repeat the procedure but this
    time inserting the suppository after the bath with these [added? or
    substituted?]: wallflower (or stock) seed, soda, and wormwood
    soaked in wine on wool pad.

Recipe 2:
2 drachmas rue leaves
2 drachmas myrrh
Soak in wine and insert.

Recipe 3: A recipe which expels a fetus of three months without any
    difficulty.
1 drachma each of
    cardamom seeds
    wallflower (or stock)
    myrrh
    wormwood
Let a woman insert it before taking a bath and drink pennyroyal
    wine.[61]

Cleopatra the Gynecologist

Late antiquity and the early Middle Ages were times very different from
our own in many respects, one of them being the attitude of writers. In
this period original writers were at pains to hide their authorship. New
works often went under the name of a former classical author or other
historic figure, probably to give authority to the contents. A work on
gynecology was written at an unknown time during late antiquity and the
early Middle Ages and passed under the name of Cleopatra.[62] As best we
know, the work is not connected in any way with the famous Egyptian
queen except possibly that someone attempted to borrow her prestige by
assigning authorship to her. Whoever it was knew and recommended a
number of abortifacients but did not explicitly note any contraceptives.

The abortifacients are clearly labeled [e.g., "it drives out the embryo [*partus*]" and "it causes at once an abortion [*statim abortum faciet*]." Ten recipes are given, most with single herbs plus a vehicle, such as water or wine. Two recipes specify amounts. One scrupulum (approx. 13 g) of the juice of iris is given with about 20 g of leek juice. Other recipes are as follows:

Suppositories
Leaves of the citron in water.
Black hellebore, chamomile, and opopanax [*Ferula*]
Orally taken
Asphaltum, silphium (= *laser*), bile of a bull, 150 grains of pepper, and rue, powdered and drunk cause an immediate abortion.[63]

The *asphaltum*'s plant identification is uncertain,[64] and it is interesting to speculate whether there actually was *silphium* left by the time the treatise was written, or whether the author was simply copying a source. Possibly another species of *Ferula*, probably asafetida, was going under the name of *laser* by this time. Other oral-route abortifacients were as follows:

Cumin pulverized with honey water
Pennyroyal with wine
Three drachmas [13 g] of dittany with honey
One obol [0.7 g] each of myrrh and opium, one scrupulum [13 g] green rue
Fig leaves cooked in water and given with one cyathus [approx. 75 ml or 0.8 pint].[65]

None of the recipes, however, appears to have come from any known authority. They may in fact be original, that is to say, derived from the folk practices of the day and recorded by the enigmatic Cleopatra.

Paul of Aegina

Paul of Aegina (seventh century) was a Byzantine medical writer who took a somewhat innovative approach to antifertility agents. He arranged them from mild to strong in his seven books on medicine. When the menstrual period is delayed, the first approach is a regimen, he advised. One should take baths and drink frequently a drink made up of sesame or roundheaded leek (*Allium shaerocephalon* L.) with rue and pepper and eaten for three to four days.[66] After a cup (cotyle) of it, one should exercise by walking, and follow this with a diet of squid, cuttlefish, and polypody, because these foods are particularly good for provoking a flow. If the condition persists, however, Paul recommended another regime consisting of bleeding with a diet of a soup made of shellfish and roundheaded leek and boiled with rue and pepper and drunk for three to four days. When the menstrual period is imminent one should drink one obol of myrrh or castor (*Ricinus communis* L.) in honey water or musk or birthwort or sage or wormwood. All during the regime, wine should be drunk.

If this procedure does not work, Paul prescribed a vaginal suppository of fenugreek, mallow, pennyroyal, rue, and birthwort. If stronger medicines (*pharmaka*) are required, one should drink Illyrian iris with wine and cyperus, arum root, cassia (a type of cinnamon), reed (*schoinos = Cymbopogon schoenanthus* Spreng.?), valerian (*Valeniana celtica* L.), calamint root, birthwort, and myrrh the size of a Greek bean with half a ladle of honeyed water and a ladle of a decoction of dittany, ammoniac (from *Ferula tingitana* L.), and Persian fennel (*Ferula persica* L.).[67] Paul declared that certain seeds are given for the same purpose, only they are inferior to those drugs above. The seeds are giant fennel (*Ferula* sp.), cumin, parsley, wild carrot (Queen Anne's lace), hartwort (*Tordylium maximum* L., of the family Umbelliferae), arum (*ammi = Arum dracunculus* L.?), stone parsley (*Sison amomum* L.), chick pea (*Cicer arietinum* L.), juniper, and "all the diuretics."[68]

Paul's account contains the elements that we saw in Soranus and Dioscorides; each of the three conveyed the antifertility plants that were found in earlier writers, and each contributed knowledge of new plants. Paul added several, including the castor plant, which contains ricin and ricinoleic acid, which is used today in contraceptive jellies. Extracts from the plant are used by modern medicine and in folk medicine because it has estrogenic activity.[69] Valerian is a well-known sedative (the drug name Valium is derived from the plant name), but it is not known as an emmenagogue-abortifacient or contraceptive.

In book 7 of Paul's work, he listed drugs in alphabetical order. For the most part he was content in this book only to list the drugs and their pharmaceutical properties (such as drying, moistening) without specific applications. For instance, rue is a calefacient (warming) and desiccant (drying), and it curbs sexual desire, but he did not specifically state that rue is an antifertility agent.[70] A physician, just the same, would know that a "drying" quality was needed to dry the sperm so that it would not be fertile. Similarly, no specific antifertility effects were given for iris, castor plant, pomegranate, and *misy*, although in the book on gynecology castor plant and iris were so specified.

In some cases, Paul gave specific usages for drugs. He listed the following as emmenagogues (without also calling them abortifacients): Queen Anne's lace, squirting cucumber, wild thyme, common madder, death carrot, caper, cassia, St. John's wort (two species), costus, *crocodilium,* cyperus, wallflower/stock, lovage, love-in-a-mist, spignel, myrrh (two kinds/species), stone bugloss, opopanax, hulwort, parsley, stone parsley, scammony, alexanders, annual woundwort, storax, phillyrea, german-der, and aster.[71] Several plants are listed as being both emmenagogues and abortifacients (e.g., for century plant: Καταμηνία γοῦν προτρέπει καὶ ἔμβρυα φθείρει τε καὶ ἐκβάλλει): century plant, myrrh, golden drop, fleabane, stock/wallflower, and fern (*filix*).[72]

Paul's account also introduced some agents not previously encountered in this book: two species of St. John's wort (*Hypericum coris* L. and, possibly, *H. crispum* L.), *crocodilium* (possibly *Eryngium maritimum*), stone parsley, *sium* (*Sium angustifolium* L.?), alexanders (*Smyrnium* sp. / Umbell.), annual woundwort (*Stachys*), storax (*Styrax officinale* L.), phillyrea (*Phyllurea latifolia* L.), and aster (*Aster linosyris* L.). Dioscorides, however, named all of these plants or ones closely related. Of these St. John's wort and lovage have reported abortifacient activity.[73] In the case of aster, Dioscorides said that it "cleans the uterus," but not specifically as an emmenagogue/abortifacient.[74] The animal drug castoreum, from the beaver, was said by Paul to provoke menstruation and aborts the afterbirth (*choria ekballei*).The wording makes it difficult to determine the action. Scammony, Paul said, was an abortifacient as a suppository; storax, he added, was good both orally and applied. The other plants, it would appear, were taken orally. In summary, Paul revealed himself to be knowledgeable about antifertility measures and innovative, although much of the information is found in earlier sources.

Early Medieval Herbals

Other late Roman and early medieval medical works popular in the Middle Ages not only reveal a continuous knowledge of contraceptive and abortifacient works but also introduce into medicine some new antifertility drugs. The popular herbal by Pseudo-Apuleius, a product of the fourth century, failed to give fertility effects for artemisia, birthwort (*aristolochia*), the great century plant, or the fern *filix*, although these plants were discussed. Emmenagogic properties were prescribed for rue and squirting cucumber. The cucumber has more explicit language: "Ad abortum."[75] Emmenagogic plants (all taken orally) are *mercurialis* or annual mercury (*Mercurialis annua* L.), blackberry (*Rubus fruticosus* L.), and pennyroyal (*Mentha pulegium* L.).[76] Mercury is reported in modern folk medicine as an emmenagogue and is known to be severely poisonous to grazing livestock.[77] A closely related species of blackberry, *Rubus idaeus*, has antigonadotrophic activity in rats.[78] There is still another species, *Rubus ellepticus* Smith, where an extract of the plant without the root was prepared, and in animal tests the extract was 70–90 percent effective in blocking implantation.[79]

Pseudo-Dioscorides' *Ex herbis femininis*, an herbal of the sixth century, has a somewhat similar pattern. It lists fewer abortifacients and no truly explicit contraceptives, and prescribes no new emmenagogues/abortifacients. *Ex herbis* recommended birthwort, shepherd purse or death carrot (*Thapsia garganica* L. and *T. avense* L.), ploughman's spikenard (*Inula conuza* DC + sp.), friar's cowl (*Arisarum vulgare* L.) or arum (*Arum dracunculus* L.), colcynth, and opopanax as abortifacients, just as did Dioscorides, except that Dioscorides did not have the antifertility use for shepherd purse.[80] Moreover, the language is often explicit; for instance, on ploughman spikenard: "Its juice placed on wool and into the genital causes an abortion in a pregnant woman."[81]

Friar's cowl or arum is reported in modern pharmacognosy as an abortifacient.[82] Germander, Dioscorides said, "draws out the menses and embryo," while the *Ex herbis* said "it expels a dead fetus."[83] Two plants that Dioscorides recommended as an abortifacient were soapwort (*Saponaria officinalis* L.) and wallflower or stock (*Cheiranthus cheiri* or *Matthiola incana*). *Ex herbis*, however, omitted the claim despite a discussion of the plants' medicinal effects.[84]

The herbals of Pseudo-Apuleius and Pseudo-Dioscorides were partly translated into Old English, the oldest manuscript being from the ninth century. Fertility effects for artemisia, "fern," birthwort, rue, ivy, lupine, and mandrake were omitted. Dittany was said to expel a "dead fetus."[85] This statement is in Dioscorides but not in Pseudo-Apuleius, and it is in the section of the Old English herbal attributed to Apuleius.[86] Blackberry, pennyroyal, ploughman's spikenard, and Florentine iris are emmenagogue/abortifacients (while iris is contraceptive, as well),[87] and two plants (sneezewort or yellow milfoil [*Achillea* sp.] and nettle [*Urtica* sp.] are both in Dioscorides but not in Pseudo-Dioscorides' *Ex herbis*.[88] The fact that the Old English translator was adding and adapting his text reveals a continuous process in adding and subtracting agents, very possibly taken directly from folk usage and not texts. A recent animal test of *Urtica dioica* L. showed a 33 percent activity in preventing implantation in albino rats, and it is known in medical reports as an emmenagogue.[89] Yellow milfoil is cited in medical reports as an abortifacient,[90] although one test on animals yielded no significant antifertility affects.[91]

Anonymous recipe manuscripts written and copied at monastic scriptoria contain abortifacients (as menstrual regulators) and contraceptives. A ninth- or early-tenth-century manuscript has a prescription for cleaning the belly of a woman who cannot purge herself. It includes colocynth, black pepper, saffron, and myrrh among its ingredients.[92] Another manuscript about the same time inscribed a recipe for moving a woman's menses that consisted of parsley, hartwart, rue, black pepper, lovage, thyme, and celery seeds.[93] Still another manuscript was more explicit when it gave two prescriptions "For Women so that They Will Not Conceive." The first recipe consisted of the *vulva leporis* (of a leopard?) and the liver of an ass that are taken as a drink with wine, and the other one was a mule's *sarcus* (translation uncertain) with ten grains and wine.[94] While it is unclear what the substances intended were, the purpose for taking it was entirely clear. Some medieval peoples, even monks, knew about birth control. These monastic recipe collections were not copying exercises for monks from classical sources, because the recipes are largely original; some of them have new drugs not known in classical antiquity.[95]

Syriac "Book of Medicines"

A long medical treatise exists in Syriac that was translated partly from Greek. The work contains numerous prescriptions, many of which reminded the modern translator, E. A. Wallis Budge, of those in the Ebers Papyrus. The work appears connected to teaching purposes, perhaps at a medical school, and borrows heavily from various Galenic works.[96] Curiously, there is little treatment of gynecology or women's problems. No antifertility prescriptions are so named, but there are recipes that likely had that effect. One recipe is called "The Caesar Antidote," which was given for "palpitation of the heart, and for evil winds . . . for delayed menses and for headache and for the medicine of death." Caesar's Antidote consists of the following:

> 3 drachmas each of castoreum, licorice juice, cassia, costus, round peppercorns, long peppercorns, styrax, opium, crocus/saffron, and spikenard
> 1 drachma of opopanax
> ½ drachma each of musk, zôrbadh [= zedoary?], dornagh [*Doronicum pardalianches* L. + sp.], and unpierced pearls
> 8 drachmas of myrrh
> honey, as much as sufficeth

The dose is given as one chick-pea size in a drink as "convenient for disease."[97]

Most of the ingredients are familiar to us as antifertility agents: castoreum, licorice, cassia, costus, pepper, styrax, crocus/saffron, spikenard, opopanax, and myrrh, with myrrh supplying the largest in amount. The amount specified—a pill the size of a chick-pea—would not be enough to cause death either to a mother or, perhaps, her fetus. A larger amount possibly would, and this flexibility in amount could differentiate its various purposes, such as in dealing with heart palpitations or headache and functioning as an emmenagogue and, lastly, "medicine of death." Even with the opium, the prescription would unlikely endanger a mother, but it would likely induce a miscarriage or abortion.

The Syriac Book contains a second explicit emmenagogue. It is a tablet consisting of three drachmas of crocus and four drachmas of castoreum, myrrh, seed of rock parsley, hyoscyamus (henbane), dûk̲ôn, opium, and styrax. The instructions say, "Make into tablets with water and administer half a drachma in extract of myrtle berries." Again, most of these substances are antifertility agents, primarily abortifacients, including the myrtle berries, which appear to be the prescription's base.[98] This is particularly true if the Syriac *dûkôn* is same as the Greek and Latin *daucos,* or Queen Anne's lace.

The Syriac Book of Medicines reveals a continuation of the medical lore regarding antifertility agents, but, here under the labels of emmenagogues and "medicine of death." Internal evidence indicates that a portion from Greek was connected with the school at Alexandria. Its contents indicate less concern with gynecology than in previous medical writings, although it retained some elements of women's problems as part of medical training.

Summary

From the British Isles to the eastern Mediterranean, late antiquity and the early Middle Ages knew about antifertility measures both from classical texts and from their own contributors. The question still becomes, how much did the common folk know, and how did they use what they knew? These questions are easy to pose, but so difficult to answer. In the following chapter, I summarize church fathers and monks who spoke against the use of contraceptives and against abortions; the mere presence of their condemnations gives evidence of their use. A similar picture emerges in the Germanic law codes.

If antifertility means were freely and openly discussed in medieval sources, one might expect to find information—even if it concerned things to avoid taking. Such information is not there, however. For example, the great Carolingian educator and writer Hrabanus Maurus (c. 776–856), archbishop of Mainz, wrote extensively about plants in his encyclopedia *De universo.* Hrabanus discussed a sequence of plants— squirting cucumber, celery, cow's parsnip, parsley, fennel, ligusticum, coriander, and rue—but his discussion is about the symbolism of their names, not their medical qualities. Similarly under trees, he placed in sequence cypress, juniper, willow, and myrtle, but other than the association, he did not allude to their antifertility qualities.[99] There is no botanical or medical reasons for these plants to be associated, however, other than the antifertility properties they all share.

Even more allusive is the herbal written by Walafrid Strabo (c. 807– 849), who discussed the herbs in his monastic garden in Germany. There grew in his garden rue, squirting cucumber, wormwood (*artemisia*), mint, and pennyroyal, all of which he praised. Not only are there no antifertility usages given, (although he discussed their other medical qualities), but he gave no gynecological usages at all.[100] His garden, it appears, was for men. Do such references as these from Hrabanus and Walafrid indicate a diminution in the knowledge and usage of contraceptives and antifertility agents? Considering who these men were and why they wrote, one would think not.

CHAPTER TEN

The Middle Ages: The Church, Macer, and Hildegard

Si aliquis . . . (If someone . . .)
First two words of canon law on contraception

S cribes modified classical texts to include antifertility information that the ancient authorities had for whatever reasons excluded from their works. Inexplicably, Dioscorides had failed to cite rue's antifertility quality, so a medieval scribe added the comment, "It calls forth the menses and expels the embryo/fetus" [κινεῖ δὲ καὶ καταμήνια, τὰ δὲ ἔμβρυα φθείρει]."[1] Writing between 1307 and 1311, Peter of Padua wrote a marginal note beside the entry for *asarus* in the Latin text of the Alphabetical Dioscorides. In it Peter commented that the herb is taken by uninformed people before coitus.[2]

New uses were found for old drugs. An example is found in a Byzantine emendation, made between the tenth and early fourteenth centuries, to Dioscorides' text. On the discussion about asparagus, a scribe added that a decoction of it in a drink causes inconception (ἀτόκιος) and infertility (ἄγονος).[3] Apparently no classical or earlier medieval authority made such a claim about asparagus. A Hippocratic work, on the contrary, said that asparagus seeds were used in a suppository to promote conception, not to prevent it.[4] In 1952, Russian investigators reported a decoction of asparagus (*Asparagus actuifolius officinalis*) is employed in folk use for its contraceptive effect.[5] In 1975, asparagus was mentioned in the *Journal of Pharmaceutical Sciences* as a candidate for future testing of antifertility agents in natural products.[6] The emendation indicates that new information about oral contraceptives was derived from folk experimentation and observation, perhaps in ways resembling what Theophrastus related about the wild carrot's fertility effects on cattle.

Although the Middle Ages knew contraceptives and abortifacients and even discovered new ones, there was an important factor present during this era that did not exist during antiquity: the church and to some extent secular law now sought to control sexual behavior and antibirth controls. The interrelationship between ethical principles as revealed in church doctrine, in canon and secular law, and in medical works of the same period is complex.

Early Medieval Law and the Church

The Germanic law codes of the early Middle Ages protected the fetus to a greater extent than had the law codes from Hammurabi to the Civil Law of the Romans; but even so, the principle of some of the early church fathers that abortion was homicide was not accepted in secular law. The Salian Law made under the Merovingian king Guntram (567–593) said that "if someone administers [something] to a free-born, pregnant woman [*feminam genuinam gravidam*]" so that she is killed, he is fined 700 *solidi*. If the child is killed, the fine is 200.⁷ In the section on *maleficia,* there is a provision seemingly against contraception: "If a woman has committed *maleficium,* so that she cannot have infants, she will be judged liable to a fine of sixty-two gold *semis.*"⁸ The woman herself is held liable, but it is not clear whether the prohibition is because of the magical element or contraception per se. Roman law and subsequently Germanic Law held magicians liable and increasingly attempted to control them through legislation. Still, it represented a step toward legal control of fertility when the woman who was the perpetrator was held responsible.

At least some of early Germanic law made a distinction between early and late pregnancy. On this accord, however, the Germanic law codes are based on principles derived from Roman law.⁹ An Allemanian law (c. 600) said: "If someone gives an abortion to a pregnant woman so that one cannot tell if it is a male or a female, he ought to be fined 12 *solidi* as if it were a male; if, however, a female with 24. If one cannot tell the gender and already it has not formed in the womb [*jam non fuit cormatus in lineamenta corporis*], he is fined 12 *solidi.*"¹⁰

While the gender distinction is interesting in itself, our concern here is the law again distinguishing early and late pregnancy, à la Aristotle. Who would bring the indictment was unstated, but given the culture, it would be reasonable to suppose that it was the husband who was aggrieved.

Bavarian and Ostrogothic law codes were even more detailed concerning birth control, but the same principles applied. The Bavarian Code (seventh century) said, "If a woman gives to another a drink [*potionem*] so that it makes an abortion, if she is a slave, she should receive two hundred lashes."¹¹ Westgothic law had much the same provision except it did not specify that it was a woman who gave the drink.[12] These laws made the fines based on the status of the person—in the Bavarian law, we observe, the third party was specified as a woman. By inference, the expectation was that the third party who gave birth control drugs would be a woman. Nowhere was there mention of a physician (*medicus* or the other words current for medical people). The expectation that these were women's actions might explain to a greater degree the association with magic (namely, *maleficia*); we also could say that men, who made the laws, were trying to protect their interest. The disregard for women was found in the Frisian law concerning men who had died "without compensation" (*sine compositione*), among whom were infants (*infans*) who were snatched from the womb and murdered by the mother." [13] The code had nothing to say about the woman.

About 830 Regino, an abbot of a monastery at Prüm in Lorraine, wrote, "If someone [*Si aliquis*] to satisfy his lust or to make deliberate hatred does something to a man or woman so that no children be born of him or her, or gives them to drink, so that he cannot generate or she conceive, let it be held as homicide." [14]

Almost a century later in his *Decretum,* Burchard repeated Regino, but he cited Regino's quotation as canon 30 from the Council of Worms.[15] Whether a Council of Worms had enacted Regino's statement is uncertain, but it is certain that Regino's opinion became canonized as church law.[16] What was being condemned was contraception. As we saw in Chapter 1, abortion was always rejected, although the point varied at which ending a pregnancy was considered an abortion. Interestingly Burchard referred to "the conceptus being excluded from the uterus by *maleficia* and by herbs." [17] By *maleficia* he meant black magic, which was used by other writers to include and, in some cases, to equal the use of herbs. The question about abortion arises as to when in a pregnancy a person potentially could have an abortion. Depending on the interpretation, the time could range from coitus to the time the fetus had formed or quickened, perhaps at the beginning of the second trimester, certainly by the third.

Generalizations about almost everything during the Middle Ages are perilous, especially about birth control attitudes. For example, we have statements like the following from Columban: "If through this [i.e., *maleficium*] one has removed from a women her fetus [*partum quis (que) deceperit*], on that account let that person increase his penance by six terms of forty days, lest he be guilty of homicide." [18] Because the section began with the phrase "if anyone has destroyed someone by his magic art [*maleficio*]," the implication is clearly that abortifacients are part of the "magical" or "evil" arts. The statement condemned the person who gave them but not the woman who received them. Not entirely so with women being absolved from sin. Caesarius of Arles (bishop from 503 to 543) condemned the woman who took a "potion to prevent conception," or one who took "potions for purposes of abortion." Thus, in comparing the two saints, Caesarius both condemned contraceptives and abortifacients, and Columban spoke only against abortifacients. The penalty for abortion was the same as for stealing an ox, a horse, or a sheep.[19] For those women who wanted no more children, Caesarius suggested that they make a contract ("religious agreement") with their husbands to abstain from sexual intercourse.[20] But Columban went further. He condemned (with the same penalty) not just abortifacients but also anyone who took a *maleficium* in order to enhance conception when sterility is indicated.[21] God, not herbs, should determine fertility. Martin of Braga expanded the condemnation of contraception outside of marriage to include contraception within marriage ("sive ex adulterio sive ex legitimo conuigio"), which condemnation he said had been pronounced by a council at Ancyra.[22]

Many of the monastic fathers cited Jerome's statement against "sterility drinks" and, like him, compared those actions to homicide. John Noonan's review of the penitentials establishes that there was widespread recognition that women and, in some cases, men were prone to control their fertility by *veneficii* or *maleficia* or *sterilitas*.[23] For one example, Pseudo-Bede asked of a person in confession, "Have you drunk any *maleficium,* that is herbs or other agents so that you could not have children?"[24] If the answer was positive, a forty-day penance was indicated; for some Fathers it was more, for some less. In the written word, the church fathers spoke; mothers did not. In some cases, the penance for intentional homicide was equal to, or less than, that for anal and oral intercourse. Pseudo-Bede said, and later Burchard repeated, that the motivation for the antifertility actions must be considered. "It makes a big difference whether she is a poor little woman and acted on account of the difficulty of feeding, or whether she acted to conceal a crime of fornication."[25]

The early medieval church continued the ancient distinction, as stated by Aristotle, that there was a difference when an antifertility measure was administered. An old Allemanian sacramentarium around the year 1000 used the word "homicide" and applied it to the mother who aborted a child whose members (that is, appendages) had formed. A woman "who has fornicated and neglected her fetus [*qui fornicantur et partes suas negant*]" and "cuts off her fetus [*uteros conceptos excutiant*]" should be given a penance of ten years. But a woman who "kills her child [*filium suum*] in her uterus before forty days [after conception]" should receive only one year of penance. For one who kills her child forty days after conception [*a conceptione*], this was homicide, and she was given a three-year penance.[26] Unclear is whether the woman who "fornicates" does so within a marriage or whether the act is a wanton act outside of marriage. Two things are certain: (1) the woman was held responsible, there being no mention of a third party who administered a *maleficium,* or magical potion; and (2) there were varying degrees of sin in abortive measures, just as Pseudo-Bede said. This text did not consider motivation per se.

Pregnancy termination in the first forty days was a considerably lesser offense. The Irish Canons of around 675 clearly borrowed from the Aristotelian tradition when they stated, "The penance for the destruction of a child in a liquid state [*liquoris materiae filii*] in the mother's womb, three and a half years." [27] Even after forty days, when it was homicide, the penalty was not the same as for premeditated murder. An old Irish penitential around A.D. 800 makes three levels of distinction: the earliest period (time unspecified), the formation of the flesh, and when the soul enters, each with varying degrees of penalties.

> (5.6) A woman who causes miscarriage of that which she has conceived after it has become established in the womb, three years and a half of penance. If the flesh has formed, it is seven years. If the soul has entered it, fourteen years' penance. If the woman die of the miscarriage, that is, the death of body and soul, fourteen cumals [are offered] to God as the price of her soul, or fourteen years' penance.
> (5.7) Anyone who gives drugs or makes a bogey or gives a poisonous drink so that someone dies of it, seven years' penance, as for a homicide. If no one dies of it, three years' penance.[28]

Distinction between the degree of sin in terminating early and late pregnancy continued from the church fathers' interpretation of Exodus 21:23 (which was mistranslated from Hebrew to Greek, as we learned in Chapter 2). In 1216 Thomas of Chobham expressed the prevailing interpretation this way in *Summa confessorum:* "For in this matter it is written in the law of Moses 'If anyone should stike a pregnant woman and she should miscarry, if the fetus has been formed let him give life for life; if, however, it is unformed, let him be amerced in money.' From this it is clear that it is a much graver sin to dislodge a formed fetus than an unformed one." [29]

Ivo of Chartres

During the eleventh and twelfth centuries the Roman church's influence extended and deepened over western Europe. The early medieval pronouncements on contraception were consolidated. The position on abortion was clearer, but what was not at all clear, and little discussed, was the question, "When is an abortion an abortion?" Despite the position taken that there is a distinction between early and late abortion, as seen by Augustine and Thomas of Chobham, there persisted the position of Basil that a Christian cannot make a fine differential. On contraception, the position taken earlier in "Si aliquis" was solemnized by Ivo, bishop of Chartres from 1091 to 1116. What he wrote on the subject was shortly thereafter adopted by Peter Lombard as the theological position and by Gratian as the rule in canon law. Because the position taken on contraception was so unambiguous, the position on abortion was clarified. Both contraception and abortion were out of order and jeopardized a person's soul.

According to John Noonan, three developments brought the issue to a synthesis: first, the traditions of earlier church councils (such as Ancyra and Worms) were repeated and endorsed by Martin of Braga and the position of Regino taken allegedly by the Council of Worms.[30] Second, there was the revival of Augustine's total works with his many statements about sexual control, some of which were not easily reconciled. In the main, there was Augustine's denouncement of poisons of sterility.[31] In addition, the bishop of Hippo had issued a number of calls to Christians, recalling the Manichean heresy on intercourse, to engage in sexual intercourse only within the marriage covenant and for the sole purpose of procreation.

The eleventh century was the right time for concern about these Augustinian statements because under the name of Cathars, the old Manichean and Gnostic heresies were revived. This movement began in Bulgaria by a bishop named Bogomil; Cathar missionaries were sent in pairs around Europe but had their greatest number of conversions in the mountainous regions of the Alps and Pyrenees. Regarding sexual intercourse, their position was that any form of intercourse was acceptable (and, according to some, celebrated), so long as it did not result in procreation.[32] The English word "bugger" comes from this movement.

The Cathars' challenge, the revival of Augustinianism, and the tradition of the early medieval monks and church councils all strengthened the stand that the church took on contraception, according to Noonan.[33] Such may have been the motivations of Ivo of Chartres, who was dissatisfied with Burchard's *Decretum,* who associated contraception with homicide. Like Augustine, Ivo judged contraception as a crime because it was against marriage's solemn purpose. He began the discussion of his position with the first word in Augustine's statement about sterility poisons—*Aliquando* ("At any time").[34] Interestingly, Ivo wanted there to be no doubt about his pronouncement of the reading: rather than condemning the killing of a *fetus,* he used two words together: *conceptus fetus.* In arguing his case against contraception, Ivo was also taking a position against early stage abortion. There was no period for which either was not a sin; or, more simply, contraception and abortion were wrong. The language and breadth of Ivo's argument lead one to the position that no form of sexual activity could be engaged in unless it had the potential to lead to conception and childbirth.

To summarize John Noonan's research on the canonists and theologians: Ivo's *Aliquando* was accepted by Gratian, whose·*Decretum* (c. 1140) adopted Ivo's position, and subsequently Gratian's *Decretum* became the law of the Roman Catholic church. Shortly thereafter, Peter of Lombard published his *Sentences* (c. 1154–57), a theological work of great importance that became the theological position of the church. Peter taught that sexual activity was for procreation alone; for any other reason, it was a sin. Like Gratian, in taking Ivo's *Aliquando*, he took with him the tradition of Basil, Martin of Braga, Regino, *Si aliquis*, and, above all, Augustine on contraception and abortion. The position of others, such as Pseudo-Bede, that the motivation for birth control should be a factor in assessing the seriousness of the sin, remained, but it was in the background, not at the forefront.

Macer's Herbal

Macer's identity is not as important for our purposes as was what he wrote about contraception and abortion. Even though it is secondary, it is interesting and possibly relevant to the issue of the church and birth control. Macer wrote what is probably the most influential and widely read herbal in the Middle Ages. The work, *De virtutibus herbarum*, is a poem about the medical qualities of seventy-one plants and herbs. It was written in the second half of the eleventh century, possibly by an obscure German named Odo of Meung, more probably by a more famous Frank named Marbode (1035–1123), who became the bishop of Rennes and wrote a similar poem on medicinal stones.[35] What is interesting about the poem on herbs is that it listed a large number of menstrual regulators (abortifacients), but it emphasized gynecological uses, and the poem was explicit about abortifacients and contraceptives. The poem's first four herbs are emmenagogues.

"The Virtues of Herbs" began with artemisia, the mother herb. The author explained that the plant was named after Artemisia (Diana to the Romans), who first discovered its uses because "mainly it cures female ailments. It stimulates menstrua and, whether drunk or applied, it produces an abortion."[36]

Under menstrual stimulators (usually *menstrua purgat*) he named the following: southern wood, wormwood, betony, camomile, fennel, lily, ligustrum, chervil, mustard, marjoram, thyme, peony, borage, cinnamon, costmary, and spikenard.[37] Clearly, Macer distinguished between a menstrual stimulator and an abortifacient, as when he wrote about Italian catnip (*nepeta,* or possibly *Mentha sylvestris* L.):[38]

> Placed or drunk it purges the menstrua by its own action [*suo cito*] . . .
> If a pregnant woman drinks it or applies its grindings, she will abort [*abortit*].[39]

About pennyroyal he wrote:

> If a pregnant woman takes this herb often, she will abort.
> It draws off the menses when taken with tepid wine.[40]

Explicitly, he said that the following were abortifacients: rue, Italian catnip, pennyroyal, savory, sage, soapwort, nasturtium, cabbage seeds, elecampane, cyperus, century plant, colubrina, white hellebore (or veratrum), black hellebore, and water germander.[41] Macer was drawing a clear distinction, but he could be interpreted as not prescribing or advocating abortion. His information could be seen as a warning not to take or eat these plants because of undesirable consequences. It is difficult, however, to see that this was his intent when he wrote about nasturtium: "The seed in the herb is strong; it causes an abortion when it is drunk with wine"; or about savory: "It provokes the urine and likewise the menstrua. It causes an abortion and purges a woman's insides." [42] These effects would appear desirable rather than something to be guarded against. No hint of disapproval is found. Generally, Macer used one of two verbs with the noun *abortum.* One verb is *pello,* and the other *depello,* the selection being based on the meter of the verse. Macer's modern translator renders both verbs into English as "to prevent an abortion." [43] Indeed, the dictionary definition for *depello* and *pello* are: to drive, drive away, expel, remove, to ward off, to drive (as to a destination).[44] Surely, Macer's intention was to say that such and such plant "causes," as in "drives to a destination," rather than prevents.[45] A woman who read the passage incorrectly, however, could very well have been taking herbs that caused an abortion when her intent was to prevent one.

Macer had one contraceptive, and possibly a second one, as something between contraceptive and abortifacient. He wrote that if the juice of spearmint (*mentha*) is "applied to the womb before the coitus, the woman will not conceive." [46] Savin, the juniper drug, he said, draws out the menstrua and expels a *conceptus.*[47] In all other places, when he wished to refer to the fetus, Macer used the word *partus.* Macer knew Latin well, and we might surmise that he used *conceptus,* not because of the necessity of his meter but because he wanted to convey that the drug's effect was only shortly after coitus during the period when, on Aristotle's authority, it was not an abortion.[48]

Coming in the second half of the eleventh century, during the height of the *devotio moderna,* Macer's herbal is a rather remarkable document in its information about birth control. The information did not, incidentally, discuss the antifertility properties (Latin, *dynamis*) of the drugs because they were not its emphasis. Perhaps if the poem had been written by Marbode, prior to his bishopric, there might have been reason not to claim authorship. We have no evidence, however, that any writer in the Middle Ages got into trouble for writing about birth control. For a modern historian, any attempt to reconcile the church's positions on abortion and contraception with the medical writings is summarily difficult and ultimately unrewarding.

Hildegard of Bingen

To many people, Hildegard (1098–1117) is Saint Hildegard, for she was a truly remarkable woman. She lived during the time when the new medical developments in southern Italy were influencing physicians around her. Even though she has been called the first German woman doctor,[49] the appellation is less deserved than that of saint because her medical knowledge was that, I suspect, of the common folk. For this reason, her knowledge of the actions of medicinal plants gives us a clue about folk practice.

Because she did not know many of the Latin names for plants, Hildegard of Bingen used many German plant names without a Latin identification in her medical work *De simplicis medicinae,* or *Physica.* Not relying primarily on texts, she described usages that she learned from her friends and neighbors. Although she lived in a cloister, she was worldly enough to know of seven plants that she said were emmenagogues and abortifacients. Asarum, what she called *haselwurtz* (*Asarum europaeum* L.):[50] "A pregnant woman will eat it, either on account she lanquishes [*morietur*], or she aborts an infant with a danger to her body, or if she has not had a menstrual period for a time period so that it hurts."[51] The "fern" (*farn,* probably *asplenon*), she said, should be used as an amulet in childbirth. Placed near the birth canal the *farn* would be the first thing that a newly born infant would smell. This odor would prevent the Devil from having the first opportunity to capture the newborn.[52] Here, Hildegard appears to transform an abortifacient into a seemingly harmless magical rite, but likely this interpretation is a case of too much modern thought being attributed to a medieval mind. It is possible that she saw the necessity for birth control, but, again, there is no direct evidence.

An emendation in Hildegard's text says that *tanacetum,* which is tansy (*Tanacetum vulgare* L.) and unknown in classical antiquity, was an emmenagogue.[53] Tansy is a well-known abortifacient in modern medicine of the type known as ecbolic.[54] This recognition of tansy's quality is the first known recorded use of the plant in the West. Feverfew (Hildegard's *metra*, or *Chrysanthemum parthenium* L.), she said, was good for regulating menstruation, without any greater specificity.[55] Similarly white helebore (*Veratrum album* L.) is a good menstrual stimulator, especially for a young girl's first menstruation.[56] She was, however, very specific about oleaster (*hirtzswam*, or *Elacagnus angustifolia* L.): "It makes an abortion to a pregnant woman with a danger to her body, should she eat this plant."[57] Hildegard's use of abortifacients, emmenagogues, and, possibly, contraceptives revealed that folk usage continued and that the knowledge was, as always, undergoing change. Pepper, mandrake, juniper, and other plants known in antiquity were passed over by Hildegard as far as fertility effects were concerned.

Hildegard, saint or not, provided an important insight into what must have been a complication in women's lives during the central Middle Ages. As abbess of her convent she stood in face-to-face encounters with the emperor, Frederick Barbarossa, and even challenged the papacy, so it should not be surprising that she had an independent spirit in her writings. On one hand, the church and secular law increasingly are protecting the life of the fetus and even the right to be conceived unencumbered by any artificial controls; on the other hand, individual women had problems, some medical, some personal, that persons of compassion wanted to address. Hildegard's writings show that they had at least some of the information.

CHAPTER ELEVEN

Salerno and Medicine through the Twelfth Century

If a pregnant woman will eat asurum, either on account she languishes, or she aborts an infant with a danger to her body, or, if she has not had a menstrual period for a time that it hurts.

Hildegard of Bingen

In the history of medicine the Salernitan period is of tremendous importance because in and around Salerno, from the tenth through the twelfth centuries, physicians established a reputation throughout Europe and were themselves writers of an amazing number of medical works. The reputation of Salerno probably exceeded its actual influence during the Middle Ages because modern historians have fastened upon Salerno as the "turning point" for the rational art of medicine. According to these historians, before Salerno there was superstition, but afterward, a return to the Hellenic, Hippocratic spirit of natural causes.[1]

Whatever the final word on Salerno's place in history, Salerno did exist as a place where a skillful guild of physicians established a reputation for practicing and training in medicine in a way we now call clinical. Perhaps the most important person, however, belongs not in Salerno but nearby at the Benedictine Abbey at Monte Cassino. There Constantine the African (d. c. 1085), newly arrived and imbued with a sense that western Christians were far behind easterners in medical knowledge, set about the task of translating and, it is suspected, modifying Arabic works into Latin. One might expect that work done in a cloister would handle contraceptive and abortifacient information gently, if at all, while the secular physicians at Salerno would be more forthright and direct. Actually, there was no such dichotomy. Constantine and, as we saw in the last chapter, Hildegard of Bingen were as direct as their medical school counterparts. A treatise attributed to Constantine, *On Sexual Intercourse,* is now known to be a part of the larger medical work, *Kitab al-maliki,* by ʿAli ibn al-ʿAbbas (Haly Abbas), called *Pantegni* in Latin. In the treatise on sexual intercourse, the Latin text has no discussion of contraceptives and abortifacients except for an intriguing statement that there are medicines "that impede and prohibit the semen and dry it out." The text says that there are "cold nutriments that suppress the libido, [and] they are lettuce, purslain, cucumber, beets, mulberry, gourd, and melons. There are in truth things that do not generate semen but dry it out and dissipate it on account of heat and dryness, and they are dill, rue, and similar things."[2] The assumption is that the reader would already know to which medicines he was referring.

In the treatise attributed to Constantine called *On Degrees* (probably adapted from a work by Ibn al-Jazzar), the medicines for abortions are clearly given; most of them, however, were cited as emmenagogues (*menstrua provocat*). Drugs were given according to the degree of intensity of their pharmaceutical actions, beginning with the weak drugs, those with one degree of action, and ending with the extremely strong and dangerous drugs of four degrees of action. *On Degrees* named these drugs as either emmenagogues or abortifacients or both.

> One degree: wormwood, chamomile, nard, valerian [*fu* = *Valeriana officinales* L.], and blackberry.[3]
>
> Two degrees: acorus [*Acorus calamus* L.], birthwort [mixed with myrrh and pepper], iris, sisymbrium, myrrh [as suppository with wormwood or rue], great century plant, southernwood [*Artemisia abrotanum* L.], a southernwood that grows in Armenia, dill, sweet almonds [*Punus dulcis* Miller, Rosaceae fam.], great burdock [*costus* = *Arctium lappa* L., Compositae fam.].[4]
>
> Three degrees: great yellow gentian [*gentiana* = *Gentiana lutea* L.], savin, cinnamon [*Cinnamomum* sp.], thyme, *cassia ligne* [a type of cinnamon], asarum, Queen Anne's lace or daucus, lavender [*sansucus* = *Lavandula* sp., Labiatae fam.], white hellebore [*Veratrum album* L.], majoram, *squinantum* [?], *sagapinum* [*Ferula persica* Willd.], opopanax, stinking fennel or asafetida, ground-pine, *chamedraeos* [germander?], reed [*canna* = *Phyragmites communis* Trin., Gramineae fam.], *ammoniacum* [*Ferula tingitana* L.], *galbanum* [*Ferula galvaniflua* Baiss. and Bushe], celery, chaste tree, bindweed, dittany, and caper spurge[5] [*lacterides* = *Euphorbia lathyris* L.].[6]
>
> Four degrees: onions domesticated and wild, parsley, *condisi,* and rue.[7]

One contraceptive was named as such: the juice of willow leaves is drunk "so that a woman will not conceive." [8] Mint augments sexual desire and, if it is drunk by those pregnant, it makes childbirth easier.[9] Calaminth extinguishes sexual desire and kills the sperm.[10] The gentian, *san-sucus,* white hellebore, opopanax, germander, and *condisi* were specifically used as suppositories. The others appear as oral-route drinks, a few so specified (e.g., birthwort, iris, opopanax, stinking ferula [asafe-tida], dittany, and rue). The great and lesser century plants were "taken with *acumine* to provoke menstruation and to draw out a dead fetus." Then, the text adds, it was good also as a suppository. The implication is that, unless otherwise stated, the default route was oral. Some plants are said to expel a dead fetus (iris, southernwood, great century plant, myrrh, gentian, and opopanax). Possessing the strongest of intensities, rue was "drunk with oxymel to dry out the sperm and kill the desire for inter-course . . . [and it] expels the menstrua." [11] In the seventeenth century a means of expressing the action of antifertility agents was "drying" the seed "without adversely affecting lust." Langham's *Garden of Health* states, for instance, that "rue eaten a certain space, drieth up natural seede in man." [12] Pepper and henbane were given as four degrees of inten-sity but with no antifertility actions listed. Pomegranate was not dis-cussed at all.

Constantine and Censorship

Constantine also translated the "Provision of the Voyager" (*Zad al-musafir*) by the same Ibn al-Jazzar who probably wrote the text for *On Degrees.* The work is a seven-book composite of medical information in a handbook, textbook format and was known in the West by Constan-tine's translation, the *Viaticum.* Book 6 of the *Viaticum* concerns "the maladies which are found in the instruments of generation." Chapter 17 concerns "On substances which induce abortion and kill the seed in the womb." In the Arabic text, Ibn al-Jazzar expressed reluctance to discuss abortion and did so, he said, on the grounds that women might know what to avoid.

> When I studied the books of the ancients who discoursed upon the force of simple medicaments and their disadvantages, I found that they had spoken of substances which kill the seed in the womb and inhibit pregnancy. I found equally that they spoke of drugs which kill embryos and cause them to fall from the womb. Thus, I decided to cite in this chapter all these drugs in order to make them known, so that women will avoid their use since they kill the seed.[13]

After discussing the specific abortifacients, Ibn al-Jazzar concluded with a more positive tone by saying that such substances were therapeu-tically beneficial when used to expel a dead fetus. "These drugs, which kill the seed and evacuate the living fetus, can be utilized in the evacuation of the dead fetus [as well], since they make it come out quickly, God willing." [14]

In the Latin translation, the entire chapter is omitted. Monica Green, who discovered this omission in Constantine's text, is uncertain whether it was a deliberate act by Constantine or whether a later scribe was responsible. Green comments, "What is more remarkable about the suppression of Ibn al-Jazzar's chapter on abortifacients at Monte Cassino, however, is that this is the first and only such suppression I have yet documented in early medieval medical literature." [15] She notes that one of the manuscripts of Cleopatra's *Gynecology* was possibly produced at Monte Cassino; even more significant, an early-twelfth-century condensation of Cleopatra's work included both abortifacients and contraceptives. [16] Were there something resembling a policy on suppression of birth control information, one would suppose that the unknown condensor of Cleopatra's text would have excluded those sections, but that did not happen. The fact, however, that Constantine did not suppress birth control information in his other works, especially in *On Degrees,* would argue that the suppression of chapter 17 of *Viaticum*'s book 6 was probably due to a scribe or copyist. It would have been incongruous for Constantine to refuse to translate Ibn Jazzar's chapter when its author was not advocating abortion but only warning women on what to avoid for the expulsion of a dead fetus. Contrary to other Arabic writers, Ibn Jazzar reflected a sensitivity to the issue of birth control. Green's finding of the suppression of birth control information must be regarded as an anomaly in medieval medicine and most likely should not be considered an act of Constantine.

Not only was he unlikely to have censored his work, but through his writings Constantine introduced several new abortifacients to Europe. Among them was caper spurge, a species that laboratory testing has shown to possess "high oxytocic [abortifacient] properties: 0.009 c.c. gives as much response as 0.003 I.U. of oxytocis without any toxic reaction." [17] Various species of spurge were employed in early Indic medicine (Vedic and post Vedic). [18] According to the written evidence, Constantine introduced this use of spurge into the West. [19] Finally, Constantine's text *On Degrees* stated that celery "provokes urine and menstruation *to the greatest extent.* Physicians [*medici*] prohibit pregnant women and those nursing to have celery." [20] Although he does not say so, I interpret his reference here to be to celery *seed.* Constantine's statement does not necessarily contradict the classification of rue as being fourth degree, while celery is third. The drug classifications were based on the intensity of pharmaceutical action for all effects, not specifically for one. In this passage on celery, as in all the other sections above, Constantine does not appear as an advocate for birth control. Certainly, he explicitly recognized that menstrual regulators (i.e., those that provoked menstruation) were also abortifacients; one cannot therefore conclude that he suppressed the section in the *Viaticum* and included such information elsewhere simply because he did not know what he was saying. Clearly he did.

Salernitan Regimen of Health and Other Works

A poem known as the *Salernitan Regimen of Health* (*Regimen sanitatis Salernitanum* or *Flos medicinae*) enjoyed enormous popularity, as evidenced by the fact that there were over three hundred editions of it. Paul Kristeller likened the composition to the Homeric question and described it as having "no definite form from the beginning, but [it] is based on a floating mass of memorial verses composed at various places through several centuries."[21] The medical lore that it contains existed before scholastic medicine developed in the universities and therefore represents a means of understanding medieval medicine before the impact of Arabic learning and scholasticism. Although most of the plants that are antifertility agents are included in verses about their medicinal values, there is only one clear abortifacient—artemisia. This "mother of plants," the one Macer selected to begin his poem, was said to "cause an abortion whether drunk or applied."[22] *Armoniacum* (= *ammoniacum* from *Ferula*) "leads out the menstrua." Plants such as birthwort and betony had no antifertility qualities mentioned.[23] Even rue, which one expects to find in birth control procedures, was only mentioned in this eliptical statement: "Rue lessens coitus in men; it increases it in women."[24] A more or less popular treatise on herbal lore is just where one would expect to find information about birth control, but by and large it is not there.

A long medical work called *On the Cures of Diseases* was written most probably in the twelfth century. Considerable attention was paid to women's diseases and problems. The treatise is pronatal, with considerable attention devoted to conception aids, stimulants for fertile intercourse, and preventives of miscarriages and abortions.[25] There is one recipe that "comforts the fetus and prohibits abortion."[26] Even so, there are antifertility measures given. Several vaginal suppositories are given to "impede conception," consisting of elderwort (*Sambucus* sp.), balsam, wormwood, artemisia, laurel oil, and "various odoriferous" things.[27] And menstrual regulators to stimulate menstruation are given that include artemisia, savin (juniper), and betony. According to the treatise, some menstrual evokers expel a dead fetus; also, a woman ought to know whether her fetus is alive before taking the recipes, because they would kill it.[28] Interestingly, one of the causes of abortion, the work stated, was "on account of a poor diet [*propter deffectum nutrimenti*]."[29]

The very same observation about the results of a poor diet was made in another treatise that Salvatore de Renzi attributed to Salerno. The work, called *The Secrets of Women,* was part of a genre of numerous, mostly anonymous works of the Middle Ages that should no more be associated exclusively with Salerno than pretty beaches are associated with Hawaii. As in the *Cure of Diseases* and *Circa instans* (see below), the version of the *Secrets* has little on abortion, and what it has is mostly on preventing abortion. On conception, considerable attention is devoted to aids for conception, not so on prevention. In the section on "the causes of abortion on account of *opilationem* poisons," are listed rue, laurel leaves, mint, calaminth, Queen Anne's lace, common germander, false bishop's weed (*ameos* = *Ammi mais* L.), and artemisia.[30] Here we have a list different from any other account and one with what appears to be a new addition, namely, false bishop's weed. The same word, *ammi,* appears in Dioscorides, but the plant is thought to be *Carum copticum* B et H. Even if it is a species of *Ammi,* Dioscorides said only that it was a provoker of menstruation.[31] Modern pharmaceutical guides also list *Ammi* sp. as an emmenagogue.[32] The paradox is that, just when a generalization appears merited (that the medieval knowledge about antifertility agents was declining), something innovative is found that shows that folk medicine was finding new drugs that probably worked. Tansy and false bishop's weed are examples. A study of other versions of *Women's Secrets* would doubtless reveal a similar pattern. For instance, one other version had a contraceptive that appeared truly innovative, certainly unpleasant, and probably ineffective: "Drink a man's urine, and it will impede conception." [33]

Even the generalization about a diminished knowledge of antifertility agents has some contradiction in the evidence. In the second half of the thirteenth century, certainly late Salernitan, a work entitled *Tables* was written, probably by Petrus Marancius, giving an extensive drug list. Under menstrual stimulators (*menstrua provocantia*) were catalogued some eighty-one drugs, almost all familiar ones, but with some additional ones, such as *stincus tori,*[34] *polycaria,*[35] and "earth apples," which is another name for birthwort.[36] Laurel was specified as "roots of" rather than the leaves. Explicitly and separately, Petrus Maranchus itemized abortifacients (*aborsum facientia*): squill, *cocula sedita,*[37] opopanax roots, henbane, bull feces, "earth apples" (birthwort), iris, cassia, century plant,[38] chamomile, and cyclamen.[39] Some unexpected omissions occur here: rue and squirting cucumber were omitted altogether; pennyroyal, artemisia, and Queen Anne's lace were listed only as emmenagogues. One might conclude that Petrus was only cataloguing, not using rational, personal medical judgment; other indications, however, argue against this conclusion. Conspicuously omitted from either listing was *silphium,* which, if only literary sources were being copied from or derived from classical sources, one would also expect to find. Could it be that Petrus knew that it was no longer available and therefore omitted it?

Another category of drugs followed the abortifacient, namely, those that "extract the fetus and afterbirth." Forty-four drugs were listed, and again, most of the same ones under emmenagogues were repeated, except this time, squirting cucumber was specified and two new ones were added: *bdellium* (an opium product) and radishes.[40]

Trotula, Female Gynecologist

The very existence of a woman doctor by the name of Trotula who practiced medicine at Salerno and wrote a work on women's medical problems is the subject of dispute. The scholarly world is now persuaded that the careful study by John F. Benton revealed that there was such a person, although he notes that there were three main treatises attributed to her and that each one may have been written by a man for male practitioners.[41] The person Trotula probably lived in the late twelfth or possibly early thirteenth century. Monica Green challenges Benton on the exclusive maleness of these works because there were female physicians at Salerno who practiced medicine; moreover, women physicians probably used these texts.[42]

As with Macer, we have the texts but are uncertain about their origin. The work has remarkably little on birth control. The text that I consulted is a sixteenth-century composite of all three treatises attributed to Trotula. While it may not say exactly what Trotula said, the text reveals what people in the Middle Ages learned about birth control from "Trotula"—in a word, little. For retention of the menstrua (which, as we have seen, was sometimes a code for early abortifacients), Trotula related a number of remedies. First, she said to drink artemisia in wine and take baths. If this does not work, take artemisia together with other herbs such as death carrot (*thapsia*), *seseli,* sage, marjoram, pennyroyal, cumin, anis, savin (juniper), balm (*melissa = Melissa officianalis* L.? mint family), betony, savory, chamomile, and lovage. These were boiled down in water and applied.[43] A drink for the same purpose was compounded by grinding hemlock, castoreum, artemisia, betony, myrrh, century plant, and sage, in equal amounts, boiled down in water and drunk in the amount of approximately one-half oz (13 g).[44] This drink is the most effective, Trotula said. The prescription appears very potent indeed and certainly would have the desired consequences—as well as unpleasant side effects. One would likely not resort to this extraordinarily strong measure if the problem were simply nonpregnancy-induced dysmenorrhea. The only

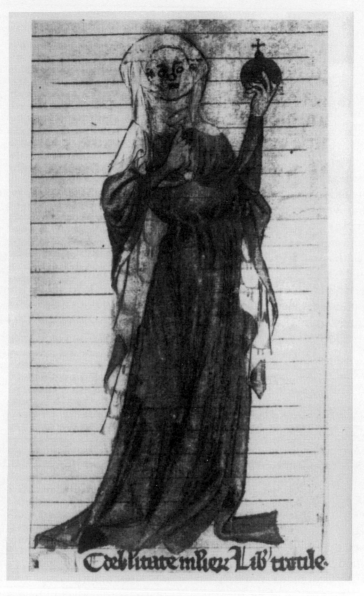

Dame Trotula. A representation of the so-called first woman gynecologist, who practiced in or around Salerno in the late twelfth or early thirteenth century, from a manuscript of the time. (Wellcome MS 554, p. 65, courtesy of the Wellcome Institute Library, London)

mention of abortion came in remedies to treat a woman who had attempted it.[45]

Other Salernitan Works

Considering the volume of medical treatises attributed to the Salernitan School, the remarkable feature is the scarcity of attention to birth control. The school was certainly secular. In such a school, characterized by its relative freedom from dogma, including Galenic medical dogma, and with an emphasis on clinical medicine, one might expect more attention to birth control; such, however, is not the case.

The most popular herbal to come from the Salernitan works is attributed to Matthaeus Platearius (d. c. 1161?). The herbal is known by the first two words of its text, *Circa instans,* and it was in the late Middle Ages more important as a medical text than was, say, Macer's more popular herbal. By legend, Matthaeus Platearius was the son of Trotula. He certainly was cautious on recommending birth control drugs. Despite a larger volume of medical uses than Macer included in his work (indeed than in most herbals), *Circa instans'* author mostly buried the issue. Rue and opopanax were recommended for "evoking menstrua, a dead fetus/embryo [*fetuum mortuum*], and afterbirth." Rue was given either orally or as a suppository, and opopanax as a suppository only and with the juice of wormwood and artemisia added.[46] Curiously, under the entries for wormwood and artemisia, Platearius said only that they evoked menstruation and did not mention a fetus.[47] Similarly, he wrote that celery seed, mallow (*malva*), and the chaste tree provoked menstruation alone.[48] As a suppository, mint was good for cleaning a tender womb (*ad matricem mundificandam teneritates*),[49] and even more inscrutably, pomegranate as a suppository with plantain was given "against menstrual bleeding."[50] As for many of the other plants that we have come to consider as being contraceptives and abortifacients, he made no mention of them in connection with fertility. He did, however, mention myrrh and balm (*melissa?*), the same plants that Trotula gave as emmenagogues. Platearius said that myrrh and balm aid conception (*conceptum adiuuvat*).[51] The question is unanswered whether Platearius was merely ill informed about gynecological matters or whether he was attempting to disguise his material. It is not out of the question that myrrh and balm could aid conception, especially if their actions were estrogenic. If timed correctly and given in appropriate amounts, estrogen assists conception, just as estrogen ingested at the wrong time or in the wrong amount can impede the same.

CHAPTER TWELVE

Islam, Arabic Medicine, and the Late Middle Ages

Each of you is constituted in your mother's womb for forty days as a semen, then it becomes a bloodlike clot for an equal period, then a lump of flesh for another equal period, then the angel is sent, and he breathes the soul into it.

The Prophet Muhammed

I n Muslim society, the evidence of continuous usages of oral contra-ceptives and early stage abortifacients is abundant—even over-whelming—as shown by B. F. Musallam.[1] In Islam, the soul comes to the conceptus at the end of 120 days (four months by lunar calendar). The authority, dating back to Hebrew scripture and Aristotle, came more directly from the Prophet.[2] All Muslim jurists accepted this, but different interprettions were taken on abortion. The Hanafi jurists permitted a woman to abort, even without the husband's permission (though she should have cause), before 120 days. Shafi'i and Hanbali jurists, however, disagreed but could not agree on a lower limit of 40 days or 80 or 120. Most Malikis prohibited abortion at any time on the basis of potentiality for ensoulment. All could agree on one thing: contraception was accept-able and not prohibited by God's law.[3] As a consequence, Arabic medical writings explored both contraceptives and early stage abortifacients, perhaps to the limits that critical, concerted medical observation would permit.

Muhammad ibn Zakariya Al-Razi (or Rhazes, c. 865–925) prescribed at least eight oral contraceptives/abortifacients, according to Musallam, with these ingredients: cyclamen juice and roots, wallflower broth, male fern, cinnamon, myrrh, willow leaves, *luffa,* and rue seeds.[4] These plants are familiar, with the exception of cyclamen, which Dioscorides recom-mended explicitly as an abortifacient when mixed with unspecified other medicines[5] and, possibly, luffa seed. Maimonides (1135–1204) said that the Arabic *luf* is the Greek *aron*.[6] Dioscorides' *aron*, or *drakontion*, is likely *Arum maculatum* L. or *Arum italicum*. Dioscorides wrote that "they say" that a smell of its flower "aborts a newly conceived embryo," which is Dioscorides' way of passing on folk reports. Dioscorides said that its root caused an abortion, however.[7] *Arum maculatum* L. and *Arisarum vulgare* L., are members of the Araceae family, which has had one of its species tested experimentally in humans as an oral contraceptive. In male and female mice it produced temporary sterility; five of its species are employed as antifertility agents in folklore reports.[8] Musallam catalogued the contraceptive and abortifacients in Arabic writings and, while new ones were reported, the same ones keep reappearing.

Ibn Sina (Avicenna, 980–1037) wrote the *Canon of Medicine,* which was a comprehensive text that had more influence in the West than the original Arabic in the Islamic world. Ibn Sina showed no inhibitions in discussing birth control measures. Indeed, he began the discussion of contraceptives with a justification as to why it was necessary for a physician to intervene even at this level. The following is a translation from the Arabic by Max Meyerhof:[9]

Prohibiting Conception:
The physician finds it necessary to prevent conception in small women, in whom it would be dangerous to have childbirth on account of a diseased womb or from a weakness in the insides. A heavy fetus causes clefts in the internal area to such a degree that urine passes involuntarily and she is unable to retain it full term. Among the measures for this situation are: [1] One should anticipate those times for coitus which are favorable for conception to occur as we have said [elsewhere]; [2] One should separate before mixing the two seeds;[10] [3] The woman should raise immediately after coitus, jump backwards from seven to nine times forcefully so that the sperm may come out;[11] [4] Another way is for the woman to sneeze;[12] [5] And also one can add slippery things to the sperm so that it is dissipated. Along these lines one could put pitch [resin] and white lead on the penis before coitus and afterwards put [in the vagina] pulp of pomegranate and alum; [6] Or one could put cabbage flowers or seed as a suppository near the time of the cleaning period and before coitus; [7] Using the same procedure before and after coitus one can use the same dipped in pitch or submerged in a decoction of pennyroyal;[13] [8] Or, as a suppository willow leaves after the menstruation period and by its property [as a contraceptive] it is especially good if [the pad] is submerged with water in which willow leaves have soaked. And the same [purpose] is obtained by [9] equal parts of colocynth pulp, mandrake, iron dross, sulfur, scammony, and cabbage seeds, collected, mixed with pitch and inserted. [10] And inserting pepper after coitus prohibits conception, and [11] so does a suppository of elephant's dung by itself or in fumigations at the times mentioned previously; [12] and it is also useful to drink

three *okas* [pints] of an infusion of sweet basil, for it prevents conception. [13] If the penis, particularly the glans, is anointed with sweet oil before coitus, conception is prevented; [14] likewise, the leaves of bindweed prevent conception if a woman inserts them after the menstruation begins.

Ibn Sina's account is a catalogue of contraceptives, the substance of which is found in ancient sources but not the specific details. Elsewhere, in the "simples" section of the *Canon,* he truly catalogued almost completely the contraceptives and abortifacients known to medicine and found in the sources.[14]

'Arib ibn Sa'id, a Muslim writer who lived in Spain in the tenth century, wrote a treatise "On the Development of the Fetus, the Treatment of Pregnant Women, and the Birth." Although the concern was with how to have healthy pregnancies and births, the author saw circumstances when an early abortion was necessary. He listed medicines that were effective in terminating pregnancies during the second and third months. They included colocynth, giant fennel, and celery seeds.[15] Similarly a formulary for hospital therapy in a Cairo hospital around 1200 by Abu l-Fadl Dawud ibn Abi l-Bayan al-Isra'ili (1161–1240) gave suppositories to expel a "dead fetus," which included the squirting cucumber, birthwort, rue, cyclamen, amoniacum (giant fennell), and mezereum (*Daphne mezereum* L.).[16] About the same time, farther to the east in Samarkand (now in the Soviet Union) and Herat (now in Iran), a writer said that the seed of the chaste tree, dittany, lichen, rue seed, and dodder (*Cuscuta epithymum* L.) are employed to promote menstruation.[17]

Other Arabic works are more detailed about antifertility agents. In the *Creation of Man,* Abu al-Hasan al-Tabib (1044–1101) has twenty-nine prescriptions for contraception, including, as oral ones, birthwort, willow, pepper, myrrh, lupine, asafetida, rue, and opopanax.[18] The Arabic writers efficiently related the heritage of antiquity's medical lore on birth control and added their own contributions.

Latin Translations of Arabic Works

Crucial in the history of the West are two developments in West Asia: (1) the Muslims based their knowledge on Hellenic and Hellenistic learning, even when they had the choice of synthesizing Indic and Chinese learning with classical western knowledge; (2) the translators of works in Arabic were faithful and, on the whole, accurate and honest in keeping the meaning. In respect to birth control, these factors largely kept the Muslims from learning East Asian medical lore, even as they brought many of the Greek works (such as Galen and the Hippocratic corpus) to the attention of excellent, gifted medical observers, such as Avicenna. The consequence is that through the Arabic writings western Europe by the thirteenth century had the knowledge of ancient medicine passed down more efficiently than it had directly from Greek to Latin. Moreover, it had new and superior knowledge regarding birth control from the Arabs, whose culture was not reticent about the subject.

Al-Razi

One of the greatest of the Muslim scholars was Muhammad ibn Zakariya al-Razi, known in the West as Rhazes (c. 865–925). His medical knowledge places him among the greatest physicians of all time. His careful, clinical description of measles was still employed as definitive in medical schools into the nineteenth century. Gerard of Cremona (b. Cremona, Italy, c. 1114; d. Toledo, Spain, 1187) rendered al-Razi into Latin, seemingly without regard to the Roman church's attitudes. This disregard was perhaps due to his commitment to *scientia,* with his remoteness from Rome in Toledo also a possible factor (although, as stated before, the church did not censure medical works). In the work, *Ad regem mansorem,* Gerard translated a section with the title "De ilis quae prohibent impregnari et quae aborsum faciunt" (Those things which prevent pregnancy and cause an abortion)." The first formula is a suppository to be used "instantly [*statim*]" after coitus, consisting of the juice of rue and pepper. Al-Razi told of other medicines that cause an abortion (*quae abortire faciunt*), such as rue juice, pulp of colocynth, savin juniper seeds (latter taken for ten days unless a fever results), mint, blackberries, and pennyroyal. Detailed information is given about preparation and amounts to be taken.[19]

In another treatise, *Antidotes,* Gerard translated al-Razi's instructions about "a preparation of myrrh for raising the fetus [*allevians partum*] and provoking the menstrua." The order of the expression is interesting: first, the action against the fetus/embryo; second, menstruation. The myrrh preparation consisted of cinnamon, myrrh, dried rue leaves (not juice as before), calamint, cardamom, pennyroyal, blackberries, asafetida, opopanax, and *serapinia* and given as a drink with a decoction of savin.[20] The *serapinia* is sagapenum gum from *Ferula persica* Willd.[21] Again, this demonstrates an active discovery of "new" but related antifertility drugs. Al-Razi's formulas are unique, but he relied on traditional drugs.

Mesuë

Another tenth-century Arabic author who had a large impact on Western medicine was Masawaih, known in the West as Mesuë. Although his work was based on the knowledge of ancient authorities—in particular,

Dioscorides and Galen—Mesuë went beyond the volume of data in his sources and classified drugs systematically by their actions, for example, beginning with "medicines that do not cause inflation." The first drug in this first category is aloes, but he made no specific reference to antifertility qualities, although they are implicit in some of the drug's pharmaceutical properties.[22] The same omission of antifertility actions occurs with wormwood, which one would not expect.[23] That the Latin translator or a later editor excluded or censored the material is unlikely.

Asarus was said in the Latin translation to increase the sperm,[24] not to interfere with fertility, as the ancient sources claimed. *Agaricus* (which Mesuë specifically called a fungus) stimulates menstruation and cleans (*mundificio*) the uterus (*matrix*).[25] Iris, he is translated as saying, "drives out the menstrua and causes an abortion,"[26] and the century plant "provokes the menstrua, makes well a diseased uterus and drives out a fetus."[27] Having omitted antifertility usage for southernwood (*Artemisia absinthium*), the texts included it for birthwort (*A. aristolochia*). Without a comparison of the Arabic text (unavailable) with the Latin manuscripts, one cannot know whether for those agents that omit antifertility information (which was in Mesuë's sources) he included it but the text edited it out, or whether the omissions were his own. Because the subject itself was not avoided, I tentatively conclude that Mesuë made discerning judgments about his material.

Gerard of Cremona also translated the work of one of Islam's earliest pharmacy writers, namely, the "Simple Medicines" (sometimes called *Breviarius*), by Yuhya ibn Sarafyun, known in the West as Serapion the Elder (ninth century). The work's influence appeared greater in the West than in the East. Serapion's approach to birth control was detailed and combined theory with practical recipes. The theoretical structure was based on the Hippocratic-Galenic models of a balance of humors, with a drying action usually being called for to prevent conception or a continuation of pregnancy.

The first section was on measures to provoke menstruation but, importantly, under this rubric were a number of drugs that he explicitly noted were abortifacients as well. For example, under calamint, Gerard translated Serapion as saying, "A decoction of calamint taken by women provokes menstruation and expels a fetus/embryo at the time of birth."[28] This wording makes it unclear whether it was intended as an abortifacient or as an aid to birth. More certain to be the former was lupine, which he said "taken with honey and myrrh expels the fetus/embryo," without mentioning the menstrua at all.[29] The menstrual regulators were virtually (but not completely) synonymous with abortifacients. The following were listed as menstrual regulators: savin juniper, myrrh, calamint, mountain pennyroyal, mint, costus (*Saururus lappa* Clarke), cassia, cinnamon, ammoniacum (*Ferula tingitana* L.), birthwort, thyme, *hasce* (*Euphorbia lathyris* L. [?], a spurge), "and others (*et aliis.*)"[30] He assumed that the list was generally known, hence there was no need to exhaust all the possibilities.

Serapion the Elder included an unusual category—"sperm medicines [*de medicinis spermatis*]," whose action it is to kill the sperm, specifically mentioning rue.[31] In the section on simple (individual) drugs, he cited Dioscorides as saying that poplar "prohibits conception when drunk with a mule's kidney."[32] Curiously, about pomegranate he noted, "In the book of ancient medicine pomegranate took away sexual desire [*abscindit libidione*]," without specifying any antifertility usages.[33] When considered with the evidence in other medical works (or in this case, the lack of it), the conclusion is justified that pomegranate had virtually ceased to be within the pharmacopoeia of antifertility measures. Elsewhere the full range of antiquity's antifertility drugs was related: for example, "willow leaves drunk prevent conception [*prohibent conceptionnem*]"; squirting cucumber "kills the fetus/embryo"; Queen Anne's lace causes an abortion; and birthwort "expels the fetus/embryo."[34] Juniper, however, had no antifertility usages listed when discussed as a simple drug.[35]

Another one writing on medicines and drugs was Yuhanna ibn Sarabiyun (fl. c. 1070?), known in the West as Serapion the Younger. He wrote a large compendium, called *Simple Medicines in Seven Books,* which was translated by Nicolaus Mutonus. Its detail about birth control devices was perhaps unrivaled. He began with menstrual "movers" from the theoretical, humoral view and then divided them into two classes according to quality. The best, he said, were savin juniper, spignel (*meum*), iris, calamint, and pennyroyal. The second group included dittany, asarum, costus, cassia, cinnamon, ammoniacum, birthwort, turnip (*bunium = Brassica napus*), and "and others of this kind [*et eius generis*]."[36] The turnip is first encountered here (although other Brassica plants were used), but the important statement came at the end: plants from both groups are safe, he said.[37]

Serapion the Younger drew heavily on Dioscorides but extended his research on drugs by surveying many authorities, including Galen. Curiously, he cited Dioscorides as having said that asparagus acted as a contraceptive, which, as we saw earlier, was an emendation in the manuscript. Since the Greek manuscripts came much later, there was obviously a manuscript tradition in Arabic that had this statement.[38] Where the Greek manuscript had the term ἀτόκιος for contraceptive, Mutonius' Latin translation of Serapion the Younger's Arabic text has *sterilitatem efficit,* thus making it clear that Jerome's "sterility poisons" were contraceptives, not abortifacients.[39] It is truly remarkable how precise the language is, having been translated from Greek to Syriac to Arabic and finally to Latin and still keeping the same meaning.

Serapion the Younger faithfully transmitted most of the antifertility drugs in Dioscorides and Galen, but he often gave more information than was in the Greek texts of his authors. For example, with the contraceptive ivy, he gave the quantities (which his Greek sources omitted) and added that it should be taken with giant fennel (*corymbus* = *Ferula* sp.).[40] Inexplicably, however, he omitted antifertility usage for cyperus, although he gave its other medicinal usages.[41] Whether the omission was a deliberate decision and a statement about its ineffectiveness or an oversight cannot be known. The fern *filix,* he said, was both a contraceptive and an abortifacient.[42] A new drug called *sandarax* made from juniper sap, he quoted Bedigoras (Burzōe) as saying, regulated menstruation.[43] He cited both Galen and Dioscorides on the chaste tree.[44] He credited Dioscorides as saying that the willow prevented conception (*conceptus prohibeat*) but omitted the part about the mule's kidney, and he quoted Mesuë as an authority for the same thing: *mulieribus ne concipiant prosuntque.*[45]

Latin Avicenna

Gerard of Cremona also translated the *Canon* of ibn Sina, known in the West as Avicenna. This work became a text of authority in medical schools, albeit more perhaps for its theoretical structure than for its practical medicine.[46] Gerard's linguistic skill was phenomenal, considering that he had no dictionaries, as he tried to find the right meanings of technical Arabic terms in Latin, including the vast array of plant nomenclatures.

In translating Avicenna's discussion of contraceptives, there were a few places that caused Gerard some problems and may have led to error. Gerard omitted white lead as one of the ingredients to be applied in a mixture on the penis before coitus. Avicenna's *futanaj,* which means (according to Meyerhof) pennyroyal, Gerard translated as *calaminti,* for calamint. If it was an error, it was either a rational error or a remarkable coincidence, inasmuch as calamint and pennyroyal were both used. Gerard did not know the meaning of *algarab* for willow, or of *berzagiesan* for mandrake, or *badruj* for sweet basil, so he transliterated the Arabic term into Latin letters, hoping, no doubt, that some of his readers would know. His transliteration methods were interesting: *badruj,* for example, he rendered as *ulbedurungi,* incorporating the article "al-." In one section, there is a line not in the Arabic translation by Meyerhof; specifically, the Gerard translation contains the observation, "inserting salt in the vagina may make the sperm weak."[47]

The Latin translation of ibn Sina's *Canon* by Gerard of Cremona does not avoid a full discussion of contraception and abortions. Included, for instance, are the conditions in women necessitating an avoidance of pregnancy.[48] In translating the section on simple medicines, Gerard was not hesitant to use words for abortion. Anise, southernwood, and asarum he called menstrual provokers.[49] Savin (juniper), however, he said, "provokes the menses and destroys the fetus/embryo inside the womb and extracts it dead [*provocat menstrua et corrumpit foetum, intra matricem et extrahit mortuum*]." Simply, cyclamen "causes an abortion [*facit abortum*]." Birthwort "provokes the menses and extracts an embryo/fetus [*provocat menstrua et extrahit foetum*]."[50]

The Arabic authorities were certainly employing their own knowledge rather than strictly transcribing the works of previous writers. Very important to the Latin West in the late Middle Ages is the fact that the knowledge available about birth control agents more than equaled the information known to the ancients.

CHAPTER THIRTEEN

Knowledge of Birth Control
in the West

To hell will I go. For to hell go the fine scholars, and the fair knights who are slain in the tourney or the great wars, and the stout archer, and the loyal man. With them will I go. And there go the fair and courteous ladies, who have friends—two or three—besides their wedded lord. And there pass the . . . harpers and minstrels, and the kings of this world. With these will I go only that I have Nicolette, my very sweet friend, by my side.

Aucassin and Nicolette, 6

The assimilation of Arabic medicine in the West was a long process that began at the same time as the development of the uniquely western institution of the university. Heretofore, it was possible for a person seeking to become a physician to learn what his master taught him, to learn the texts available, and to feel reasonably assured that he knew all there was to know in order to practice medicine.

In this chapter we shall examine the New Learning, which is what we call the assimilation of Arabic works in the Latin West. In respect to birth control during the assimilation period, the context of learning was changed without substantial changes in the information itself. We shall examine the works of three leading writers of the day: one was a leading surgeon and town physician, another was a university master who also practiced medicine, and the third was one who wrote so that he poor could benefit from the learning without the extraordinarily high medical costs that greeted the new age.

By the thirteenth century, it was no longer possible to learn all the texts because the volume of information was too great. Moreover, the thirteenth and fourteenth centuries saw the greatest change occur in medical education since medicine had divorced itself from the ancient temples.

Now in order to practice medicine and be called a physician (*medicus*), one had to have a university education. University learning was required for membership in the guild, which in turn was required for practicing medicine.

William of Saliceto

William of Saliceto (Guglielmo da Saliceto, c. 1210–c. 1280) had an illustrious career as a physician who studied and taught medicine at Bologna and later was made town physician of Verona. His fame rested mostly with his *Surgery*. Perhaps it was his experience in what we would call first aid that led him to say that there were circumstances in which a physician ought to act either to prevent conception or to produce an abortion. The information that he gave is not that unusual except that he was one of the first western physicians to borrow values derived from the Arabs. The content of his antifertility measures was mostly derived from Avicenna's *Canon*. As a physician it was normal for a writer virtually to avoid the subject, as did Platearius, or, to be more circumspect, to avoid comment and merely to list the remedies.

In his work *Summa conservationis et curationis*, William began a chapter entitled "Those Things That Prohibit Conception and [Cause] Abortion." He wrote, "Although this chapter may not be according to the strict rules of law [*de mandato legis*], nevertheless [it is necessary] for the ordinary course of medical science on account of the danger that comes to a woman because of a dangerous risk of conceiving on account of her health, debilities, or the extremity of her youth." [1] The regimens and remedies that follow were mostly from Avicenna, although he condensed Avicenna and added contraceptives; for instance, he said that dried savin juniper and *scolopendrum* (a fern) prevent conception. [2] If the period after coitus had been ten days, then she should be given three drachmas of rue seeds and savin or juniper. For abortion, other recipes followed with savin, cypress, pennyroyal, and other familiar ingredients. [3] A new word, however, is encountered: *mentastri,* which means any species of wild mint, thus helping us with the problem in the Hippocratic treatises as to what the exact species might have been. He was saying simply that it does not matter. For the fumigants, William specifically said that they were inhaled, not vaginally exposed as per the Hippocratic corpus. Finally, William's account differed from the classical counterpart inasmuch as his recipes almost all specified amounts (what we call dosage). Medieval medicine was building and improving upon classical medical knowledge and not slavishly copying, as has been supposed.

Arnald of Villanova

Arnald of Villanova (c. 1240–1311) is one of the best examples of the New Learning after the assimilation had time to mature.[4] Arnald wrote and practiced medicine in Montpellier at the medical center, which was part of the *studium generale*. At Montpellier the New Learning came both from Italy and from Spain, especially Toledo. Arnald was celebrated in his day and in frequent contact with the papacy. He was physician to two popes, but he was in and out of trouble with the Holy See, not because of his medical teachings, but because of his theological writings.

Arnald included birth control information in his works. For example, in the treatise *On Compound Medicines,* or *Antidotarium,* a recipe for caper and artemisia was given to provoke the menses, although not explicitly for abortion.[5] Arnald was concerned in his medical knowledge with sexuality because he gave recipes to increase sexual activity and to enhance conception.[6]

The work *Breviarium practice* was attributed to Arnald, but the legitimacy of Arnald's authorship has been questioned. Whether or not the work was by Arnald, the point is that during the Middle Ages and Renaissance, it was thought to have been by him, and this ascription gave added authority to its contents. The work was made part of the *Articella,* the series of works that were required reading in the medical curriculum in universities. Although not all versions of the *Articella* include this pseudo-Arnaldian work, it was included in some medical curricula. This inclusion is important because it has specific information about birth control. In those schools where it was taught, medical students learned about the prescriptions for contraception and abortions. But the point is that this is an exception to what appears a trend: namely, in most medical curricula birth control was not a part of the learning.

Breviarium practice's first section (book 3, chapter 5) discussed the extraction of a "dead fetus" and "making an abortion [*ad faciendum abor-sum*]." As suppositories, drinks, and fumigants, the treatise's author discussed castoreum, sweet flag, thyme, opopanax, galbanum, rue, scammony, blackberry, birthwort, pepper, and betony, among others. Specific quantities were given in some recipes (e.g., a prescription with "three drachmas of dried rue leaves" [approx. ½ oz]).[7]

The next chapter has a startling statement. The chapter's title is, "Things so that a woman may not conceive in order that she might be seen marriageable."[8] Heretofore, seldom have we had a hint as to the motives for taking contraceptives (with exceptions being something like Hildegard of Bingen's menstrual regulators when there was pain). The penitential literature, such as Pseudo-Bede, contrasted the poor women who had too many children to feed vis-à-vis the wanton lass whose pregnancy was a product of sin. Here, however, the author was giving information for women so they could be sexually active before marriage without consequences!

The advice the author gave was practical, but he produced another surprise: many of the recipes were more what we would call magical (e.g., involving amulets). Many, however, were the familiar drug remedies. One fumigant "so that a woman might not conceive" was the burning of a mule's hoof over hot coals. Another appears derived from Dioscorides, but it has a change: willow leaves were drunk or put in a drink with a mule's hoof (*ungula*), not the kidney. Some other recipes were grain, juniper seed, and ivy; the fern filix in a drink; elephant dung in a suppository; and frankincense, gum arabic, myrrh, and alum in a suppository.[9] He concluded his antifertility section with much the same practical advice on menstrual provokers, with one recipe containing rue.[10]

Peter of Spain

It is more of a surprise to us in the late twentieth century than it was to people who lived in the thirteenth century that a medical writer who gave birth control advice to the poor became a pope. Peter of Spain wrote an immensely popular book called *Thesaurus pauperum* (Treasure of the Poor), popular enough that, among its multilingual translations, three are in Hebrew. Born in Lisbon between 1210 and 1220, Peter was the son of a physician. His career took him to study in Compostela and Paris, later becoming the bishop in Siena and, in 1276, pope, taking the name John XXI. Thus, when Peter began his advice to the poor about birth control and started with remedies to diminish sexual desire, probably only people today would find it surprising. The first advisory was to put a plaster of hemlock on the testicles before every coitus.[11] Explicitly, then, the remedy was not to prevent intercourse but (implicitly) to reduce consequences. Among the remedies was to drink the juice of *nymphea* (probably, *Numphaea alba* L.) for forty days, with Macer cited as the authority. Herbs prescribed were pepper, rue, chaste plant, calamint, and costus.[12]

There is a large chapter on plants to provoke menstruation, where Peter quoted from Gilbert the Englishman (fl. 1250), Macer, and Dioscorides. Before relating information, however, from the authorities, he chose to give his own list: cinnamon, cardamom, sweet flag, pennyroyal, mint, sage, and *satiureia* (*Thymus capitatus* Hoffm Link?).[13] Finally, there is a chapter on abortion (*De abortu*), but the information that Peter gave was on how to prevent one, not to produce one.

The Paradox of the Late Middle Ages

Peter of Spain's reluctance to be explicit and yet, at the same time, to relate information about birth control reflects the paradox of the late Middle Ages. The knowledge of birth control devices, at least from the viewpoint of the written record, was never greater; in contrast, the Roman church took an increasingly militant stance against almost all sexual activity (except for procreative purposes within the marriage covenant) and against birth control of any sort, including contraceptives. Another example of this paradox is seen in the works of Albertus Magnus, a philosopher, natural scientist, theologian, and teacher (Thomas Aquinas was his pupil). In Albertus' theological writings, he condemned birth control. In his natural philosophy works, he related practical birth control information.[14] To us moderns, the contradiction is troublesome, but medieval theology did not draw the same conclusions as we do about when life began. According to Pamela M. Huby, who has studied Albertus on when life begins, he did not argue that the embryo possessed a soul (his position was in accordance with Aristotle's stages), but he "uses forms of words that show that life is already present and some sort of external and indeed heavenly power is at work right from the beginning."[15] Although there is probably no direct connection, Albertus' position on the potential for life is similar to classical Stoic thought.

A paradox similar to that of Albertus is found in the works by Maimonides (1135–1204), Jewish physician and theologian, who practiced medicine in Cairo, far from the cloisters of Albertus' world. In his work on Jewish law, he condemned the destruction of the seed as a means of avoiding potential conception, and yet in a regimen of health that he wrote for his monarch, he gave this advice: "Contraceptives [to be used] before intercourse. The things that prevent conception are (1) from the man's side anointing [the penis] with juice of onion, wood tar, or gall bladder of chicken, and (2) from the woman's side inserting suppositories with juice of peppermint, or pennyroyal, or the seeds of leek after purity."[16]

One might argue that Maimonides gave a stricter accountability to his brother and sister Jews than he did to his sovereign, because he was giving advice to a Muslim, not a Jew. This interpretation is unlikely because of the fact that in his *Treatise on Cohabitation,* intended, we suppose, for all people, he gave practical, mostly dietary, advice on how to avoid procreation. He listed the drugs that have the capacity to "dry the sperm and weaken coitus," namely, the seeds and juice from rue, cumin, black cumin (*Nigella sativum* L.), pepper, and cabbage. The foods that he said to avoid if one wanted a child (or to take if one wanted no child) were lentils, galban (*Lathyrus sativus* L.) and "cooling vegetables" such as worm-wood, spinach, cucumbers and melons of various sorts, and, especially, lettuce.[17]

In his *Code* of religious laws, Maimonides raised the question about whether it was justifiable to sacrifice a fetus whose birth threatened the life of the mother. He answered according to traditional Mishnah inter-pretation that one cannot sacrifice one life for another in this case because the fetus has not yet received life. In cases such as these, it is permissible to remove the fetus "either by drugs or by surgery." [18]

Thus, in principal, Maimonides was morally against contraception and abortion, but he saw circumstances where either or both were preferable to alternative choices. We cannot be certain whether this was the distinc-tion that Albertus made in a different religious code in a different culture. With this interpretation supplied, however, the positions of Maimonides in Jewish culture and Albertus in Christian were similar to that of Theo-dorus Priscianus in pagan culture. Theodorus had cited Hippocrates as saying that abortion was wrong morally but, this admonition not with-standing, there were circumstances when the physician was obliged mor-ally to perform one.

Late Medieval Law on Contraception and Abortion

The penetration of the church's stance into secular law is seen in two provisions in English law promulgated by Edward I (1271–1307).

> He who oppresses a pregnant woman, or gives to her a poison, or delivers to her a blow [strong enough] so as to cause an abortion, or who gives to her [something] that she will not conceive, if the fetus is formed and animated [*foetus erat jam formatus et animatus*], is guilty of homicide . . . Item: A woman commits homicide who so devastates an animated child through a drink [*potationem*] or similar things in the stomach.[19]

Here the law has come closer to accepting the church's position. In an-cient and early medieval law, the law protected the father from those who interfered with his children and the mother from malpractice. Here the very act of abortion (as defined after the fetus his "quickened," or been "ensouled") *or contraception* is murder whether administered by another party or the woman herself. Curiously, however, in Edward's law as stated, an early stage abortion (using the term "abortion" in its modern meaning) is implicitly not murder, only contraception and late term abor-tions being so regarded. Finally, there is the recognition of what we sus-pected in interrupting the ancient sources, namely, that when a contra-ceptive or abortifacient is envisioned, it is chemical and orally taken unless otherwise stated.

At the time when the church was extending its influence into the marriage bed, another movement pressed in the opposite direction: namely, the troubadours and minnesingers. The romance literature was spawned by the Crusades and often stood in sarcastic opposition to the piety of the church and the hypocrisy of secular life. These songs often applauded sexual wantonness, especially if "love" was present. This movement came at the very time when the message of the church was taking hold in everyday life of the western European. These literary ideas reflect at least the segment of the medieval community who sang its songs and told its tales of Lancelot and Guinevere, Tristan and Isolde, Aucassin and Nicolette, among others. Such stories expressed contempt for chastity and approval for premarital and extramarital sexual intercourse, whatever the means. To what extent the values represent a significant portion of society is conjectural. The philosophy of the troubadours and love poets may have been confined to a small elite, or it may have represented a countermovement against what some of the people saw as having too high standards for human behavior.

Danielle Jacquart and Claude Thomasset attach importance to a late medieval debate about the existence of a female seed (*semen*). Aristotle was certain that women supplied nourishment to a man's seed and that is all.[20] Some of the Hippocratic writers and Galen challenged Aristotle on this point by saying that females contribute a seed to make the fetus, but it is the weaker seed.[21] The contradiction among the leading authorities stayed, until the late Middle Ages reopened the question. The ensuing debate was important, according to Jacquart and Thomasset, because of its significance to women's equality.

A dialogue called *Placides et Timéo*, in French toward the end of the thirteenth century, deals with a popular-science approach to "secrets of the philosophers." The mysteries of conception and birth are discussed. Aristotle does not stand; the child is formed by seeds from the father and the mother.[22] Medieval writers came to accept the Hippocratic-Galenic position that the embryo was a mixture of two seeds, male and female, although most of them continued to hold that the female was colder, therefore inferior. Little attention was paid to the female's emission of seed (meaning fluid at sexual climax), whereas medical writers, whatever their persuasion (and almost all being male), emphasized the reception of the male seed. Vaginal secretion was confused and combined with ovulation and cervical secretion, with neither the Aristotelian nor the Galenic models supplying congruence between theory and experience to rationalists such as Albertus Magnus. Jacquart and Thomasset see the late Middle Ages as bringing together theoretical constructs of physiology with empirical observations to explain both physical and mental states. In the art of love, troubadours were inspired to portray intercourse to please the woman. A worthy man need not have a release with each coitus.[23]

Galen's and Avicenna's elevated placement of female sensuality did not penetrate the popular culture, which saw the female as the passive recipient of male sperm. Even so, the changed theoretical position of sexual physiology, when combined with the literary movement of the troubadours and the notion of chivalry, placed women in a different position. If the movement was toward equal partners in the sexual acts, the question becomes: did women receive more acknowledgment of rights to control pregnancy?

The culture did not move in the direction of more reproductive rights for women, however, even though it changed women's status. With certainty we know that the knowledge of contraceptives and early stage abortifacients was available continuously in the West. First, works such as by Dioscorides, Pliny, Oribasius, and Marcellus were available and were in Latin. By the eleventh century the Arabic and Greek material was being translated into Latin. New herbals in the West, such as Hildegard's *Liber de simplicis medicinae* and Matthaeus Platearius' *Circa instans,* referred to abortifacients and, much more often, emmenagogues. If anything, however, the society moved more toward a pronatal position.

The church's position was expressed by Thomas Aquinas. Fornication, whether mutually agreed on or not, violates "right reason." Nature has given humans and animals a means by which reproduction can occur. Sexual liaison is, by nature's law, for procreative purposes. If one departs from inseminating sexual intercourse by "unnatural acts," both animal nature and the love of God are violated.[24] For a good Christian, there is the necessity of a conscious procreative purpose for all sexual intercourse. The Thomistic position explained why earlier canonists could condemn both agents that impeded procreation and those that enhanced it: each was unnatural and therefore wrong. Even so, Thomas accepted the Aristotelian-Albertean position that the fetus was first an animal before it was a person, and thus that it develops in stages. His position, while differing in some details from Albertus', concerned the theological inquiry of the development of the soul; as such, he was not involved with the ethics of abortion per se.[25] Whatever may have been his intended purpose, however, his writings served as a basis for the justification by the church against both contraception and abortion.

For almost every societal trend during the Middle Ages, another one pulled in another direction. The crystallization of church doctrine during the thirteenth and fourteenth centuries was countered but not checked by the mystical Hermetic philosophy. Hundreds of treatises existed that contained practical information (in German, *Fachliteratur*), and many of those works were ascribed to the god Hermes and connected with ancient

Egyptian lore. Possessing hardly a particle of Christian ethics, the Hermetic works seemingly did not challenge church doctrines directly. The works simply revealed secrets. According to the underlying and sometimes explicit ethic, every herb, stone, and star had a purpose—a secret, as it were, embedded within it. These secrets were discoverable to virtuous people, and by their nature, the knowledge of the secrets could be useful to people. We need only learn the God-given secrets of nature for our benefit because God made the universe for people. In this sense, God made the herbs that cause contraception and abortion as well as the herbs that could increase the opportunity to conceive. When the secrets are discovered, God's will is fulfilled in that the divine order of the universe was unfolding.

James A. Brundage observed that in the late twelfth and early thirteenth century there was more attention in the documents to marital contraception. The usage of contraception to avoid children was grounds to nullify a marriage. Inasmuch as neither the canonists nor the moral writers specified the contraception employed, Brundage is of the opinion that coitus interruptus was "presumably the most effective technique available in this period." [26] The evidence found by David Herlihy about married Italian women who had but few children could be explained by coitus interruptus or, for that matter, by infanticide.[27] There is little evidence for either, however, as I discussed in Chapter 1. Inasmuch as the women were of a high social class, infanticide appears extremely unlikely, as does coitus interuptus (*amplexus reservatus*), because, among other reasons, it requires a high degree of male cooperation.

Anecdotal evidence is found throughout the medieval period for the use of birth control drugs, as we have seen. For instance, Procopius (sixth century, Constantinople) spoke of the secrets of prostitutes that Theodora employed to prevent conception.[28] A question used to teach medical students posed this query: "Why, when prostitutes have more frequent intercourse, do they rarely conceive?" [29] The formula answer was scholastic in tone and devoid of scientific details. The answer pointed to no specific agents, but at least the practice was acknowledged and, more important, the specifics were implicitly not to be a part of medical training—at least at the early level of university medical education. The church's position quite clearly had an effect on what was taught.

CHAPTER FOURTEEN

The Renaissance

"Je possède une certaine herbe. Si l'homme la porte quand il mêt son corps à celui de la femme, il ne peut engendrer; ni, elle concevoir," said Pierre.

"Et de quelle espèce est cette herbe?" replied Béatrice.

Inquisition at the Pyrenees village of Montaillou

And to sum it up in a phrase, he said that she had an ass that savored of mint and wild thyme.

A captain describing a visit to a woman's bed, in Aretino's *Dialogues* (1971, p. 85)

Eek whan man destourbeth concepcion of a child, and maketh a womman outher bareyne by drinkinge venemouse herbes, thurgh which she may nat conceyve, or sleeth a child by drinkes wilfully, . . . yet is it homicyde.

Chaucer, *Persones Tale*, 575–580

W hen the shepherd Pierre Clergue persuaded Béatrice, a village girl, to have an affair with him in the early-fourteenth-century village of Montaillou, he gave her an herb the day before the seduction that he said would prevent her conceiving. This much she told the Inquisition.[1] The Inquisition's account was preserved because its inquisitor later became pope, and therefore the trial's documents were part of his papers. Le Roy Ladurie, who studied these papers, thought maybe the herb was given as an amulet.[2] Perhaps it was, but more than likely the future papal inquisitor was not sensitive to the details because such knowledge was beyond his ken. Probably the herb was meant to be taken orally. Whatever the herb was—and we could make a fairly educated guess from among five or six indigenous plants—and however she used it, this evidence of the well-nigh silent subculture shows that contraceptives were used in the late Middle Ages and the early Renaissance. If they had been totally ineffective, would so many people—ranging from high ecclesiastical and medical authorities down to Pierre and Béatrice—have been so wrong? If the unspecified herb had not worked, would Béatrice not have told her daughter to beware of shepherd boys with herbs?

Whatever can be written about the hailed placebo effect does not apply to birth control measures. Full-term pregnancy simply cannot be psychosomatic. If a person takes a drug and has potentially fertile intercourse, he or she cannot know whether it worked if pregnancy is not an outcome. If she becomes pregnant, on the other hand, she knows that it did not work. Scientific studies aside, a reasoned argument for the effectiveness of the contraceptives and early stage abortifacients in this study is their persistent presence in the records. If they were not effective, would people have had confidence in them generation after generation, from the time of the earliest Egyptian medical records? Would the historical data have shown such vitality and variability in the medical works, such as judged by the discovery of new agents and the fact that most writers wrote innovatively about the experiences with drugs? If, in contrast, the agents were merely placebos at best, magic at worst, would not the documents have been stylized, inelastic, and static, with one writer copying from the other (as did some times happen, more often in works on magic)? If we are correct about the usage of birth control agents being sufficiently effective and widespread as to give people some control over reproduction, how then do we explain the apparent near loss of this information in the modern period?

Commentators and Doctors

Had it been left without religious and moral restrictions, the Renaissance should have been a great period for increased knowledge and awareness of birth control agents. First and foremost, there were the humanists, whose zest for classical lore led them further and further back to the Greek and Latin classics with such fervor that they produced the Renaissance. Hippocrates, Galen, and Dioscorides were studied with such enthusiasm that the humanists wanted to know the exact words of the original text, just the right nuance, and in the case of plant drugs, they wanted to be sure that they were identifying the same plant that the original authors described. Texts, long lost in the West, such as those by Soranus and Theophrastus, were recovered and explored. The Arabic writers, most especially Avicenna, were culled for all their valuable learning. Even Pliny received close scrutiny for all his information that might be useful. Formal gardens were founded in Padua, Pisa, Florence, and Naples, where a new profession was founded: custodian of botanical gardens. With impressive energy and great expense, expeditions were outfitted to track down plant species and bring them back to the gardens so that their medicinal usages, lost during the misnamed "dark ages," could be regained. A new verb entered the vocabulary of European tongues: "botanize," meaning to explore for plants. The purpose was not the plants qua plants but plants qua medicines. The result was the divergence and ultimately separation of two fields: botany and pharmacy.

The second factor that should have stimulated birth control information was the discovery of the New World and the suddenly enlarged number of plant species that could have contributed new agents, especially with information from the American Indians. Antonio Brassavola (1500–1555) attacked the authority of Dioscorides by saying that the Greek herbalist could not have known one plant in a hundred of those on the earth. Nicolaus Monardes (1493–1588) said that Dioscorides could not possibly have known the New World plants.[3]

A third factor was the secularization of the northern Italian urban states. The city-states were areas of contention between papal and imperial authority, but mostly they were independent of either. Many of the larger cities—Venice, Florence, Pisa—had their own universities that were not controlled by the local bishop, who otherwise would have insisted on some degree of doctrinal compliance. The issues of the day, religious and political, swirled around and through these relatively free universities.

Finally, the university culture emphasized the rational forms of human behavior and decried the mystical, magical, and superstitious. While historians question the success of the Renaissance's ideal in reviving Plato's clarion call for the preeminence of the intellect, its rhetoric pressed for the rational over the superstitious. These factors (humanism, New World discoveries, secularization, and emphasis on the rational) should have produced an atmosphere that would have reinforced the ancients' attitude toward birth control: if one wanted it, one need only know how to do it. Permission to practice it was not a critical issue.

Hermolaus Barbarus

"I was born for science; to science I have devoted myself," wrote Hermolaus Barbarus, one of Venice's leading figures of the fifteenth century. Born of a renowned family, Hermolaus received the best of educations and was devoted to the study of what he called science, what we now call letters. Hermolaus' love of words was perhaps equaled only by his love of plants. His career took a nearly disastrous turn when he accepted a papal appointment to be patriarch of Aquileia, and appointment that his fellow Venetians did not accept lightly. First, Hermolaus studied Pliny and wrote a celebrated two-volume work called *Castigationes Plinianae* (The errors of Pliny; first ed., Rome, 1493), in which he corrected not so much Pliny as what medieval scribes and editors had done to his text. Fresh from this study, Hermolaus undertook a translation of Dioscorides in the early 1480s. In a letter, he described how he ended his day: after supper, "close to eleven P.M., I go down into the garden or into my neighborhood; in either place, we contemplate the herbs there and we think about Dioscorides (which no doubt we will publish soon [or sometime (*aliquando*)]. In this I use half an hour. Then I go to bed."[4]

Hermolaus translated Dioscorides and demonstrated considerable care in getting the right meanings for the plant descriptions, but he was not as diligent on the medical usages, especially those involving birth control. For instance, he said that the leaves of the willow tree "per se vero ex aqua conceptionem potu adimunt" (remove conception as a drink by themselves with water).[5] The action of the chaste tree, he translated, as "ciunt et menses poti" (as a drink it excites the menstrua) and "semen potum cum pulegio et suffitum et appositum feminas purgat" (its seed as a drink with pennyroyal both fastened and applied purges the menses).[6] The translation is very poor. Dioscorides' Greek said that the chaste tree "destroys generation"; in other words, it is a contraceptive, an intent Hermolaus did not grasp.[7]

Hermolaus composed a small commentary called the *Corallari,* which accompanied his translation. For the most part his attention was directed toward identifying the plants. Most of Dioscorides' contraceptives and abortifacients were not the subject of his comments (e.g., he passed over rue, birthwort, and pennyroyal). On the fern *asplenon,* however, Hermolaus added some information: women take the plant to become sterile. Possibly he learned this from local folklore.[8] In one place, he truly added to Dioscorides. The leaves of round and long ivy, he said, cause sterility, but its fruit does not, whereas Dioscorides had said only that the berries had the action.[9] A curious selection of words in his translation of the chapter on the squirting cucumber betrayed his gender and background: he wrote, "Abortum gravidis facit" (it causes an abortion in pregnant women).[10] Hermolaus Barbarus' knowledge was that of a philologist, not a medical person. As a churchman, his knowledge of women's matters appears slight. As learned as he was, his knowledge did not extend deeply into the substance of birth control. It was not that he feared to relate the information (clearly he did not); it is just that he knew little.

The Translators

Other translations of Greek into Latin during the Renaissance showed that, generally, the translators knew their languages well enough but, in some instances, they were not very familiar with the medicine, especially in female matters. A Latin translator of Hippocrates' *Diseases of Women* clearly was bothered by the passages on birth control, as he noted in his commentary. The translator and commentator was Maurice de l'Corde (Maurius Cordaeus, fl. 1570s), who was a strong Protestant physician in Paris, where he studied. The term for contraceptive, ἀτόκιος, he properly translated into the Latin as something that hinders conception (*conceptio*), but he did not translate or seek to translate *misy*, the copper compound.[11] Where the Greek text read ἐκβόλιον ὑστέρων ("uterine abortifacient"), de l'Corde translated it "eliicit secundas medicamentum" (the medicine ejects the afterbirth), which is hardly a translation at all.[12] For ἔμβρυον ἀπόπληκτον ("embryo destroyer"), he was closer to the point with "embryonem perculsum" (embryo knocker).[13]

Jean Ruel (1474–1537) was one of the best of the humanistic translators because, in translating Dioscorides, he brought to bear three talents: classical studies, medicine, and botany. His translation was published in Paris in 1516, just after the posthumous translation by Hermolaus Barbarus, but Ruel was unacquainted with Hermolaus' work. For the willow tree, Ruel's translation was: "Sumpta per se [i.e., perforated leaves], et cum aqua praestant mulieribus, ne concipiant" (Taken by itself or with water, they are responsible for women not conceiving).[14] Thus Dioscorides' curious word ἀσυλλημψία became *ne concipiant*.[15] His choice of words was different in his translation of white poplar: "Sterilitatem inducere tradunt si cum mulino rene bibatur" (They relate that they [poplar barks] cause sterility if drunk with a mule's kidney).[16] Thus, Dioscorides' precise word, ἀτόκιος (contraceptive), becomes *sterilitas* (sterility). Ruel kept Dioscorides' critical words, "It is reported that . . . ," which was his way of not embracing folklore that he had not tested. Ruel was literally correct when he translated the passage on the fern *asplenon:* "Conceptum adimere creditur, per sese, aut cum muli liene appensa" (It is believed to take away conception either by itself or hung with a mule's spleen).[17] On abortion, Ruel did not avoid the correct terms. For savin (juniper), he translated: "Foetum etiam viventem interficit, et mortuum eijcit" (It also kills a living fetus and ejects a dead one).[18] On cabbage, however, his translation was crude: "Flos post conceptionem in pesso subditus, partum abortu vitiat" (The flowers placed in a suppository after conception spoils a birth by abortion).[19] Dioscorides' text said that cabbage was a postcoital contraceptive (ἀτόκιος).[20]

The translations into the vernacular of Peter of Spain's *Treasury of Health* were more definitive than Ruel's translations. The Italian translation published in 1518 included the section on menstrual regulators ("A provocare lo tempo delle donne") but completely omitted the chapter on contraceptives.[21] In contrast, the English translation, published about 1560, was more literal, as these selections demonstrate. "Against great desyre to fleshly lust . . . Hemlockes bounde to a mans stones, take utterly awaye all desyre of copulation . . . All men and inespecially Dioscorides sayth that Peper, Rue, Tutsayne, Calamint, Castoreum, wast the sede of generacyon (by dryuynge it up) of there propertie and strong heate . . . If a man eate the flowers of a sallowe or wyllowe tre, or of a Popler tree, thy wyl make cold al the heate of carnall lust in him." [22]

In another way the humanist translators contributed their talents to medicine and science: they interpreted the works, especially those originally written in Arabic. For example, in the beautiful Juntine edition of Avicenna, Andrea da Belluno (Bellevensis) supplied a glossary of terms that Gerard of Cremona could not translate for lack of knowing the Latin equivalent of the Arabic. Gerard merely transliterated the Arabic for willow into the Latin as *algarab;* Andrea added that this was *salix,* or "willow." [23] In the recipe for contraception, Avicenna said to take three pints of *badruj.* Not knowing what this was, Gerard simply transliterated the word as *albedarungi.* Andrea said that it was a species of *ozimus* (basil).[24] Without the scholarship supplied by Andrea da Belluno, it is unlikely that many Western physicians used Avicenna's text to prescribe or compound the drugs, simply because their knowledge of Arabic would have been either nonexistent or far less extensive than Gerard's vocabulary.

The humanists' genius during the Renaissance is revealed in their commentaries. Believing that the classical texts incorporated both wisdom and useful information as well as aesthetically stimulating experiences, scholars during the Renaissance sought to explain and to explicate the texts. Many of the commentators were knowledgeable about medicine in addition to their philological pursuits. Perhaps the greatest (in terms of contemporary recognition and success) was Petrus Andreas Matthiolus. While serving as town physician in Gorizia, he wrote a commentary in Italian on Dioscorides that was published in 1544.[25] Perhaps owing to the obscurity of his publisher, the edition did not receive much circulation. It was enough, however, for a Florentine publisher in 1547 and another edition in Venice in 1548, this one by the Valgrisi firm. Matthiolus' fame was made. He revised and expanded his work and wrote in Latin for a wider audience. Over the years, he brought out revisions that were printed in eleven editions in Latin. There were later two German translations of his commentary (with printings of the first translation in 1562 and of the second in 1590, 1598, 1600, 1626, and 1678), two French (printings of the first in 1561, 1566, 1576, 1579, 1605, and 1680; of the second, in 1572), and one Czech (1562, 1596).[26] His reputation spread throughout Europe, but for most of his years, he remained a practicing physician in Venice.

One would believe, then, that Matthiolus, as the acknowledged leading scholar on Dioscorides, himself a physician, and living in secular Venice, would have been expansive in relating birth control information. While there was no hint that he felt restricted in any way, he knew little about such information, or if he did, he did not give it away.

Women's matters were definitely not his specialization, although, given his extraordinary ego, he would doubtless take issue with this statement. In his lifetime, he seldom owned up to error, almost never to doubt. In his commentary on rue, Matthiolus wrote: "It moves the urine. This in this sense, it extinguishes birth and flatulence [*partium faltusque extinguit*]."[27] Similarly, he said that ligusticum roots and seeds "have warming faculties, thus they stimulate the menses, provoke urine, and cut off flatulence [*ex calefacientium sunt, adeò ut menses cieant, et urinas provocent, flatusque discutiant*]."[28] Whether this was a way of referring to abortion is unclear from his words. Generally, his commentary neglected birth control information altogether, and where he mentioned it, the contents repeated Dioscorides without adding knowledge. Given his own and his time period's prejudice for the rational and against the superstitions of the Middle Ages, one would think that he would have corrected the text in certain places, as where Dioscorides said that the white poplar taken with a mule's kidney caused contraception. In his commentary, however, Matthiolus devoted his energy to discussing trees, and of this matter, he said only that it causes "sterility, [that is] not bearing fruit [*sterilis haec, nec fructum ferens*]."[29] Similarly, when Dioscorides related the folklore about the fern asplenon being used as an amulet with a mule's spleen to prevent conception, Matthiolus repeated the information without challenge, but he did attempt to identify the fern. He said that physicians and pharmacists (*pharmacopoles*) both consider asplenum the same as scolopendrium, but the common people called it *cetrach* (a fern).[30]

It was not that Matthiolus would not write the words for "abortion" or "contraception"—he would. It was just that he seemed to have little to add to what Dioscorides had already said. This reluctance did not extend to most matters, because Matthiolus was typically verbose. On the squirting cucumber he wrote, "Elaterium is the most harsh of all medicines, and it is one of the best because it is the oldest." He told how a "certain physician, a quite arrogant man," had made much money on it. Among its medical virtues, he said, it provokes the menses and "kills the fetus."[31] Matthiolus had the opportunity to show his erudition while commenting on the chaste tree. Writing on Ruel's translation that the products of the chaste tree are drunk with pennyroyal, Matthiolus recounted the ancient festival of Thesmophoria where the women put branches beneath their beds. He made the connection between the ritual and the effect of the drug, but he did not understand that it is a contraceptive rather than an abortifacient.[32]

Amatus Lusitanus

Born in Portugal of Jewish parents who had escaped the 1492 persecutions in Spain but were forced to be baptized in Portugal, Amatus went to Salamanca to study medicine. After practicing medicine, probably in Lisbon, he was forced to flee by a threatening Inquisition. He immigrated to Antwerp, established a good reputation, and began writing notes on Dioscorides in connection with his medical practice. He moved to Ferrara in 1540 and developed a friendship with a circle of physicians and humanists interested in plants. He negotiated for a position as city physician at Ragusa (Dubrovnik) and, anticipating the successful completion of a contract, resigned his position at Ferrara. What he did not know was that his newly published commentary on Dioscorides had angered Matthiolus in Venice.

In a letter addressed to a friend, Matthiolus wrote on July 13, 1553, "Soon your Lordship will see an Apologetic Epistle in print at the end of Latin Dioscorides addressed to a certain Amato Lusitano, a Marrano physician, for whom it was not enough to have stolen the entire commentary from my work but who has also had the effrontery to write against me in more than twenty places in his wretched commentary on Dioscorides." [33] Living hand to mouth, Amatus could not bring Ragusa's city council to make a decision. At the end of his 1558 Latin edition of Dioscorides, Matthiolus wrote a vitriolic attack on Amatus' work, entitling it *Apologia Adversus Amathum Lusitanum cum Censura in eiusdem Enarrationes*.[34] In 1559 Amatus wrote to his Venetian publisher: "Since there is a law in Venice that nothing can be printed without license of the Church, I do not know whether anything may have been added or deleted. I believe that the clergy has completely destroyed my defense written against [the attack of] Matthiolus; for everyone must know that I would promptly answer this Apologia." [35] Persecuted in Italy, his home ransacked, and unable to publish his reply to Matthiolus, Amatus eventually migrated to Salonika, where a community of Jews had fled the Hispanic persecutions. His life was a tragedy, but his commentary on Dioscorides was, from a medical viewpoint, superior to Matthiolus'.

If he did not know about a drug or could not add to Dioscorides' account, Amatus was content not to comment. For many of the plant drugs, he gave no antifertility usages (e.g., for iris, myrrh, cyperus, poplar, willow, pomegranate, myrtle, pepper, birthwort, liquorice, aloe, sage, dittany, mint, and artemisia). The omissions meant that he could not add to Dioscorides' account. Savin (juniper), he said, "kills a living fetus and expels a dead one." [36] Common juniper did the same thing in the same manner, but also its seed, if administered at the time of coitus, worked the same way, provided it was modestly applied.[37] While Amatus gave no explicit antifertility usages for the chaste tree other than what Dioscorides had already said, he developed a very interesting and detailed discussion of the similarities and contrasts between the qualities of rue and the chaste tree.[38] Ivy, he said, is drunk to cause sterility (which we know means contraception).[39] Pennyroyal "moves the menses" (*menses movet*): there is no mention of a fetus, but thyme "stimulates the menses and plucks out the fetus [*menses provocat, foetum evellit*]."[40] In contrast, calamint (*nepeta*), he said, "kills the *conceptus* and evicts it."[41] Because Amatus was so careful with his words, he obviously intended to distinguish here between a late stage abortifacient (which involves a *fetus*) and an early stage one (involving a *conceptus*).

Silphium is found only in Libya, Amatus said. He quoted Hippocrates, who described the unsuccessful attempts to transplant it in Greece and Syria. Then he related what was suspected as happening during late antiquity and the early Middle Ages (see Chapter 2), namely, that what was once called *silphium* was called by Amatus' time asafetida.[42] Ligusticum and Queen Anne's lace were menstrual stimulators, he said, without explicitly mentioning abortion, but the squirting cucumber was both an emmenagogue and an abortifacient.[43]

Amatus' scholarship was vigorous in trying to identify the plants. The reader may recall that the only male oral contraceptive encountered in this study was the *periclumen* plant in Dioscorides, which was difficult to identify. There is no doubt, however, about the plant that Amatus thought it was; he thought it to be our honeysuckle. As he often did, he began the chapter with the names of the plant in the various languages that he knew: "Graece περικλυμενον: Latine, periclymenos, volucrum maius, mater sylva, vinciboscum; Hispanice, madre sylva; Italice, matri selva; Gallice, cheuvrefueille; Germanice, geyszblatt, speek oder valdgilgen et zeunling."[44] With this much to go on, our identification is certain: *Lonicera periclymenum* L., or honeysuckle. Our certainty, however, is confined to Amatus and the sixteenth century, for he does not necessarily tell us what Dioscorides' plant was. Amatus possessed information, however, about honeysuckle's properties not found in Dioscorides. He said that its seed induces sterility if drunk in large quantities.[45] What he did not say or comment on was Dioscorides' statement that it was for males. Another commentator on the same text, Marcellus Vergilius (1464–1521) in Florence, however, gave a full account of honeysuckle. Marcellus said that if honeysuckle seeds (amount unspecified) were drunk by a male for thirty days with white wine, he would be sterile.[46]

In his commentary on Hippocrates' *Diseases of Women*, Maurice de l'Corde (Maurius Cordaeus) mostly correctly translated the Greek text on contraceptives and abortifacients, but his Protestant religious values caused him difficulty in his commentary to the text. De l'Corde noted that a contraceptive is different from an abortifacient by stating that the Hippocratic oath had specified abortive suppositories but did not proscribe contraceptives. A contraceptive must be superior to that which terminates pregnancy, and de l'Corde noted that Dioscorides as well as Hippocrates named a number of agents that caused abortions. He said, though, that he did not wish to comment on contraceptives because of an uncertainty as to what was being described. He made no attempt to identify *misy*, the copper compound, although his knowledge of Greek almost certainly would have made its identification in Latin known to him.[47] When the Hippocratic text discussed abortifacients, de l'Corde said that there were good uses for these agents, such as to give relief from menstrual retention; however, he was aware of a limited number of other uses. In fact, he used the term *oxytocia* for abortifacient, a meaning unmistakably clear. A physician (*medicus*) should imitate nature, he said, but he ought to do that which does good (*sed eius etiam minister affectus bene, hoc est benevolus*).[48]

The World and Europe

Knowledge of antifertility measures in Europe increased with the new plants found during the sixteenth-century expansion. A very effective interceptive agent was zoapatle 1 from *Montanoa tomentosa* Cerv. A Spanish monk, Fray Bernardino de Sahagún (1529–90), described it as an antifertility plant. The plant was included in a Latin herbal in 1552 called *Libellus de medicinalibus indorum herbis*.[49] Similarly, Europeans learned the use of Peruvian bark, or Jesuit bark (what we call quinine), as an abortifacient, as a physician writing in Virginia in 1734 described it.[50] Garcia d'Orta (c. 1550–c. 1568) was a Portugese physician who lived in Goa and wrote extensively about the plants that he found in India. He reported on *bletre* (*Bletia* sp.), an eastern herb, that women eat it before having commerce with men.[51]

Mayan recipes were recorded mostly by Jesuit priests, who doubtless because of who they were, did not record antifertility agents as such. From these records, however, there are a number of recipes to provoke menstruation. One recipe is for a plant called *ah-chicam-kuch,* which is not further identifiable. Another recipe is familiar: take rue leaves and roots, boil them until the liquid boils away, put the concentrate in wine, wrap it in cotton-wool and apply into the vagina.[52]

No doubt many other new agents were introduced to the European pharmacopoeia as it became worldwide, or perhaps it is better to say, as the Europeans became better informed about the nature of drugs around the world. Mediterranean and European drugs had always been shared across continents, at least across Europe, Asia, and Africa. For instance, the new drug camphor, discovered and manufactured by the Chinese sometime before the ninth century, reached Europe and became part of its regular drug repertoire by the tenth century, long before the first Arabic-to-Latin translations of medical-pharmacy works.[53]

This study has a conspicuous omission: Chinese and İndian medical uses of antifertility agents. The great study of Chinese science headed by Joseph Needham has yet to publish its findings on medicine. There are indications that the Chinese and Indian medical writers knew of many agents we have already described.[54] In a preliminary study, Joseph Needham reported that the Chinese medical authorities had discovered the use of androgens and estrogens to treat sexual disorders as early as the eleventh century.[55] Placental tissue, a source of estrogens, was employed for amenorrhea, which we know could be for an early abortion as well.

Artemisia was a traditional emmenagogue (abortifacient) in the Philippine Islands, according to a report in 1901.[56] Rue was not native to southeastern Asia but came to the area from the Mediterranean area, but by the early part of the twentieth century, rue was planted in "almost every garden" in Bombay.[57] In Indian medicine rue was given both as a contraceptive and an abortifacient.[58]

Khou Tsung-Shih (fl. 1110–1119), author of *Pen Tshao Yen I* ("The Meaning of Pharmacopoeia Elucidated"), discussed mercury drugs but warned pregnant women not to take them because they caused sterility.[59] Norman Himes's history of contraception catalogued few references in Chinese medicine and concluded that since Chinese culture always stressed large families, they appeared to want to know little about agents to limit conception and birth.[60] Himes's generalization appears unmerited because, no matter what a culture's emphases may be, there will always be circumstances where there are human and medical needs to regulate reproduction. Among the reasons, there is the one observed explicitly by Avicenna; namely, the problem of pregnancy in an extremely young girl when her skeletal development has not matured for natural childbirth. An account of Chinese medicine, written by a Presbyterian missionary at the beginning of the twentieth century, contains no explicit mention of contraception or abortifacients. He was naive enough, however, to include information about emmenagogues, such as cyperus.[61] Like this missionary, who did not know what he was disclosing, the information about the Chinese use of birth control agents is likely in the sources and awaits only modern scholarly attention.

Summary: The Broken Trail of Learning

The surprise about the Renaissance sources is that they knew so little about birth control compared to classical and medieval authorities. The influence of the church and secular law must have been a factor, but how much is questionable because, as we have seen in the earlier period, the information had a continuity from culture to culture, cutting across periods when religion and societal values placed great stress on bearing and raising children. Chaucer's likening abortion to homicide in the Parson's Tale is an indication that the church's teachings had some effect.[62]

Increasingly during the fourteenth and fifteenth centuries medical writings were in the vernacular. A late medieval herbal in English gives this recipe as an abortifacient: "Take the rotes of *madir* whil it is grene." A German herbal of the same period for the same purpose reads, "Nim vnitige rocholter ber, daz sint die grinen ber."[63] Unlike these explicit abortifacients, a fifteenth-century English leechbook indicates a more veiled way by which knowledge of contraceptives and abortifacients was transmitted in written documents. It contains a number of recipes "for that sickness which is in the womb or in the body, that ever shall be helped with any medicine." The recipes contain many of the familiar herbs such as this one: "Take rue [*ruw*] and sage [*sawge*] and drink it with water."[64]

Premodern parents probably had a good grasp about the food supply and how far it could be extended. The data show that some form of fertility regulation appeared to anticipate bad times. They had a vital need to control family size. Reasonably, such persons, pagan or Christian, living in the first or the fourteenth century, would have a number of options and may have used them seriatim. As clearly explained and viciously denounced by Augustine, "they even procure poisons of sterility [*sterilitatis venena*], and, if these do not work, extinguish and destroy the fetus in some way in the womb, preferring that their offspring die before it lives, or if it was already alive in the womb to kill it before it was born."[65] The first step was timing within the menstrual cycle, tricky at best. The medical theorists, at least, were wrong, believing that the most fertile period was when menstruation was ending and immediately thereafter.[66] A woman could take her herbs—willow, rue, birthwort, or whatever was available locally that she knew—according to instructions from her mother, her adviser, or, less likely, her physician.

Many of the antifertility plants fall into the category of pot herbs, the mints (e.g., pennyroyal, dittany, and sage) and rue, and were served in salads or placed on meat. The woman's salad may have been her control over her own life and her family's life, while the men and nonchildbearing women ate from the same bowl and saw it as simply a nourishing, tasty meal course. If the salad was prepared correctly and eaten in the correct amounts, a woman would likely avoid pregnancy. Rural people in India cook the roots of *Echinops echinatus* as part of their diet but put there to control fertility. And control fertility it does, according to a 1988 laboratory study that found that the plant had "very significant anti-estrogenic activity." [67] The table use of this root in India parallels how Gargilius Martialis had said that women eat rue with their meals and do not have children. [68]

As best we know, the degree of efficacy was dependent on the right herbs, harvested at the right time, prepared the right way, and taken in the right amounts and, importantly, at the proper time. One needs to know whether to use the root, sap from stem, flowers, seeds, fruit, or other morphological sites for extraction. Sometimes heating such as in a tea destroys or reduces the active ingredients, and sometimes it does not. In the case of toxins, a reduction in efficacy is desired. Even the time of day can be important: herbs are best harvested in the mornings (or so say herbalists). Extraction methods are very important details. Some drugs are soluble in water and are effective only if extracted with water. Others are effective only if extracted by alcohol. Even soil conditions and the climate in which a plant was raised can affect drug potency. Such details are not in the documents of the period except as generalized rules. [69] Normally the information is not precisely given in other medical prescription literature.

By and large, a person learned the information as orally transmitted lore, just as one would learn recipes for cooking. The cookbooks of the Middle Ages related vague instructions, such as "take cloves, ginger, pepper, cinnamon, sugar, [and] vinegar." [70] The only practical way for the information to be learned was through experimentation. Aretino, a sixteenth-century Italian author, placed in the mouth of a courtesan a statement about fertility measures: "I experimented with as many herbs as would fill two meadows." [71]

Just to be sure, in case the woman was determined, as well as knowledgeable, she might prepare a vaginal suppository prior to bed. If the oral herbal contraceptive and/or the suppository did not work and a woman missed her monthly period, she would take an herb or herbs that provoked menstruation and, with it, an aborted fetus—though she would not have known for certain. Even more certainly, her husband and her priest would be unknowing.

The question we face is, Why were the Renaissance writers seemingly less informed about birth control agents than were their classical and medieval predecessors? I know no single answer but propose a possible explanation that is multifaceted. By the twelfth century, medical training moved from the apprenticeship method to the universities. By the fourteenth century, to practice medicine one had to be a university graduate in most of the towns and cities of Europe because of the controls by guilds. The university curriculum was geared toward medical theory and less so toward the clinic. Increasingly the compounding and dispensing of drugs fell out of the realm of the physicians' offices and into the domain of the pharmacists' guilds. From the beginning the university was mostly for males and became even more gender biased by the late Middle Ages. An important fact, however, is that many of the plants were common and could be gathered near the home or from the garden. Even the knowledge and cooperation of the pharmacists was not critical.

Gynecology fell more and more to midwives, who received no formal training from the university. The physicians had their place only when female medical problems called for drastic or nonroutine action. By the fifteenth and sixteenth centuries, few physicians knew about birth control agents, simply because it was not part of their training in becoming doctors, nor was there a ready means to learn about them during regular practice. The chain of learning broke, and the chain of folk knowledge nearly broke. Heretofore, physicians such as the Hippocratic writers, Dioscorides, Galen, and al-Razi learned about the agents from the practices of people who knew what and how much to take. Physicians of the Renaissance, however (such as Matthiolus), distrusted folk medicine and had no occupational or professional means to acquire the knowledge.

How much of a factor the pronatal policies of societies and the opposition to birth control by the Christian church were is difficult to determine, but they must have had some effect. The knowledge about the plants, as we have seen, is not as simple as a blanket directive to take this or that plant for contraception or abortion. One had to learn the proper amount, the time within the menstrual cycle, the relation to coitus (before or after), the means of application (suppository or oral), the frequency, and many other details for each agent. One mother failing to tell her daughters about what she had learned would be enough to break a chain that was, in many cases, thousands of years old. In addition, some women and men surely took seriously the pronouncements of the church and did not resort to chemical means to regulate fertility.

A desire for large families was perhaps another factor in breaking the efficiency of orally transmitted lore. Also, one wonders if the psychological impact that virulent syphilis had on sexual practices might have also retarded the transmission of information about birth control agents. During the sixteenth century, it was not just a matter involving sexual activity and reproduction. The possibility of contracting syphilis meant that there was no safe way to have sex. Some daughters may not have been told about the drugs to take to avoid pregnancy for fear that this assurance could lead to sexual activity and potentially fatal consequences.

As explored in this chapter, the evidence indicates that the Renaissance writers knew less about birth control than did their medieval, Islamic, and classical forerunners. The chain of learning was breaking but in fact survived into the modern period, when finally, in this century, the rediscoveries of modern science confirmed the insights of the earliest recorded medical writers.

CHAPTER FIFTEEN

Later Developments

Some there are who hold conception to be a curse, because God laid it upon Eve for tasting of the forbidden fruit, I will greatly multiple thy conception.

Mrs. Jane Sharp, *The Midwives Book* (1671)

T ried in the Winchester Assize in 1871, *The Queen v. Wallis* was an important case in the annals of jurisprudence. Since 1803, England had a criminal abortion law, known as Lord Ellenborough's Act.[1] Prior to 1803, common law restricted abortion only after quickening, or perceived fetal movement. In all the court cases tried on this statute, there had not been a case like this one. Mr. Wallis was accused of "administering or causing to be administered" to a woman, pregnant by him, a "noxious substance." Testimony at the trial quickly established what the noxious substance was: an infusion of pennyroyal and a quantity of Griffith's Mixture, a drug compound readily available in the stores. The defense did not contest this, nor did they challenge the fact presented by the queen's prosecution that the woman, then in her sixth month of pregnancy, aborted and "recovered without any bad symptom."[2] Testimony established that she took no other drugs during this period and that no violence or "mechanical" injury had occurred on her body. She was, however, in the habit of horseback riding on a regular basis up to the time of the abortion. Readily she agreed that she took two doses of Griffith's Mixture, which the court learned consisted of iron and myrrh. Witnesses for the queen's prosecution contended that although not labeled as such, the ingredients in Griffith's Mixture were "clearly abortive in their character" and that the amount taken of pennyroyal tea was "sufficient to procure abortion."

At this point in the proceedings the queen's prosecution and defense contested the evidence. Medical expert after expert was called by both sides, but neither could establish whether pennyroyal and Griffith's Mixture could cause an abortion. The defense's experts denied that pennyroyal was a "noxious substance." Three witnesses—Hicks, Tyler Smith, and Barnes—particularly impressed the court. They said that Griffith's Mixture was just as good, "chalybeate" tonic, although it was often given to nonpregnant women as an emmenagogue. The woman testified that she had asked Mr. Wallis to purchase Griffith's Mixture for her. She had not made or taken the pennyroyal tea, however, as she claimed she still had the dried leaves. Defense witnesses said that there were no instances in medical history of the ingredients in Griffith's Mixture having "any effect on the uterus." The queen's prosecution contended that both the mixture and pennyroyal, which it believed was taken, were indeed "noxious remedies."

The court became confused. Most witnesses agreed that both substances could be considered emmenagogues and, in the case of pennyroyal, probably was "used for the purpose by ignorant women, but it had no effect in producing an abortion." The court attempted to find experts who could define the difference between an emmenagogue and an abortifacient. Some witnesses said that any agent that provoked menstruation was thereby ecbolic, or abortive; others said that they were different. Unable to get medical experts to agree on whether the substances caused an abortion or whether an emmenagogue was the same as an abortifacient, the court ruled that the abortion was caused by the daily horseback rides.[3]

The Queen v. Wallis was an important case in English and American jurisprudence because it demonstrated the difficulty in making legal distinctions about menstrual regulators and abortives. The case as presented in the law books reveals an important historical shift of opinion. In the 1865 account in *Taylor's Principles and Practices of Medical Jurisprudence,* pennyroyal is accepted as an abortifacient. Taylor observed that an infusion of pennyroyal "is more powerful than the decoction since the poison, being a volatile oil, is dissipated by long boiling."[4] By the 1905 edition of the same work, however, Frederick J. Smith, its new editor, said that while pennyroyal may have been popularly viewed as an emmenagogue and abortifacient, it is, "we believe, never used at the present day by medical men. It has neither emmenagogue nor ecbolic properties."[5] In Smith's view, it was all superstition.

In the 1970s, when James C. Mohr was researching a book on abortion in nineteenth-century America, he encountered in his documents references to women who had taken abortifacient drugs. Baffled about the discrepancy between the historical documents and modern medical authorities, he asked colleagues at the Johns Hopkins Medical Center about the possible efficacy of the abortifacient drugs. He was told that the psychological pressure on some women who took these agents was probably sufficient to induce abortion but that the drugs themselves could not have been effective. Mohr concluded, "The nineteenth century had no preparations capable of directly producing abortions, though contemporary physicians and the public believed otherwise."[6] Mohr's book remains the best study of the subject, but on this point he was misled by modern medical specialists. In the case of Mohr, then, a historian was led to disbelieve his documents.

Early Modern Knowledge of Birth Control Drugs

In the seventeenth and eighteenth centuries, the knowledge of contraceptives and abortifacients continued to decline.[7] Francis Mauriceau (1637–1709), the greatest authority for the period on gynecology and obstetrics, condemned abortion and would not write about contraception. He even failed to list those foods and drugs that a woman should avoid in order to prevent a miscarriage.[8] Herbalists, in contrast, continued to relate information about antifertility, albeit at a significantly reduced level. The *Compleat Herbal* of 1787 said of rue, "There is little use made of it now."[9] In actual practice, however, its usage did not disappear altogether.

Great herbalists, such as Jacobus Theodorus (d. 1590) in Germany, John Gerard (1545–1612) in England, and Joseph Piton De Tournefort (1656–1708) in France, mentioned antifertility plants not as a means for birth control but as warnings about unwanted consequences.[10] De Tournefort told of meeting an "old doctoress in Salamanca in Spain" who used the root of the death carrot to produce abortions, but it was done "in great hazard of their lives."[11] As director of the botanical gardens in Paris, De Tournefort traveled internationally, searching for plants, but his writings reveal little knowledge about birth control. A decoction of horehound (*stachys*), he said, brings on menstruation and causes an abortion—"in women," he added.[12]

While the amount of information in popular herbal literature declined, it never disappeared altogether. The 1886 *Dictionary of Plant-names* said that savin (juniper) derived its name from its "being able to save a young woman from shame."[13] Folk experimentation even continued in finding new substances. An eighteenth-century guide gave information on a new menstrual regulator, Peruvian bark, claiming that "we know none preferable."[14] In 1671, Jane Sharp's *Midwives Book* specified things to avoid for women who wanted to conceive or for women who, once pregnant, wanted to carry their child. One should not drink the wine from Holland known as *stum* because it prevents conception, and one should not eat *eringo* (*Eryngium alpinum* L.) because it causes an abortion.[15] This is the first mention of this plant, whose reported abortifacient activity is confirmed in modern scientific studies.[16]

There is every reason to believe that even in this century new agents continue to be found. A 1939 French guide to natural product remedies listed as emmenagogues artemisia, wormwood, parsley, rue, savin (juniper), saffron, and—mentioned for the first time—groundsel (*Senecio vulgaris* L.).[17] Groundsel shares the same abortifacient qualities as other members of the same plant family (Compositae), such as artemisia and wormwood.[18] The past is present today, faintly, as the same plants are used today for the same antifertility purposes.[19]

Innovative antifertility means continued to be related in both medical and popular literature. Some physicians, such as Joseph Brevitt, who wrote a book in 1810 advising "female practitioners and intelligent mothers," felt that abortion was wrong.[20] He refused even to mention contraceptives or abortifacients, although he did give a number of emmenagogues: asafetida, black hellebore, bitter apple (colocynth), savin (juniper), cantharides (Spanish fly), and—a new item to the list—electricity.[21]

Two recent studies on birth control, one on early modern England, the other on Germany, report numerous instances where women were taking the same plants as their medieval counterparts: aloes, asafetida, myrrh, rue, ginger, sage, myrtle, hellebore, nutmeg, common juniper, savin, laurel, pennyroyal, pepper, wormwood, thyme, tansy, willow, "fern," mint, and dittany.[22] Medicine, however, increasingly excluded antifertility drugs from its realm. An article in a medical journal in 1760 illustrates this point. A physician reported on a woman who had a dead fetus but could not abort it. He said that he found in the works of Aëtius of Amida a statement that a fern (*fougère* = *filix* = *Aspidium filix mas*) was effective in such cases. Trying it, the patient aborted and regained her health.[23] The very fact that his experience was considered sufficiently new to medical practice as to merit a journal article reveals how far medicine in the eighteenth century was removed from classical learning on the pharmacy of birth control agents.

In the nineteenth century, the criminalization of abortion added another reason for forgetting this information. The Ellenborough Act of 1803 made abortion illegal, declaring that it was a crime for anyone to "unlawfully administer to, or cause to be administered to or taken by any of his Majesty's subjects any deadly poison, or other noxious and destructive substance or thing, with intent [for] . . . his Majesty's subject or subjects thereby to murder, or thereby to cause and procure the miscarriage of any woman, then being quick with child."[24] Note here that the

expected means of abortion were chemical. In the courses of the nineteenth century, however, the definition of the earliest time of abortion
changes from quickening, as in this 1803 law, to conception.

Criminalization of abortion drove medicine to keep a greater distance
from birth control. In 1852 in the region of Cornwall, Dr. Pascoe was
prosecuted for administering oil of savin to a woman who aborted. Even
though she told the doctor that she had disease of the heart and liver, the
court found Pascoe guilty because he should have conducted an examination to determine pregnancy.[25]

Among 1,000 patients examined in a late nineteenth-century clinic in a
large London hospital, 183 women had amenorrhea, of whom 156 were
pregnant.[26] These statistics demonstrate the extent of the problem and
suggest the difficulties that medical practitioners faced. In 1847 Dr.
Whitehead observed that the examination of potentially pregnant women
who might want a menstrual regulator and (while he did not say it) an
abortion was "one of the most delicate positions in which either a patient
or practitioner can be placed." Dr. Whitehead's opinion was, "however
culpable his patient may be, to shield her fame, as far as is practicable." [27]

Because of such a situation as the Pascoe case, physicians risked reputation, license, and personal freedom when they gave abortifacients
knowingly or unknowingly. While some physicians, like Whitehead, continued the centuries-old practice, others were unwilling to take risks as a
matter of conscience, expediency, or knowledge. Dr. Burns, an English
physician in 1808 after criminalization of abortion, said, "Many people
at least pretend to view attempts to excite abortion as different from murder, upon the principle that the embryo is not possessed of life, *in the
common acceptation of the world*." [28] Traditional views, however, were
eroding. Forty years after Burns's statement, Dr. Charles D. Meigs wrote,
"The stupidest thing a physician can do is to be misled by such com-
plaints to the administering of drugs and medicines, which may bring on,
not the menses, but an abortion, or a premature labor." [29]

In 1869 Pope Pius IX declared the new church position on ensoulment,
namely, that it occurs at conception. Any termination of pregnancy from
that moment was considered abortion. Angus McLaren believes that the
medical communities in Western countries did not oppose Pius IX's bull
largely because defining ensoulment at conception relieved the physician
of the legal and moral responsibility of determining when quickening
happened. By and large, in keeping with Aristotle's position on the formation of the fetus, quickening was a determination in a woman's realm,
not a physician's.[30]

Whatever their legal responsibility, physicians in the nineteenth century knew less and less about antifertility drugs, as we saw, for instance,
in the case of *The Queen v. Wallis,* when medical experts could not decide

whether an emmenagogue was the same as an abortifacient or whether the drugs were effective. Dr. Whitehead doubted that the emmenagogues that some women took actually worked for menstrual stimulators or for abortion, except when "some powerful predisposing cause was already prevailing." [31] Drug contraceptives, especially oral ones, virtually disappeared from medical literature.

Legislators assaulted the use of birth control drugs. In many jurisdictions of the United States laws prohibited the dispensing, advising, or publication of any information about, in the words of a Colorado law, "recipes or prescriptions for drops, pills, tinctures, or other compounds, designed to prevent inceptions, or tending to produce miscarriage or abortion." [32] The important point is that whenever the means were identified in the laws, they specified chemical means. The state of Iowa was much more specific; a 1924 law specified the drugs: "No person shall sell, offer or expose for sale, deliver, give away, or have in his possession with intent to sell, except upon the original written prescription of a licensed physician, dentist, or veterinarian any cotton root, ergot, oil of tansy, oil of savin [juniper], or derivatives of any said drug." [33] Louisiana's law against contraception and abortion was more vague, proscribing "sale or advertisement of . . . any secret drug or nostrum purporting to be exclusively for the use of females or for preventing conception or for procuring abortion or miscarriage." [34] The law's authors must have been cognizant of the use of menstrual regulators, because it forbade the sale or advertisement of any drug "for the use of females."

Whereas the written works lead one to believe that physicians knew little about birth control drugs in the late nineteenth and early twentieth centuries, legislators and lawyers must have known better about them, otherwise the laws cited above would not have appeared. A famous case in England in 1898 involved a suit against the proprietors of Allen's Mixture, which advertised: "Important to Ladies—Especially to those who require ABSOLUTE CERTAIN and speedy remedy; a remedy to which in thousands of cases has never failed to afford COMPLETE RELIEF." [35] Writing in the *Times* about the advertisement, Justice Darling said that the court found that the intent was to convey the information that "the medicine would procure miscarriage or abortion," something the law clearly had forbidden. [36]

Summary

We have seen indications in all periods that folk experimentation led to the discovery of new drugs to contracept and to abort, while some of the drugs, which were judged less effective or available and more dangerous, were dropped from use. Folk experimentation and observation took place in ways resembling what Theophrastus related about the wild carrot's fertility effects on cattle. In the same way, modern science's recognition of plant hormones came from animal science.[37] Bernard de Gordon (c. 1258–1320) said that in testing drugs, one should first try them out on birds, then on mammals, next in hospitals, then on Franciscans, and finally on people.[38] Aretino, a sixteenth-century Italian author, placed in the mouth of a courtesan a statement about fertility measures: "I experimented with as many herbs as would fill two meadows."[39] People observed the effect that plants had on animals and on themselves and learned what to take to prevent or end pregnancy at the same time that they learned how to avoid unwanted terminations.

Right up to the twentieth century, women have affirmed their right to take menstrual regulators, even when it aborted pregnancy, up until the fetus moved or quickened.[40] If pregnancy continued, there were stronger, late stage abortifacients and manipulations or surgical procedures, which were dangerous and risky. Before and after coitus, there were regimens of exercise, bath, and diet, the details of which fill many a parchment leaf in medical and gynecological works.[41] There was advice on what to do in order to conceive, what not to do, and what to eat and what not to eat. Following a lengthy discourse on regimens and diet to prevent miscarriage, Soranus said that if one wanted to abort, one should simply do the reverse of what he said to prevent miscarriages.[42] Folk wisdom was rich in such details.

Were contraceptives and early stage abortifacients a significant part of birth control? If they were not, how can we explain the indications of planned parenthood in fifteenth-century Florence or the low fertility of first-century Romans or fifth-century Constantinople? A number of anthropological-historical studies from Nigeria,[43] China,[44] Korea,[45] the Soviet Union,[46] Haiti,[47] New Mexico,[48] Egypt,[49] Malaysia,[50] and India[51] reveal that traditional societies are employing various antifertility agents. If modern populations can regulate their fertility by plant drugs, surely so could premodern societies, because there is strong evidence that similar methods and agents were being used then.

In the late nineteenth century, the birth control movement had begun, and new devices for contraception were making their way into working-class bedrooms (and even more pervasively, it would appear statistically, into those of the upper class).[52] These devices included the modern diaphragm, spermicidal jellies, and the latex rubber condom.

The extent to which natural-product drugs are responsible for population limitation and family birth control is unquestionably declining and, in much of modern industrial society, probably well-nigh extinct. There are a few exceptions reported, such as three women in Colorado in 1978 who took pennyroyal oil for abortion after reading about it, one of whom died.[53] One can find earlier cases as well, such as the death of Mary H., age nineteen, who in 1877 took one ounce of oil of cedar and died twenty-six hours later in Boston City Hospital.[54] The fatalities involving Mary H. and the Colorado woman were not caused by their learning directly about the folklore of abortifacients. In both cases they took concentrated oil instead of a weaker tea, which indicates that the folklore reports that they received were inefficiently transmitted.

Tommy Bass is a contemporary Appalachian herbalist whose knowledge of herbs is probably about the level that many once had during the Middle Ages. Bass was reluctant to learn about "women's medicine." He would not recommend emmenagogues. He said of one reputed emmenagogue/abortifacient, "People shouldn't know about it." [55] Bass's reluctance to disclose women's matters comes at the end of a long period where people become increasingly reluctant to discuss birth control.

The trend began prior to Christianity. It was slow, but the direction was toward restricting artificial birth control information. Although women may have acted throughout all periods to some degree as if prevention and early termination of pregnancy were within their rights, there were steady encroachments on women's authority in this area. Roman and German law gave limited rights to a head of household to have children. Christian church doctrine, canon law, and eventually the laws of states came to restrict women's claims that they should regulate reproduction. By the nineteenth century, because of a combination of religious, moral, and economic factors, many countries were protecting the fetus. Modern medicine excluded drug controls for conception and pregnancy from its province and eventually relegated the folklore regarding such control to small, mostly nonindustrial population groups. Physicians, in part because of a mistaken notion of what the Hippocratic Oath said, were no longer expected to have such knowledge. The evidence is abundant, however, that the ancients had knowledge of chemical means to control birth. It is intriguing to ponder why so few now know what so many once did.

However, the history of the nineteenth and twentieth centuries is written, however the vexing questions regarding rights, morals, and birth control are worked out by ours and future generations, the historian can understand the distant past better when the historical population data are understood as the product of millions of people making deliberate, calculated, and largely rational decisions about when to have and not to have children. Because of the various modern medical and animal sciences, biochemistry, pharmacy, and anthropology, we have reason to believe our historical documents in the matter that premodern peoples could limit family size. Surely the Greeks, Romans, and medieval peoples practiced some infanticide and more sexual restraint. There is no need to believe, however, that the scale of these practices was sufficient to produce the demographic profile that existed. What they did—which we know because they told us—was to take drugs and to be as careful as possible.

ANF	*Ante-Nicene Fathers: Translation of the Writings of the Fathers Down to A.D. 325.* Alexander Roberts and James Donaldson, eds. 10 vols. Grand Rapids, Mich.: Eerdmans, 1950–.
CCSL	*Corpus Christianorum: Series Latina.* Turnhout: Brepols, 1958–.
CHED	*Complete Hebrew-English Dictionary.* 3 vols. Tel Aviv: Massadah Publ., 1986.
CSEL	*Corpus Scriptorum Ecclesiasticorum Latinorum.* Joseph Zyche, ed. Vienna and Prague: Tempsky, 1887–.
DGRBM	*Dictionary of Greek and Roman Biography and Mythology.* 3 vols. Boston: Little, Brown, 1859.
DUSA	*Dispensatory of the United States of America.* 25th ed. Arthur Osol et al., eds. Philadelphia: Lippincott, 1955.
FC	*Fathers of the Church.* Washington, D.C.: Catholic University of America Press, 1947–.
FE	*Flora Europaea.* 5 vols. Cambridge: Cambridge University Press, 1864–1980.
IH	*Index Hippocraticus.* 4 vols. Josef-Hans Kühn and Ulrich Fleischer, eds. Göttingen: Vanderhock & Ruprecht, 1986.
IK	*Index Kewensis Plantarum Phanerogamarum.* Supplement 9 [Supplement 13 (1956–1960)].
LS	Liddell and Scott, *Greek-English Lexicon.* 9th ed. Compiled by Henry George Liddell, Robert Scott, Henry Stuart Jones, and Roderick McKenzie. Oxford: Clarendon Press, 1968.
MM	*De Materia Medica.* Dioscorides. Max Wellmann, ed. 3 vols. Berlin: Weidmann, 1958.
OCD	*Oxford Classical Dictionary.* Oxford: Clarendon Press, 1961.
OLD	*Oxford Latin Dictionary.* P. G. W. Clare, ed. Oxford: Clarendon Press, 1982.

PG   *Patrologiae Cursus Completus . . . Series Graeca.* J. P. Migne,
              ed. 161 vols. Paris, 1857–1866.
PL   *Patrologiae Cursus Completus . . . Series Latina.* J. P. Migne,
              ed. 221 vols. Paris, 1879–1890.
Pharmacopeia *Pharmacopeia of the United States of America.* 18th rev. ed.
              Bethesda, Md.: U.S. Government Printing Office, 1970.
Statutes   *Statutes of the Realm. Annon regni quadragesimo tertio
              Georgii III.* London: H.M. Stationery Office, 1950.
Taber   *Taber's Cyclopedic Medical Dictionary.* 6th ed. Philadelphia:
              F. A. Davis, 1954.
TLG   *Thesaurus Linguae Graecae.* Lucille Berkowitz, ed. Rev. ed.
              New York: Oxford University Press, 1986.
TLL   *Thesaurus Linguae Latinae.* Leipzig: Teubner, 1956.

1. Population and Sex

1. Polgar 1972, pp. 203–211; see also Hollingsworth 1969, esp. pp. 375–388, and bibliography.

2. The Augustan legislation to increase fertility in 18 B.C. (*Lex Julia de maritandis ordinibus*) and A.D. 9 (*Lex Papia Poppaea*) was followed by the Alimentary Laws, which are discussed in Chapter 2. Russell (1985, pp. 161–176) speaks of the first millennium A.D. as a period of "population stability."

3. Russell 1985, pp. 111–138, 169–172; in an earlier work, Russell (1948, pp. 92–117) published statistics showing that the complete recovery from the Black Death (beginning in 1347) occurred only between 1475 and 1556, but in part this long delay is attributable to recurrences of the plague; see also Hollingsworth 1969, pp. 375–388. Thrupp (1965, pp. 101–109) notes that in England the plague of 1361 "looks almost worse" than the first plague (p. 109). On the plagues during the sixth and seventh centuries, see Russell 1976, pp. 64–78.

4. Notably Pirenne 1937 and 1946.

5. A good discussion of fluctuations in early modern Europe with comparative data from Asia is in Braudel 1979, pp. 31–103.

6. Herlihy 1974, p. 37.

7. Two recent studies are Foucault 1984 and Brown 1982. See also Cameron 1986, pp. 266–271.

8. Brown 1988; Jacquart and Thomasset 1985; and Bullough and Brundage 1982.

9. Rouche 1987, p. 535; Nardi (1971) sees progressively changing attitude in Roman society against abortion and infanticide.

10. Pomeroy 1988, 3:1311; Shaw 1987, pp. 30–46; Hopkins 1964–65, pp. 309–327.

11. Gies and Gies 1987, pp. 33, 183–184, 207–208, 233, 283; Hanawalt 1986, pp. 95–100.

12. Herlihy 1985, pp. 144, 146–149; 1965, pp. 236–237; 1969, p. 1350; 1970, p. 96, where Herlihy quotes Bernardine of Siena as attributing a low fertility to late marriages for men, reluctance of some to marry at all, and contraception practices with marriage; 1972, pp. 1–24; 1973, p. 111, where an examination of records for Verona showed that poorer households had fewer children than did wealthier households.

13. For example, Hopkins 1965–66, pp. 143–150; Veyne 1987, p. 13.

14. Noonan 1986, p. 95, citing Epiphanius, *Panarion* ("Medicine Chest"), 63.1.4. The passage can also be found in *PG*, 41:1063.

15. References to *Yebamoth* ("Sisters-in-Law") 34b, in *The Babylonian Talmud,* (Epstein ed.), *Seder Nashim,* 1:215–216; *Niddah* ("The Menstruant") 13a, in *Seder Tohorroth* (p. 89); cited and discussed in Noonan 1986, pp. 10–11, 50; Preuss 1978, pp. 458–459; Himes 1936, pp. 70–71.

16. Flandrin 1985, p. 117, and Biller 1982, p. 19.

17. Ladurie 1973, p. 328; also strongly accepting the position is Ariès (1948, pp. 496–497).

18. Scarborough 1969, p. 209n.

19. Himes 1936, pp. 100, 186–206.

20. It is generally assumed that the first mention of a contraceptive technique in Greek comes from Herodotus (*Histories,* 1.61.1), who describes Peisistratus as not wanting children and therefore having wrongful sexual intercourse with his wife.

21. Ariès 1953, p. 467; on ancient sexual practices, see Foucault 1984.

22. Jacquart and Thomasset 1985, pp. 124–125.

23. Soranus, *Gynaecology,* 1.62 (Temkin trans., pp. 34–35; Burguière et al., ed., pp. 60–61); Noonan (1986, pp. 16 and 120) notes that the only form of birth control that Augustine specifically prohibited is intercourse during the sterile period. Augustine's position came in part because he reacted against the Manicheans, who employed this method but who regarded the optimum sterile period as "after the purification of the menses when a woman is likely to conceive" (*Morals of the Manichees,* 18.65 [*PL,* 32:1373]; cited in Noonan 1986, p. 120). On the notion that the most fertile period was near the end of the menstrual cycle, see Dean-Jones 1989, pp. 188–190.

24. Hopkins 1965–66, p. 135; see Himes 1936, esp. p. 100.

25. Gourevitch 1984, pp. 198–199.

26. Fontanille 1977; Keller (1988) contends that some of the agents were effective in producing abortions; Nardi (1971) lists ancient literary texts. On Nardi, see the extensive review by Dickison (1973, pp. 159–166); a broader perspective is Devereaux 1976.

27. Soranus, *Gynaecology,* 1.60–61 (Temkin trans.). On surgical instruments, see Moïssidés 1922, pp. 59–85; Jackson 1988, pp. 105–109; Milne 1907, pp. 81–82; for the details of an abortion to remove a dead fetus, see Celsus, *De medicina,* 7.29 (Spencer ed., 3:454). See also Waszink 1950, 1:55–60, and Waszink's earlier commentary on an edition of Quintus Septimus Tertulianus's *De anima* (1947, esp. pp. 15*–20*, 423–428, and passim). The

Hippocratic work *De mulierum affectibus,* 1.91.1–28 (Littré ed., 8:218–220), lists the treatments as postabortion (l. 25) but states that it is after the expulsion of a dead fetus. The ancients used interchangeable terms for the abortion of a dead or deformed fetus and for induced abortion of an otherwise healthy fetus.

28. The first translation is from Edelstein 1967, p. 6; the second is in the Chadwick and Mann translation (p. 67); the third is in the Jones translation (1:299). Nardi (1971, p. 60) supports Jones's reading: "similmente non darò ad una donna un pessario abortivo."

29. I base this conclusion on two statements by Jones (1924, p. 49) who, when he summarizes medical etiquette for physicians, says that the doctor "ought not . . . to cause abortion." In the preface to his translation of the oath (1:295–296), Jones observes that the author of *Nature of the Child,* by listing abortion means, "unblushingly violates the spirit, if not the letter of the Oath." By inference, Jones (like Littré) believed that the spirit of the oath prohibited all abortions, not merely those administered by suppositories.

30. Scribonius, *Compositiones,* Praef. 5.20–23 (Sconocchia ed., p. 2); my translation. See also Pellegrino and Pellegrino 1988, pp. 22–38.

31. Ibid., 5.23–24.

32. Oxyrhynchus Papyrus, 2547; Lichtenthaeler 1984, p. 150. Discussion of this section of the oath is on pp. 143–152.

33. Jones 1924, p. 31.

34. *Khalq al-insan,* translated and quoted by Musallam (1983, p. 70). It is not clear from the context whether the author is referring to the Hippocratic oath or to the Hippocratic treatise *The Nature of the Child;* in either case, the Arabic author thought Hippocrates advocated abortion.

35. Jones 1924, pp. 35, 37. The former reads, "Neque praegnanti mulieri ad interficiendum conceptum fetum potionem porrecturum."

36. Theodorus Priscianus, *Euporiston,* 3.6 (Rose ed., p. 240): "Abortivum dare nulli umquam fas est. Ut enim Hippocratis attestatur oratio, tam duri reatus conscientia medicorum innocens officium non decet maculari. Sed quoniam aut matricis vitio aut aetatis impossibilitate, sub qua causa praepropere frequenter partus evenit, feminae periclitantur, expedit praegnantibus in vitae discrimine constitutis sub unius partus saepe iactura salutem mercari certissimam."

37. Tertullian, *A Treatise on the Soul,* 25 (Holmes trans., *ANF,* 3:206).

38. Soranus, *Gynaecology,* 1.60 (Ilberg ed.; Temkin trans., p. 63).

39. Ibid.; Hippocratic corpus, *De natura pueri,* 7.490 (Littré ed.; and Joly ed., 11:55).

40. Soranus, *Gynaecology,* 1.65.

41. Ibid., 1.64.

42. See n. 27 above.

43. Dixon 1988, p. 94.

44. Hammurabi, *Laws,* 209–214 (Pritchard ed., p. 162). In addition, Hammurabi's laws gave a woman the right, if she had just cause as determined by the city council, to refuse to have sexual relations with her husband (law 142).

The next law (143) adds, "If she was not careful, but was a gadabout, thus neglecting her house [and] humuliating her husband, they shall throw that women into the water."

45. *Babylonian Laws* (Driver and Miles ed., 1:313).

46. United Nations 1953, p. 75.

47. The important principle in ancient codes is that a physician, layperson, or "magician" who administered a poison, enchantment, spell, or other form of treatment could be held liable if harm occurred to the mother. These laws, clearly stated in Roman legislation by the second century A.D., can be seen as protecting adult life, not that of the fetus. See *Digest,* 48.19.39; 48.8.8.; 47.11.4; 48.19.38.5. On the subject of law, the fetus, and the newborn, see Noonan 1986, pp. 26–28 and passim; Dickison 1973, p. 161; Nardi 1971, pp. 354–367, 413–479.

48. A biological explanation for the male-to-female ratio is presented in Bullough and Campbell 1980, pp. 317–325. Evans (1980, pp. 112–120) denies that any factor favors males over females.

49. Engels 1980; in answer to Harris, see Engels 1984, pp. 386–393.

50. Harris 1982, pp. 114–116.

51. Golden 1981, pp. 316–331.

52. Pomeroy 1975, pp. 46, 69–70, 127, 140, 227–228; 1985, p. 25; Feen 1983, pp. 283–300; Oldenziel 1987, pp. 87–107.

53. Pomeroy 1984, p. 111; the document gives a widow the right to abandon a child born after the death of her husband, such permission being granted by her mother-in-law. I assume that the papyrus document to which Pomeroy refers in her earlier study (1975, p. 127) belongs to another period. (See papyrus references in the following note.)

54. Oxyrhynchus Papyri, 744 (Lewis and Reinhold 1955; 2:404); another papyrus (Berlin No. 1210, approx. A.D. 150) speaks of adoption rights for rearing a child exposed on a "dung heap" (2:382).

55. Another papyrus acknowledges infanticide as part of an understanding regarding the separation of a couple: if the woman has received her dowry and is pregnant, she has the right to expose the child and to find another man (Oxyrhynchus Papyri, 744, and discussed in Lewis 1983, pp. 54–55).

56. Tacitus, *Germania,* 19; and discussion in Herlihy 1985, pp. 53–54.

57. Russell 1985, p. 222.

58. Brissaud 1972, p. 251 n. 91; Brissaud, however, assembles impressive anecdotal and archival records showing that there was at least some practice of infanticide during the Middle Ages.

59. Kellum 1973–74, p. 367.

60. Hanawalt 1986, pp. 101–103. Hanawalt believes that the skeletal remains on which much of the evidence depends could be explained by sex-differentiated burial practices. See also Coleman 1974, p. 325. Rejecting the data that Coleman presents from St. Germain, on the basis of records beginning in the early ninth century, Herlihy (1985, pp. 63–65) says that the ratio of 135 males per 100 females "breaks the bounds of credibility," and he offers reasons other than infanticide that would explain the statistical results.

61. Hanawalt 1986, pp. 95, 101–103. In an earlier article, however, Hanawalt (1977, pp. 9–10) took a somewhat different stance, commenting that "the extraordinarily low incidence of recorded infanticide and child murder does not necessarily mean that it was rare. A plausible argument can be made that infanticide was not consistently illegal in the Middle Ages." Helmholtz (1975, pp. 382–390) finds evidence for infanticide in Canterbury Church court records, but there is no indication of the scale of the practice.
62. Boswell 1988.
63. Mols 1955, 2:288–289.
64. Chaddock 1956, p. 450.
65. Sieff 1990, p. 25; Thomlinson 1965, p. 429.
66. Willigan and Lynch 1982, pp. 65, 84; Hawley 1959, p. 363.
67. Chen, Quq, and D'Souza 1981, p. 55. In citing this study, I am mindful of Engels's lament (1984, p. 390) that in "the simplistic comparison of Greeks or Romans to Bengalis or other modern primitive or developing societies, the assumption that because something is done in Bangladesh, it must also have been done in Greece and Rome, is fast becoming a nuisance in the writing of classical social and economic history."
68. Pavlík 1990, p. 41; Gupta 1987, pp. 77–100; Scrimshaw 1978, pp. 383–399.
68. Voland and Siegelkow 1990, pp. 42–43, indicating that the data are published here for the first time. It is not clear from this report how "live births" were recorded. If the figures are generated from a registration procedure, usually baptismal records, then there is opportunity for discrepancies between birth and registration.
70. Angel's bibliography is in Stewart 1979, pp. 509–516; Grmek's many publications are well summarized and most of them listed in his important work, Grmek 1989.
71. Angel 1969, pp. 430–431; also see Angel 1972, pp. 88–105.
72. Angel 1969, p. 431; 1972, pp. 94–95; Grmek 1989, pp. 99–107; Brothwell 1972, pp. 75–87.
73. Amundsen and Diers 1969, pp. 125–132.
74. Angel 1972, pp. 9–95; Grmek 1989, p. 97.
75. Reported in Hanson 1989, p. 89.
76. Suchey et al. 1979, pp. 517–540.
77. Steele and Bramblett 1988, pp. 202–206.

2. Evidence for Oral Contraceptives and Abortifacients

1. Himes 1936, p. 100.
2. Brunt 1971, p. 147.
3. Himes 1936, esp. p. 97; Knodel and van de Walle 1979, p. 227: "Indirect evidence leads us to conclude the family limitation was not a form of behavior known to the majority prior to the fertility transition period and thus was not a real option for couples"; Ariès 1948, pp. 495–498, 514–521.
4. Fontanille 1977, p. 195. More recently Suder (1988, pp. 161–166) argues that the data of the Roman Empire show that the female mortality rate was

highest between the ages of fifteen and twenty-nine, the most fertile period; this finding identifies the factors as those associated with childbearing: accidents during pregnancy and childbirth and problems involving hygiene, contraceptives, and abortions, all connected with the expected high number of pregnancies.

5. Ariès 1948, pp. 494–531; in a later article (1953, p. 466) Ariès wrote, "C'est la thèse de l'impensabilité que j'ai défendue." Landurie 1973 also views the late eighteenth century as the time when contraception became a demographic factor.

6. Noonan 1986; additional evidence was gathered by Flandrin (1969, pp. 1370–90).

7. Hopkins 1965–66, p. 150.

8. Gourevitch 1984, pp. 198–199; Brundage (1987, p. 26n) agrees that premodern contraceptives were ineffective; McLaren (1984, p. 75) says, "One presumes that most [early contraceptive efforts] did not have the desired physiological effect but it is possible that some were successful." See also Veyne 1987, pp. 9, 12–13, a discussion of contraceptives that does not address the issue of their efficacy.

9. Matossian 1989, pp. 38–41, 53–58.

10. *DUSA,* pp. 512–526.

11. Matossian 1989, p. 67.

12. See below, chapter 14.

13. Plato, *Laws,* 5.740.

14. Plato, *Theaetetus,* 149c–d; see analysis in Tomen 1987, pp. 97–102.

15. Aristotle, *Politics,* 7.16.15.1335b19–26.

16. Polybius, *Histories,* 36.17.5.12.

17. Translated by Hopkins (1965–66, p. 141), based on text in Musonius, frag. 15a; Hopkins 1965, pp. 72–74.

18. Brunt 1971, pp. 558–566; Hopkins 1964–65, pp. 126–127, 141.

19. Chrysostom, *Homily 24 on the Epistle to the Romans* (PG 60:626–627): "Τί σπείρεις ἔνθα ἡ ἄρουρα σπουδάζει διαθεῖραι τὸν καρπόν; ἔνθα πολλὰ τὰ ἀτόκια; . . . πολλαὶ γὰρ ὥστε ἐπιχαρεῖς γενέσθαι, καὶ ἐπῳδὰς καὶ σπονδὰς καὶ φίλτρα καὶ μυρία ἕτερα μηχανῶνται. . . . Καὶ γὰρ θαρμακεῖαι λοιπὸν κινοῦνται, οὐκ ἐπὶ τὴν νηδὺν τὴν πορνευομένην, ἀλλ' ἐπὶ τὴν ἠδικημένην γυναῖκα"; this passage is translated and discussed by Noonan (1986, pp. 98–99).

20. Jerome, *Letter 22, to Eustochium,* 13 (PL 22:401): "Aliae vero sterilitatem praebibunt, et necdum sati hominis homicidium faciunt. Nonnullae cum se senserint conceptisse de scelere, abortii venena meditantur, et frequenter etiam ipsae commortuae, trium criminum reae, ad inferos perducuntur, homicidae sui"; see also discussion of passage by Noonan (1986, pp. 100–101).

21. Mincius Felix, *Octavius,* 30 (Wallis trans., ANF 4:192).

22. On the Alimentary Laws, see Duncan-Jones 1974, pp. 291–310.

23. Preuss 1978, pp. 412–416; Noonan 1986, pp. 30–36 (Old Testament), 49–55; Himes 1936, pp. 69–78.

24. *Yebamoth* 65b, in *The Babylonian Talmud* (Epstein ed.), *Seder Nashim,* vol. 1, pt. 3, pp. 436–437).

25. *Yebamoth* 65b, in *The Babylonian Talmud* (1973, 5732). The English translation is from the Epstein edition (*Seder Nashim*, 1:439). I am grateful to Gordon Newby, history department, North Carolina State University, for the English translation. The Hebrew indicates that a certain type of plant was orally taken.

26. *Yebamoth* 65b, reported by Gordon Newby, to whom I am grateful for the Hebrew translation.

27. *CHED* 3:1955; I am grateful to Gordon Newby and Cindy Levine for assistance in reading and interpreting the Hebrew.

28. Keil and Delitzsch 1983, 1:135; see discussion in Waszink 1950, 1:58–60; Dunstan 1988, p. 42.

29. Augustine, *Quaestiones Exodi*, 80.1439–45 (in *CCSL* 33, pt. 5); based on translation found in Dunstan 1988, p. 44.

30. Quoted in Dunstan 1988, p. 44, citing Gregory's *Adversus Macedonianos*.

31. Basil, *Epistolarum*, 188.2 (*PG* 32:671; Way trans. FC 2:12–2).

32. Aristotle, *History of Animals*, 7.3.588b (Bekker ed.); accepting the 40–90 day interpretation is Jöchle (1974, p. 426) and Noonan (1986, p. 90); rejecting it is Feen (1983, pp. 293–294). Cf. also Aristotle, *Generation of Animals*, 736a–b (Bekker ed.), where he avoids stating a definite point at which a rational soul is endowed. The best study of Aristotle on this subject is Balme 1990, pp. 20–31. See also Boylan 1984, pp. 83–112.

33. Marcus Aurelius, *Meditations*, 12.24.

34. Plutarch, *De stoicorum repugnantiis*, 41–43 (1052–53) (Cherniss ed. 13, pt..2, pp. 568–578); see also Sandbach 1940, pp. 20–25; Tertullian, *A Treatise on the Soul*, 25 (Holmes trans., *ANF*, 3:206).

35. Augustine, *Quaestionum in Heptateuchum*, 2.80 [On Exod. 21:22] (*CSEL* 28, pt. 2, pp. 146–147); cf. Noonan 1986, p. 90.

36. *Yebamot* 4:11, in *The Talmud* (Neusner trans., 21:158–159).

37. *Sanhedrin* 91b (Epstein ed.), in *Seder Nezikim*, 3:612.

38. Newmyer 1988, pp. 108–123.

39. *Sanhedrin* 91b.

40. Fontanille 1977, p. 194. For a Christian, historical perspective of the "foetus animé" and the "foetus inanimé," see Riquet 1949, pp. 615–630, esp. pp. 620–621.

41. *Shabbath* 135b (Epstein ed., in *Seder Mo'ed*, 1:683); on Hebrew law and abortion, see Preuss 1978, pp. 413–416.

42. *Niddah* ("The Menstruant") 3.1, in *Mishnah*, p. 747.

43. Published in Nardi 1971, pp. 133–134: "Αἴ κα γυνὰ ἐγβάληι, αἰ μέγ κα διάδηλον ἦι, μ[ι] αἴνονται ὥσπερ ἀπὸ θανόντος, αἰ δέ κα μὴ διάδηλον ἦι, μιαίνεται αὖτα ἀ οἰκία καθάπε[ρ] ἀπὸ λεχός." See also Sokolowski 1962, no 115, p. 189.

44. Feen 1983, pp. 290–292.

45. Noonan 1986, pp. 44–91.

46. More recently, see Gorman 1982, p. 16; Noonan 1986, p. 25 and passim. See also Dickison 1973, pp. 159–166.

47. Sokolowski 1955, no. 20 [pp. 53–55], ll. 14–22; see also Dittenberger 1920, 3:113–119; Nardi 1971, pp. 193–194, who places the inscription in error in the second or third century B.C. Sokolowski says of the inscription:

"La tendance universaliste et morale des préceptes dérive d'un esprit oriental plutôt que grec." The text reads:

(14) . . . πορευ]-
(15) όμενοι εἰς τὸν οἶκον τοῦτον ἄνδρε[ς καὶ γυναῖκες]
(16) ἐλεύθεροι καὶ οἰκέται τοὺς θεοὺς [πάντας ὀρκούσ]-
(17) θωσαν . . .
(19) . . . μὴ θίλτρον, μὴ φθορεῖον,
(20) μὴ [ἀτ]οκεῖον, μ[ὴ ἄλλο τι παιδο]-
(21) φόνον μήτε αὐτοὺς ἐπιτελεῖν μήτε [ἑτέρωι συμβου]-
(22) λεύειν μηδὲ συνιστορεῖν, ἀποστερ[οῦντες δὲ μη]-
(23) δὲν εὐνοεῖν τῶι οἴκωι τῶιδε . . .

48. Soranus, *Gynaecology*, 1.60 (Temkin trans., p. 62); for the Greek text, see
    Ilberg ed., p. 45; Burguière, Gourevitch, and Malinas ed., p. 59; and Rose
    ed. Unless otherwise indicated, future citations to the Greek text are to the
    Ilberg edition.

3. Soranus on Antifertility Agents

1. Soranus, *Gynaecology*, 1.63 (Temkin trans., pp. 65–66).
2. Ibid., 1.62 (Ilberg ed., pp. 46–47).
3. Saha, Savini, and Kasinathan 1961, p. 140; Watt and Breyer-Brandwijk
   (1962, pp. 875–876) note antifertility uses in Mauritius and Sumatra.
4. Heftmann, Ko, and Bennett 1966, pp. 1337–39; Dean, Exley, and Goodwin
   1971, pp. 2215–16, report smaller amounts of estrogens than those found
   in Heftmann et al. and conclude that there may be seasonal variations;
   Farnsworth et al. 1975, p. 718. Another test on animals showed that pomegranate was 50 percent effective in preventing fertilization in rats (Prakash
   1986, pp. 21, 23).
5. Gujral, Varma, and Sareen, 1960, p. 50. In somewhat different results, another experiment isolated the uterus of the albino rat to test compounds and
   found that pomegranate caused a "moderate increase in amplitude and frequency of contractions without appreciable alteration in tone" (Dhawan
   and Saxena 1958, p. 811).
6. Prakash et al. 1985, p. 447.
7. *DGRBM*, 3:204; *OCD*, pp. 236, 666; *Bulfinch's Mythology* 1894, pp. 64–
   71; cf. Ovid, *Metamorphoses*, 5.523–550.
8. Soranus, *Gynaecology*, 1.63; my translation is based on Oswei Temkin's
   translation (p. 65), with some changes based on the Greek edition by J.
   Ilberg (p. 47).
9. Ibid. (Temkin trans., pp. 65–66; Ilberg ed., p. 47).
10. King 1990, p. 11, with refs. to works in the Hippocratic corpus.
11. Elujoba, Olagbende, and Adesina (1985, pp. 281–288) report that this
    plant is used as an abortifacient in Nigeria but is actually an anti-
    implantation agent. All the women who took 5 g/kg of the fruit pulp
    aborted or failed to conceive.
12. Columella, *De arboribus*, 23.1; Pliny, *Natural History*, 21.17.33 (W. H. S.

Jones et al., ed. and trans., 6:184; unless otherwise noted, all future citations to *Natural History* will be to this edition).

13. Oswei Temkin's translation as "Cyrenaic balm" hardly helps with identification. The various translators of Pliny translate it as a variety of saffron because Pliny says that a type of saffron from Cyrene is darker and deteriorates rapidly (*Natural History*, 21.17.33 [Jones trans., 6:185; André 1969, p. 37; and the new Einaudi translation, by Aragosti et al. 1985, p. 171]). Isidore (*Origines*, 17.9.27) has: "laser herba . . . cuius sucus dictus primum lacsir quoniam . . . hoc et a quibusdam opium Cyrenaicum appellatur." The Hippocratic treatises use the term σίλφιον, often ὀπὸς σιλφίου but sometimes as ὀπὸς κυρηναικός (see *De morbis*, 3.16.64 and numerous entries in the computerized *TLG*). The *TLL* points to the gloss in Pliny (*Natural History*, 19.15.38): "laserpicium quod Graeco silphion vocant, in Cyrenaica provincia repertum, cuius sucum laser vocatur [cf. *Gloss.* sucus herbae ferulae]." Pliny (*Natural History* 19.15.35) says that it has not been found in Cyrene "for many years." On *silphium*, see Gemmill 1966, pp. 295–313; and Scarborough 1984, p. 76, which proposes that the plant be called *Ferula cyrenaica* Diosc., in honor of Dioscorides.

14. Herodotus, *Wars*, 4.169, 199; Theophrastus, *Enquiry into Plants*, 3.1.6, 6.3.1–5; Hippocrates, *De morbis*, 4.34 (Littré ed., 7:546).

15. Aristophanes, *Knights*, 893–894; Pliny, *Natural History*, 19.15.39–41; see also Gemmill 1966, pp. 295–313, and Andrews 1941–42, pp. 232–236.

16. Scribonius Largus, *Compositiones*, 67.175.177 (Helmreich ed. 1887; Sconocchia ed. 1983), in three references to *laser Cyrenaicum* in prescriptions, said that if it was not available, one could substitute *laser Syriacum*, which is likely another species of *Ferula*, perhaps asafetida.

17. Dioscorides, *De materia medica*, 3.80. (1.3) (Wellmann 1906–14; repr. 1958; hereinafter abbreviated as MM and all citations to Wellmann ed.).

18. Farnsworth et al. 1975, pp. 554, 590. The medicine enjoys a British and an Indian patent (British pat. 1,025,372 [Cl.A 61k], April 6, 1956; Indian Appl., July 25, 1963). In the human experiment the following were taken in equal doses daily for twenty-two days while abstaining from sexual coitus: 4 drams of the active principle of *Embelia ribes*, 4 drams of *Piper longum*, 2 drams of asafetida, and 4 drams of borax (soda). Ferula plants contain both ferulic acid and valeric acid.

19. Farnsworth et al. 1975, p. 576; Saha, Savini, and Kasinathan 1961, p. 136; Singh et al., 1985, pp. 268–270, which reports that when an extract of *F.j.* is given to female rats from one to five days after coitus, pregnancy is prevented.

20. Singh et al. 1985, pp. 268–270. The statistical reduction was significant: P < 0.01 in implantation number. See also Farnsworth et al. 1975, p. 576, and Duke 1985, pp. 191–195.

21. Keller 1988, p. 174.

22. Berendes 1902, p. 297; the modern taxonomy is *Opopanax chironium* (L.) Koch (the same plants as *Pastinica opopana* L., in an admittedly confused taxonomy). See Mabberley 1987, p. 413. The descriptions of *F. opopanax* Spr. closely resemble *Ferula palmyrensis* Post and Beauverd (*Index Kewensis*

1938, p. 114) and may be the same plant. In any case, the important fact is that its chemistry would be similar.

23. Flückiger and Hanbury 1879, p. 327; quotation from Gildemeister and Hoffmann 1900, p. 488.

24. Farnsworth et al. 1975, p. 576, on the basis of ten separate studies; the veterinary use of philocarpine is in *Merck Index* 1960, p. 818; on its use as a uterine stimulant, see Dhawan and Saxena 1958, pp. 808–811.

25. Conway and Slocumb 1979, pp. 247–248.

26. Guerra and Andrade 1974, pp. 191–199.

27. Prakash et al. 1985, pp. 447–448.

28. Kong, Xie, and But 1986, p. 4.

29. Farnsworth et al. 1975, p. 561; Casey 1960, pp. 593, 596; Saha, Savini, and Kasinathan 1961, pp. 134, 139.

30. Used as both an abortifacient and an emmenagogue; see Farnsworth et al. 1975, p. 569; Casey 1960, p. 594; Saha, Savini, and Kasinathan 1961, p. 139.

31. As an abortifacient, see Farnsworth et al. 1975, p. 557; Casey 1960, p. 594; Saha, Savini, and Kasinathan 1961, p. 139. *Commiphora myrrha* (Nees) Engl. = *Balsamodendron myrrha* L. Other species of the genus can also be a source for what is called myrrh.

32. Farnsworth et al. 1975, p. 571; Malhi and Trivedi 1972, p. 1926.

33. Atal, Zutshi, and Rao 1981, p. 231; cf. *Merck Index* 1976, p. 1129.

34. Duke and Ayensu 1985, 1:484.

35. Farnsworth et al. 1975, p. 736; Tuskaev 1971, pp. 295–298. This plant is cited in *Index Kewensis* 1956–1960, p. 66.

36. Duke 1985, p. 417; Terra 1980, p. 113; Leung 1980, p. 409; Malhi and Trivedi 1972, p. 1927.

37. Terra 1980, p. 113.

38. Soranus, *Gynaecology,* 1.36 (Temkin trans., p. 34).

39. Ibid., 1.61 (Ilberg ed., p. 46; Temkin trans., p. 64).

4. Terminology in Dioscorides' De materia medica

1. *MM,* 1.81 (1.3).

2. Ibid., 2.120 (3.4). The ancients' wild cabbage was different from the horticultural varieties of today.

3. Ibid., 2.159 (3.4).

4. Ibid., 2.179 (3.6).

5. Ibid., 3.134 (2.7). André 1985, p. 29, identifies Pliny's and Dioscorides' *asplenos* (*-on*) as *Ceterach officinarum* Willd., but also passing under the same name were the ferns he identified as *Adiantum capillus-veneris* L. and *Asplenium adiantum nigrum* L.

6. *MM,* 1.103 (2.1–2).

7. Ibid., 1.77 (2.7).

8. Ibid., 1.104 (1.4).

9. Ibid., 2.109 (1.7–8).

10. Ibid., 3.45 (1.5): ἐμμήνων ἀγωγά.
11. Ibid., 3.80 (6.1–2).
12. Ibid., 3.7 (2.7).
13. Ibid., 4.185 (1.6–7). For the uncertainty of identification, see Chapter 8 in the discussion of Pliny. The fern *Pteris neruosa* Thunb. is used in traditional Chinese medicine as a contraceptive (Kong, Xie, and But 1986, p. 22).
14. *MM*, 4.19 (1.9).
15. Ibid., 2.166 (2.3–4): τῶν ἄρτι συνειλημμένων ἐμβρύων φθόριον εἶναι. The text appears confused. The Wellmann edition provides this reading and says that a smell of the roots is sufficient. The seventeenth-century John Goodyer translation (1934, p. 206), which was based on a text from the 1598 Frankfurt edition, says that thirty of the plant's seeds are taken in a drink. The Old Latin translation, done in the sixth century, has a reading close to Wellmann's: "si a[d] mulieri pregnanti fuerit ordoratu, abortum facit," thus omitting from the Greek "the newly conceived" (Latin text, Stadler 1896, p. 237). Later in the same Wellmann text (5.3) there is the phrase ἐμβρύων κομιδήν, which I interpret to mean oral administration.
16. *MM*, 3.48 (4.3–4).
17. Ibid., 1.64 (3.8–9).
18. Ibid., 3.123 (1.6).
19. Ibid., 1.112 (2.1–3).
20. Ibid., 2.140 (rocket); 3.76 (parsnip); and 1.110 (rue).
21. Skarzynski 1933a, p. 766; 1933b, p. 323 [abstracts of paper given before the Polish Academy].
22. Butenandt and Jacobi 1933, pp. 104–112.
23. Part of the reason for the skepticism was that the first attempts to reduplicate the findings of estrone in pomegranate and date palm were negative, but in 1965 and 1966 the experiments were successful in confirming Butenandt's and Jacobi's findings. See Heftmann 1966, p. 1137, and Bennett, Ko, and Heftmann 1966, pp. 231–235.
24. Bygdeman 1981, pp. 301–318; Csapo 1976, pp. 705–718.
25. Skarzynski 1933a, p. 766; 1933b, p. 323; see also *Merck Index* 1960, p. 418.
26. Chaudhury 1966, pp. 12, 15.
27. Kamboj and Dhawan 1982, p. 200.
28. *MM*, 1.81 (1.3).
29. *Pharmacopoeia*, p. 242.
30. *Merck Index* 1960, p. 418.
31. Jean Ruel's translation was first published in Paris in 1516, but for this citation, I used the edition with Petrus Matthiolus' commentary (Venice, 1554), fol. 88 (for white poplar): "sterilitatem inducere tradunt si cum mulino rene bibatur."
32. de Laszlo and Henshaw 1954, p. 628.
33. Farnsworth et al. 1975, p. 557, citing M. Guto, T. Noguchi, T. Watanabe, I. Ishikawa, M. Komatsu, and Y. Aramaki, *Takeda Kenkyuscho Nempo* 16 (1957): 21; the plant species is listed in the *IK* 1931–35, p. 103.

34. *MM*, 2.130; Farnsworth et al. 1975, pp. 561, 735; Casey 1960, p. 595, as an abortifacient; *Brassica napus* and *B. pekinensis* exhibit estrogenic activity. Vague et al. 1957, pp. 745–51; see also Keller 1988, p. 195.
35. *MM*, 2.179 (5.1); see Brondegaard 1973, p. 168, for reports on ivy's use in Iran as a contraceptive.
36. *MM*, 2.159 (3.5).
37. Aristotle (*History of Animals*, 7.3.583a23–24 [Bekker ed., 1:583]); Hippocrates, *De natura pueri*, 13.1 (Joly ed., 11.56), says six days; Galen, *De semine*, 1:7 (Kühn ed., 4:537), says that the sperm may live many days. Modern medicine has developed postcoital oral contraceptives. See Bubio et al. 1970, pp. 303–314.
38. Bubio et al. 1970, pp. 303–314.
39. As a contraceptive, see Duke 1985, p. 224; as an abortifacient, see Watt and Breyer-Brandwijk 1962, pp. 117–118. As a poison for animals, see Lewis and Elvin-Lewis 1972, p. 49.
40. Gujral, Varma, and Sareen 1960, pp. 48, 51; Farnsworth et al. 1975, p. 554; Keller 1988.
41. Casey 1960, p. 594, reporting on a related species, *V. trifolia* L.
42. Kamboj and Dhawan 1982, p. 192.
43. Prakash 1986, p. 22.
44. For a historical and etymological review of juniper, see Brøndegaard 1964, pp. 331–351.
45. Prakash et al. 1985, p. 447 (under pomegranate).
46. List and Horhammer 1969–79, p. 256.
47. *MM*, 4.172 (3.4); cf. 4.170 (4.8–9).
48. Kong et al. 1985, p. 304; Kong, Xie, and But 1986, p. 4; Bingel and Fong, 1988, pp. 78–80.
49. *MM*, 4.146 (1.10).
50. Lin et al. 1981, pp. 319–329.
51. *MM*, 1.1 (3.1–2).
52. Kong, Xie, and But 1986, p. 5. Pallasone A has neither estrogenic nor anti-estrogenic activity.
53. *MM*, 1.1 (2.6–7): σὺν οἴνῳ δὲ ποθεῖσαι ἄγουσιν ἔμμηνα.
54. Ibid., 2.152 (3.9).
55. Qian et al. 1986, pp. 295–302.
56. Fontán-Candella 1960, p. 12; other tests, however, have somewhat disquieting results: both *Allum cepa* and *A. sativum* taken orally pass through the placenta, resulting sometimes not in abortion but in abnormal births. Possibly this action can explain the alleged contraceptive effect (see Goswami 1978, pp. 515–516).
57. Casey 1960, p. 594; Saha, Savini, and Kasinathan 1961, p. 131.
58. Dioscorides' drug affinity theory is explained in Riddle 1985.
59. Kong, Xie, and But 1986, p. 19.
60. André 1985, p. 7, noting that by the sixth century the name had transferred to bryony (*Bryonia dioïca* Jacq.); in his German translation of Dioscorides, Berendes (1902, p. 261) proposes *Boletus laricis* Jacqu., *Polyporus officinalis* Fries, or *Agaricus albus,* the latter a fungus. Near the beginning of the

twentieth century, the substance called surgeon's agaric, which came from the fungus *Agaricus albus*, N.F., was a cathartic and used by surgeons also as a styptic in hemorrhaging. See Sayre 1917, p. 82.

61. Usher 1974, p. 260.
62. *MM*, 3.2 (2.5).
63. Duke 1985, p. 404.
64. *MM*, 3.3 (2.6).
65. Duke 1985, p. 207, as emmenagogue; Jöchle 1974, p. 432; Trease and Evans 1978, pp. 509–511.
66. *MM*, 3.4 (4.4).
67. De Laszlo and Henshaw 1954, p. 627; Brondegaard 1973, p. 168; Farnsworth et al. 1975, p. 542.
68. Palma 1964, p. 166; Saha, Savini, and Kasinathan 1961, pp. 132, 150; Angeles et al. 1970, pp. 139–148; Farnsworth et al. 1975, p. 556.
69. Kamboj and Dhawan 1984, pp. 194, 206, testing *Aristolochia indica*. Another species, *A. bracteata*, was found to possess little oxytocic properties, but the potassium chloride in its extract is a uterine stimulant. See Saha, Savini, and Kasinathan 1961, p. 150, where the authors say that *A. indica* is thought to have more active oxytocic qualities. They found no toxic side effects.
70. Kong, Xie, and But 1986, pp. 5–6. See also Wang and Zheng, 1984, pp. 405–409, through *Index Medicus* 05631595 85247595. Much the same results but with more chemical analysis are reported by Che et al. 1984 pp. 331–341.
71. Reiners 1966, p. 359; Duke 1985, p. 215; Farnsworth et al. 1975, p. 718.
72. Sharma et al. 1983, p. 185. The substance glycyrrhizin, which is sweet tasting, is shared by another plant, *Lippa dulcis* Trev., which is used as an abortifacient in Mexico. See Compadre 1986, p. 99. Plant vendors in Mexico were reluctant to specify the action, often simply saying, "Used by women."
73. *MM*, 3.6 (3.1), 7 (2.7).
74. On great century plant, see Palma 1964, p. 610, and Jöchle 1974, p. 433; on feverwort, see Jöchle, p. 431.
75. On *Convolvulus althaecoides*, see Trease and Evans 1966, p. 587; this assertion was dropped in the 11th edition (1978). The gladiolus and iris are reported in Farnsworth et al. 1975, p. 718, where the action of isoflavonids is discussed as well.
76. On ginger, see Farnsworth et al. 1975, p. 577; on water pepper, see de Laszlo and Henshaw 1954, p. 629; Garg and Mathur 1971, pp. 421–423; East 1955b, pp. 252–262; and a folklore report, Casey 1960, p. 593.
77. Farnsworth et al. 1975, p. 559.
78. Duke 1985, p. 10.
79. Jöchle 1974, p. 135.
80. Saha, Savini, and Kasinathan 1961, p. 135; Casey 1960, p. 594; Palma 1964, p. 406 (as emmenagogue).
81. See n. 15 in this chapter. In addition, an alternate reading in the manuscript tradition related to the El Escorial manuscript (Wellmann's RV) has an entry for the "smaller arum," which Behrendes and Goodyer read as Dioscorides

text and Behrendes identifies as *Arum italicum,* with the reading that the plant "kills in the first stage of pregnancy the embryo [im ersten Stadium der Schwangerschaft den Embryo tödten]" (p. 244). Possibly the meaning points to an early stage embryo, although neither the text nor the lexicon are clear.

82. Steinegger and Hänsel 1968, p. 388. A member of the same family, *Caladium sequinium,* was employed in German prison camps to produce temporary and permanent sterility; see Farnsworth et al., 1975, pp. 542, 547; Price 1965, pp. 3–17.

83. *MM,* 1.18 (1.7, 10–11).

5. Early Stage Abortifacients in Dioscorides and Soranus

1. Soranus, *Gynaecology,* 1.64 (Ilberg ed., pp. 47–48; Temkin trans., p. 66); Dioscorides (*MM,* 2.103 [1.12]) recommended linseed with fenugreek as a clyster in the womb, without giving a specific function.

2. Dioscorides discusses fenugreek in a vaginal suppository as a mollifying agent (*MM,* 2.102 [2.3]) and considers artemisia as an emmenagogue and abortifacient (3.113 [2.5–6]).

3. Soranus, *Gynaecology,* 1.65 (Ilberg ed., p. 48; Temkin trans., p. 67); cf. Hippocrates, *Aphorisms,* 5.31 (Jones ed., 4:166).

4. Soranus, *Gynaecology,* 1.65 (Ilberg ed., p. 48; Temkin trans., p. 67).

5. Ibid., 1.65 (Ilberg ed., pp. 48–49; Temkin trans., pp. 67–68 [with my modifications]).

6. *MM,* 2.109 (1.7–8).

7. Mazur et al. 1966, pp. 299–309, reported in *Chemical Abstracts* 65 (1966):11163q.

8. Sizov 1969, pp. 44–46, as reported in *Chemical Abstracts* 72 (1970):119957u. See also *Chemical Abstracts* 78 (1973):66914t and Farnsworth et al. 1975, p. 566.

9. Saha, Savini, and Kasinathan 1961, pp. 138, 140; Casey 1960, pp. 592, 596; Duke 1985, pp. 271–272.

10. *MM,* 1.78 (2.8).

11. Duke 1985, p. 271.

12. *MM,* Praef. 9; cf. Riddle 1985, pp. 70–73.

13. *MM,* 5.107 (2.1).

14. Ibid., 3.23 (2.2), employed both orally and as a suppository.

15. Duke 1985, p. 66; reporting numerous medical studies is Casey 1960, p. 592 (for *Artemisia siversiana*).

16. Farnsworth et al. 1975, p. 549. See also, Weniger, Haag-Berrurier, and Anton 1982, pp. 73–74.

17. *MM,* 1.6 (1.12); Saha, Savini, and Kasinathan 1961, p. 136; Casey 1960, p. 596.

18. Soranus, *Gynaecology,* 1.65 (Ilberg ed., p. 49; Temkin trans., p. 68).

19. Hippocrates, *Aphorisms,* 5.31 (Jones trans., 4:166–167).

20. *MM,* 3.121 (2.5–6), 3–32 (1.7).

21. For laboratory study, see Chaudhury 1966, p. 11; see also Farnsworth et al. 1975, p. 560; Palma 1964, p. 563, for the use of spikenard as an emmenagogue.

22. Jöchle 1974, p. 434.

23. Woom et al. 1987, pp. 399–401. The tests revealed that the active compound (fraxinellone) did not have estrogenicity but appears to be active in the inhibition of implantation.

24. Fischer 1927, pp. 6–7, observes that Dioscorides used the phrase (or similar) "it aborts a dead fetus [τεθνηκότων ἐμβρύων ἐκβόλιον] in these chapters of *MM*: 2.70 (6.12–13), 3.32 (1.7: τὰ τεθνηκότα ἔβρυα ἐκτινάσσει), 83 (2.2–3: ἐκβάλλει δὲ καὶ τὰ τεθνηκότα ἔμβρυα ὁμοίως λυφθεῖσα), 112 (2.6–7: ἔμβρυα τεθνηκὸς ἐκβάλλει). In the following chapters the wording is "it expels/kills the fetus [ἔμβρυα κτείνει]": 1.78 (2.8), 4.172 (3.5); and "it destroys [φθεῖρον]" in: 2.155 (1.4: ἔμβρυα φθεῖρον καὶ ἔμμηνα κινοῦν), 156 (2.4: κινεῖ δὲ καὶ καταμήνια καὶ τὰς ἔμβρυα φθείρει), 3.35 (3.2: φθείρει δὲ καὶ ἔμβρυα καὶ ἔμμηνα ἄλει), 48 (4.4–5: ἔμμηνά τε ἄλει καὶ ἔμβρυα φθείρει), 81 (2.2), 4.148 (2.5), 162 (3.3), 170 (4.8: ἔμβρυα φθείρει [without mention of menstrua]), 176 (2.5–6: ἔμβρυα τε φθείρουσι προστιθέμεναι), and 5.72 (3.8–9: φθείρει δὲ καὶ ἔμβρυα, καὶ πρὸς τὰς ὑστερικάς). Fischer notes that Pliny uses the Latin equivalents to "expelling a fetus (ἔμβρυα κτείνει . . . ἄλει, etc.]" by stating, "Partum (partus) stimulat, extrahit, pellit" in *Natural History*, 23.53.99 and 24.92.146; see other references below in Chapter 8.

25. See Chapter 8 below for a full discussion of the phrase "dead fetus."

26. Cited in Brøndegaard 1964, p. 338.

27. Galen, *Hippocratis aphorismos libri V* (Kühn ed., 17b:858).

28. *MM*, 1.10 (2.2): ἄγουσι δὲ καὶ ἔμμηνα.

29. Farnsworth et al. 1975, p. 542; de Laszlo and Henshaw 1954, p. 627; and Brøndegaard 1973, p. 168.

30. *MM*, 1.4 (2.4).

31. Farnsworth et al. 1975, p. 735.

32. Arenas and Azorero 1977, p. 304.

33. *MM*, 3.130 (1.6); on Dioscorides and folklore, see Riddle 1985, pp. 82–85.

34. *MM*, 1.93 (1.8–10).

35. *DUSA*, p. 1710; Ullsperger 1953, pp. 43–50; Abdul-Ghani, Amin, and Suleiman 1987, pp. 216–220.

36. *Merck Index* 1960, pp. 292–293, reports that large doses result in diarrhea, abdominal pain, and nervousness.

37. *Chinese Herbal Medicine Materia Medica* 1986, p. 320.

38. *MM*, 1.93 (1.6–7).

39. Harborne 1977, p. 85.

40. Tyler, Brady, and Robbers, 1981, pp. 191–192.

41. *MM*, 1.69 (1.7–8).

42. Ibid., 1.67 (2.4): *bdellion* = gum of *Hyphaene thebaica*.

43. Ibid., 1.109 (5.2–3).

44. See Chapter 8 below.

45. Hippocrates, *De mulierum affectibus,* 1.78.17 (Littré ed., 8:17); Aëtius, *Peri tōn en mētrai pathōn,* 16.17 (Zervòs ed. 1901, p. 19; hereinafter cited as *Iatricorum*).

46. Wolfgang Jöchle, chap. 2, n. 34, pp. 425–439. The two pharmacognosy guides are E. Steinegger and R. Hänsel, *Lehrbuch der Allgemeinen Pharmakognosie* (Berlin: Springer, 1963), and G. E. Trease and W. C. Evans, *A Textbook of Pharmacognosy,* 9th ed. (London: Baillière, Tindall and Cassell, 1966). I have checked Jöchle's references using Steinegger-Hänsel's 2nd ed., 1968, and Trease-Evans' 11th ed., 1978.

47. Farnsworth et al. 1981, pp. 330, 338.

48. In 1949 (in Polish), Jan Lachs published a thirty-two-page study, but Lachs does not refer to the discoveries of his countryman Skarzynski, nor does he relate Dioscorides to science studies. Lachs discussed Dioscorides' Greek terminology and related the agents that were applied to each term, such as "ecbolic" and "contraceptive drugs" (esp. pp. 24, 28–29). I found no indication in Skarzynski or in Butenandt and Jacobi that they were aware of Dioscorides' recommendations.

49. *MM,* 3.110 (1.4–5, hulwort); 36 (2.3, thyme); 23 (2.1–3, sage); 4.1 (4.6, *kestron* = betony); 3.27 (1.9, marjoram).

50. For thyme, see Duke 1985, p. 483; Farnsworth et al. 1975, p. 550; Chaudhury 1966, p. 13, reports a negative result in one rough screening test. For sage, see Duke 1985, p. 420; Farnsworth et al. 1975, p. 550; Casey 1960, p. 597; and Duquénois 1972, pp. 1841–49; for marjoram, Farnsworth et al. 1975, p. 550; de Laszlo and Henshaw 1954, p. 629; Chaudhury 1966, p. 6.

51. For hulwort, see Farnsworth et al. 1975, p. 565 (as uterine stimulant); for betony, see pp. 564–565.

52. *MM,* 3.31 (1.2).

53. *Morbidity and Mortality Weekly Report* 1978, pp. 511–513.

54. The calculation was made by Norman Farnsworth and related to me by personal communication from Mark Blumenthal (May 3, 1990).

55. Farnsworth et al. 1975, p. 564; Watt and Breyer-Brandwijk 1962, p. 523.

56. Jöchle 1974, p. 430.

57. Farnsworth et al. 1975, p. 549.

58. *MM,* 4.148 (2.6) for *Veratrum;* 4.162 (3.3) for *Helleborus.*

59. Van Kampen and Ellis 1972, pp. 549–560; Farnsworth et al. 1975, pp. 568, 736.

60. Duke 1985, pp. 506–507.

61. Duke 1985, p. 227; Casey 1960, p. 593; Saha, Savini, and Kasinathan 1961, p. 137.

62. As a regular drug, see *DUSA,* pp. 1711–12, and an abortifacient, de Laszlo and Henshaw 1954, p. 629.

63. Albert-Puleo 1979, pp. 193–195.

64. *MM,* 4.14.

65. In his 1902 translation of Dioscorides (p. 373), Berendes believed it to be a species of *Lonicera,* and he gave several candidates. Gunther, editor of the Goodyer translation (1934, p. 410), tentatively proposes *Convolvulus arvenis.* Because the identification is so uncertain and the documentary evi-

dence is inconclusive, laboratory work on the chemistry and pharmacy of the many candidate species proposed might be the only way to determine the plant Dioscorides intended. In Chapter 14 there is discussion about the Renaissance interpretation of the plant.

66. *MM*, 3.45 (rue), 48 (opopanax), 123 (wallflower/stock); 1.64 (myrrh given with rue), 2.159 (pepper).
67. Ibid., 1.112 (myrtle), 2.140 (rocket), 3.76 (cow parsnip).
68. Ibid., 2.102 (2.3–4), 4.68 (4.4).
69. Jöchle 1974.

6. Ancient Society and Birth Control Agents

1. Ovid, *Metamorphoses*, 10.500–502 (lines 310–533 for the full story). On the legend, see Lehner 1960, p. 72.
2. Personal interview with Mary Reichle, public health nurse, in Watauga County, North Carolina, in July 1990.
3. *MM*, 3.72 (2.6).
4. Scribonius Largus, *Compositiones*, 121 (Sconocchia ed., p. 64).
5. Farnsworth et al. 1975, p. 554; Kamboj and Dhawan 1982, p. 207; Garg and Garg 1971, pp. 302–306.
6. Sharma, Lel, and Jacob 1976, pp. 506–508. On days 8–10, however, the implantations remained in 61 percent of the animals. The test results show that, as the early sources indicated, the plant's effect is good as a postcoital antifertility agent.
7. Kaliwal, Ahamed, and Rao 1984, pp. 70–74.
8. Kong, Xie, and But 1986, pp. 18–19; see also Kaliwal, Ahamed, and Rao 1984, p. 74.
9. Kant, Jacob, and Lohiya 1986, pp. 36–41.
10. Aristophanes, *Peace*, 706–712 (Rogers, ed. and trans., 2:64–65).
11. Scholia, 712a, in *Scholia in Aristophanes* (Holwerda ed., 2:110).
12. Aristophanes, *Lysistrata*, 87–89 (Rogers ed. and trans., 3:14–15).
13. Rogers ed., *Aristophanes* 1927, p. 14.
14. Aelian, *On the Characteristics of Animals*, 9.26 (Scholfield ed., 2:246); Pliny, *Natural History*, 24.38.59; Wagler 1894, s.v. *agnos*.
15. Frazer 1935, 2:116.
16. Pliny, *Natural History*, 24.38.62.
17. Ibid., 24.38.62; *MM*, 1.103.
18. *CHED*, 3:1955.
19. Zohary 1982, see pp. 74–75 for Triticum plants; see also, Zohary 1966, Löw 1934.
20. Farnsworth et al. 1975, pp. 563–718, 732.
21. A study of some chemical characteristics was reported in Nakai and Sakamoto 1977, pp. 269–276.
22. *CHED*, 3.1955.
23. Aelian, *Varia historia*, 2.7 (Dilts ed., pp. 19–20; trans. by Feen 1983, p. 289 [quotation only]).
24. The term *atokion* was used as an adjective with the word *pharmakon* ("drug") by Pollux (2nd cen. A.D.), *Onomasticon*, 2.7 (Bethe ed., 1:82).

25. Fragment printed by Nardi 1971, pp. 87–88, and translated in Feen 1983, pp. 290–291.
26. Feen 1983, p. 291.
27. Cicero, *Pro Cluentio*, 11.32 (Hoedge trans. [ed.]).
28. *Digest*, 48.8.8, 19.39 (Mommsen-Watson eds., 4:820, 854; Scott trans., 11:61 [Ulpian], 124 [Tryphonius]).
29. Marcianus, in *Digest*, 47.11.4 (Mommsen-Watson eds., 4:754–755; Scott trans., 10:328).
30. Russell 1972, p. 5.
31. *Digest*, 48.19.38.5 (Scott trans., 11:123).
32. Nardi 1971; Noonan 1986; Fontanille 1977.
33. Plautus, *Truculentus*, 1.97, 200–201 (Nixon trans., 5:234, 244–245).
34. Juvenal, *Satirae*, 6.592–598 (Green trans., p. 149).
35. Ovid, *Amores*, 2.13–14; *Fasti*, 1.621–624; *Heroides*, 11.37–42.
36. Philo, *De congressu querendae eruditio gratia* (Manqucy ed., p. 539).
37. Lucretius, *De rerum natura*, 4.1277.
38. Seneca, *Fragments*, No. 84 (Haase ed.).
39. Noonan 1986, pp. 56–106; Crutchfield 1989, pp. 34–38.

7. Egyptian Papyrus Sources

1. In a letter to me dated April 10, 1990, Robert K. Ritner, of the Oriental Institute of the University of Chicago, reports to that the sign here is for "male" or "sexual intercourse" but is used in an ideogram in P. Berlin 192 for the phallus/semen that the woman was not to receive. He agrees with the editors of the *Grundriss* (n. 2 below) that the translation "pregnant" is justified here.
2. *Grundriss der Medizin der alten Ägypter* 1958, 4, pt. 1, p. 277; 4, pt. 2, p. 211; 5:476–478 (hierglyphs text; hereinafter cited as *Grundriss*).
3. Ibid., 4, pt. 1, p. 277; note pt. 2, p. 211; 5:477 (hieroglyphs text). The word *shm* suggests, according to Robert Ritner (see n. 1 above) "fluid derived from pounding/extract." In the context here with soda, a fluid does not appear likely. The ancients had a variety of substances called by the Greek term *nitron* (as corresponds to the Egyptian term), but in almost all cases it was some form of sodium carbonate/saltpeter or cautic soda (such as borax). The context here suggests a pulverized powder or, if a fluid is called for, soda with water added, causing a greater caustic action. The term *h* appears to refer to a measure.
4. *Grundriss*, 4, pt. 1, p. 277; note pt. 2, p. 211; 5:477.
5. Musallam 1983, pp. 79, 84, 102, 104.
6. Ibid., p. 79. In the sixth century Aëtius of Amida (see Chapter 9 below) lists *crocodilum* as an emmenagogue, but this is believed to be a plant, probably *Eryngium maritimum*.
7. So say Frey 1985–86, pp. 82–83, 85–86; Himes 19–36, pp. 63–68.
8. Te Velde 1967, pp. 28–29.
9. Ritner 1984, p. 221.
10. *A Guide to the Egyptian Collections in the B.M.* 1909, p. 126. For this

observation I am grateful to Jeffrey Compton, a student in one of my lecture classes who recognized the depiction from a slide.

11. See Chapter 8.
12. *The Leyden Papyrus,* col. 12 (Griffith and Thompson, eds., pp. 86–89).
13. Frey 1985–86, pp. 80–81; Himes 1936, pp. 59–63.
14. Ras. IV C 2–3, in *Grundriss,* 4, pt. 1, p. 277; 5, pp. 476–477 (hieroglyphs text); *Five Ramesseum Papyri,* Barns ed. 1956, pp. 24–25.
15. According to Robert Ritner (letter to author, April 10, 1990), the hieratic sign here—*rnp.t*—generally means "year" but can also mean "season" or "time period." He suggests that in this context the sense points to pregnancy periods. The Egyptians had three seasons of four months each.
16. *Grundriss,* 6:277; 5:476 (hieroglyphs text).
17. *Grundriss,* 4, pt. 2, p. 211, and *Five Ramesseum Papyri* 1956, p. 25, n. to C. 3.
18. *Grundriss,* 4, pt. 1, p. 277; pt. 2, p. 210; 5:476. Note another translation, apparently of this same passage: "To bring about abortion, only one remedy is given: Dates, Onions, and the Fruit-of-the-Acanthus, were crushed in a vessel with Honey, sprinkled on a cloth, and applied to the Vulva. It ensured abortion either in the first, second or third period" (Bryan 1924, p. 83).
19. See *Grundriss,* 6:200–201, 503–504, 563; Manniche 1989, pp. 65–67 and passim. Acacia is employed in a variety of ways in Egyptian gynecology. See *Papyros Ebers,* Joachim ed. 1890, repr. 1973, pp. 175–179.
20. *Grundriss,* 6:590; Manniche 1989, p. 89.
21. *MM,* 4.176 (2.4).
22. Gopinath and Raghunathan 1985, pp. 22–23.
23. De S. Matsui et al. 1971, pp. 67–68; Farnsworth et al.1975, pp. 550, 565.
24. Watt and Breyer-Brandwijk 1962, p. 547.
25. Chowdhury, Kaleque, and Chakder 1984, pp. 372–374.
26. Farnsworth et al. 1975, p. 740, with many references.
27. Watt and Breyer-Brandwijk 1962, p. 349; also see Duke 1985, p. 128.
28. Prakash et al. 1985, p. 447 (pomegr. dis., c. II).
29. Watt and Breyer-Brandwijk 1962, p. 342.
30. For pointing out this term to me I thank Robert Ritner.
31. *Grundriss,* 4, pt. 1, pp. 278–279, pt. 2, p. 212 (notes): 5:478–479 (hieroglyphs texts).
32. Kopcewicz 1971, pp. 1423–27.
33. This may be the same preparation that is mentioned in Kahun Papyrus 17 as a cure for staunching blood coming during childbirth with the separation of the placenta. See *Grundriss,* 4, pt. 2, p. 213.
34. Ibid., 4, pt. 1, pp. 279–280; pt. 2, p. 212; 5:480–481 (hieroglyphs text).
35. The sign can also mean "phallus," but the context points to "semen."
36. Berlin 192 (Rs. 1, 2–2), in *Grundriss,* 4, pt. 1, p. 277; pt. 2, pp. 211–212; 5:478; and Manniche 1989, pp. 76, 152.
37. Manniche 1989, p. 108.
38. Casey 1960, p. 592; Chaudhury 1966, pp. 4, 14; Watt and Breyer-Brandwijk 1962, p. 1033.
39. Farnsworth et al. 1975, p. 554.

40. Sharma et al. 1983, p. 185.
41. For instance, celery is discussed by Dioscorides (*MM*, 3.64).
42. See Chapter 10 below.

8. Greek and Roman Medicine from Hippocrates to Galen

1. Hippocrates, *De natura muliebri*, 98 (Littré ed., 7:414): Ἢν μὴ θέλῃ κυΐσκεσθαι, μισους ὅσον κύαμον διεὶς ὕδατι, δίδου πίνειν, καὶ ἐνιαυτὸν οὐ κυΐσκεται.
2. Hippocrates, *De mulierum affectibus*, 1.76 (E. Littré ed., 8:170): Ἀτόκιον. ἢν μὴ δέῃ κυΐσκεσθαι, μίσυος ὅσον κύαμον διεὶς ὕδατι, πίνειν διδόναι, καὶ ἐνιαυτόν, ὡς ἔπος εἰπεῖν, οὐ κυΐσκεται.
3. *MM*, 5.100.
4. Galen, *De simpl. med. temp. ac fac.*, 9.35 (Kühn ed., 12:241).
5. Theophrastus, *On Stones*, (Caley and Richards eds. and trans. 1956, pp. 126–164 for commentary on copper).
6. Pschera et al. 1988, pp. 341–348; Gupta and Devi 1975, pp. 736–739; Hagenfeldt 1972, pp. 37–54; Bull et al. 1987, pp. 49–55. Copper is absorbed from the intestinal tract of people. On copper, see Goodman and Gilman 1941, p. 1118. Wolfgang Jöchle (1971, p. 8) says that the action may be because of chronic intoxication, but given the small amount of research, his explanation is inadequate. In searching for an explanation of the use of copper, I wrote to a number of fertility experts, some of whom were experts on the copper uterine device, but no one who replied could supply an explanation. The American Fertility Society was helpful in recommending experts (letter to author, November 17, 1988).
7. Zhu 1981, pp. 248–264.
8. Oster and Salgo 1975, p. 433.
9. Ibid., pp. 433–435.
10. Levinson 1978, p. 779.
11. Oster and Salgo 1975, p. 432.
12. I am indebted to Samuel Tove, a friend and former chair of the Department of Biochemistry at North Carolina State University, for this suggestion.
13. Another copper product, called "flowers of copper [ἴον χαλκοῦ], is found in a drink to be taken "when the fetus and the insides are bad" (Hippocrates, *De mulierum affectibus*, 1.78 [Littré ed., 8:186, 2–4]). In another, copper filings (χαλκός) appear in a vaginal suppository (Ibid. [Littré ed., 8:186, 4–5]).
14. This identification was proposed by E. Littré, one that I cannot confirm or deny (Littré 8:179, 7).
15. Hippocrates, *De mulierum affectibus*, 1.78 (Littré ed., 8:178, 1–12).
16. Scarborough 1979, p. 21.
17. Hippocrates, *De mulierum affectibus*, 1. 78 (Littré ed., 8:178, 12–14).
18. On his treatise, see Grensemann 1982, 1987, and a review of this volume by Smith (1988, pp. 649–651).
19. Littré 8:179.

20. Hippocrates, *De mulierum affectibus*, 1.78 (Littré ed., 8:178, 14 and 180, 10).
21. Ibid. (Littré ed., 8:180, 14–18).
22. Ibid. (Littré ed., 8:180, 18 through 8:182, 5).
23. *MM*, 2.124 (purslane), 175 (buttercup).
24. Saha, Savini, and Kasinathan 1961, p. 140; Casey 1960, p. 595.
25. Feng et al. 1962, pp. 556–561.
26. André 1985, p. 81.
27. Hippocrates, *De mulierum affectibus*, 1.78 (Littré ed., 8:182, 20 through 8:184, 2).
28. Indira et al. 1956, pp. 202–204; Farnsworth et al. 1975, p. 735.
29. *MM*, 3.54 (1.5), 55 (1.3).
30. Pliny, *Natural History*, 8.50.112.
31. Hippocrates, *De mulierum affectibus*, 1.78 (Littré ed., 8:184, 2–5).
32. Ibid. (Littré ed., 8:184, 5–14).
33. *MM*, 3.63 (coriander).
34. Al-Said et al. 1987, pp. 165–173.
35. Dierbach (1824, p. 167) believed the plant to be *Mentha sativa* L. or *M. crispa* L.
36. Kamboj and Dhawan 1982, p. 192; Conway and Slocumb 1979, p. 253, calls *Mentha arvensis* pennyroyal mint.
37. Kanjanapothi et al. 1981, pp. 559–567.
38. Farnsworth et al. 1975, p. 736; Sharaf and Goma 1965, pp. 289–290; Duke 1985, p. 375.
39. Hippocrates *De mulierum affectibus*, 1.78 (Littré ed., 8:184, 15–18).
40. Ibid. (Littré ed., 8:184, 19–22).
41. Ibid., 1.91 (Littré ed., 8:218, 13–15).
42. Ibid. (Littré ed., 8:218, 15 and 219, 19).
43. Ibid. 1.78 (Littré ed., 8:184, 19–24).
44. Ibid. (Littré ed., 8:184, 24 and 186, 2).
45. Ibid. (Littré ed., 8:186, 2–4).
46. Ibid. (Littré ed., 8:186, 4–6).
47. Ibid. (Littré ed., 8:188, 13–14).
48. Ibid. (Littré ed., 8:188, 18–21).
49. *MM*, 4.162 (3.3).
50. Duke 1985, p. 227; de Laszlo and Henshaw 1954, p. 629; Casey 1960, p. 593, noting three other studies.
51. Watt and Breyer-Brandwijk 1962, pp. 306, 778.
52. Hippocrates, *De mulierum affectibus*, 1.78 (Littré ed., 8:188, 21 and 189, 3).
53. Ibid. (Littré ed., 8:188, 14).
54. Ibid. (Littré ed., 8:188, 13).
55. Ibid., 1.91 (Littré ed., 8:220, 16–18).
56. Ibid., 1.78 (Littré ed., 8:188, 8–13).
57. Pliny, *Natural History*, 24.32.47 (poplar); 24.37.56–58 (willow).
58. Ibid., 29.27.85.

59. Ibid., 24.11.18: Pliny's *cedrus* is likely *Juniperus excelsa,* whose activity would be approximately the same as Dioscorides' *Juniperus communis.*
60. Ibid., 20.51.143.
61. Ibid., 27.17.34, 55.80. André 1985, p. 29, identifies Pliny and Dioscorides (*MM,* 3.134) as *Ceterach officinarum* Willd., but two other ferns he believes passed under the same Greek-Latin term: *Adiantum capillus-veneris* L. and *Asplenium adiantum nigrum* L., as well as two flowering plants: *Iris pseudacrorus* L. and *Pimpinella saxifraga* (L. A. Carnoy (1959, p. 41, simply mentions *Ceerach officinarum* plus other ferns). The *OLD* (s.v.) simply says *Ceterach officinarum* and considers *felix* (al. *filix*) a generic term for a large fern. André (1985, p. 105) identifies Pliny's and Dioscorides' plants (*pteris,* in *MM,* 4.184) as *Polystichum filix mas* Roth, but also passing under the same name in other sources are *Pteris aquilina* L. and *Polypodium vulgare* L. In the British Pharmacopoeia the male fern is called *Dryopteris filix-mas,* which is a generic term for a complex of three related species: *Dryopteris filix-mas* (L.) Schott., *D. borrei* Newm. and *D. abbreviata* (Lam. and D.C.). After studying the identification of these ferns, I believe that *asplenon* is likely either *Asplenium adiantum nigrum* L. or *Adiantum capillus veneris* L. or both; that *thelupteris* is *Pteris aquilina* L. and that *filix* is *Dryopteris filix mas.* On the subject of the early-twentieth-century use for these (and related) ferns, see Sayre 1917, pp. 84–86, and more recently, *DUSA,* pp. 121–124, where it is said that the active chemical substances are suspected to be similar among those ferns known as the male fern.
62. Brøndegaard 1973, p. 168.
63. Murthy, Basu, and Murti 1984, pp. 141–144, through *Chemical Abstracts* CA101(3): 17582t. Isoadiantone was isolated from *Adiantum capillus.*
64. Kong, Xie, and But 1986, p. 16.
65. Pliny, *Natural History,* 20.34.86 (cabbage), 34.89 (rue), 54.154 (pennyroyal); 21.84.146 (hulwort), 89.156 (thyme), 22.48.100 (*silphium*), 71.147 (sage), 24.13.22 (*galbanum,* for *Ferula galbaniflua* Boiss. et Buhse); 26.90.153 (lesser century plant and dittany), 90.154 (birthwort), 90.156 (mandrake), 90.159 (artemisia), 90.151 (wormwood), 90.157 (Queen Anne's lace), 90.154 (myrrh and pepper), 90.158 (scammony), and 90.152 (opopanax).
66. Albert-Puleo 1979, pp. 193–195.
67. Pliny, *Natural History,* 20.41.248; cf. *MM,* 2. 128. On the identification of Pliny's *sisymbrium,* see André 1985, p. 241. If, however, the plant is *Nasturtium officinale* L., that plant of the Crassulaceae family has abortifacient qualities (see Farnsworth et al. 1975, p. 561).
68. Pliny, *Natural History,* 20.30.74 (chicory); 22.26.54 (chamomile); 24.20.30 (ground pine); and 26.90.153 (false dittany).
69. Farnsworth et al. 1975, pp. 559 (chicory), 561 (water mint), 564 (false dittany).
70. Verma et al. 1980, pp. 561–564; Gupta, Tank, and Dixit 1985, pp. 262–267, through *Chemical Abstracts* CA107(9): 70981x.
71. Gupta 1985, pp. 262–267; Joshi et al. 1981, pp. 274–280.
72. Kholkute, Mudgal, and Udupa 1977, pp. 35–39. Malva and the hibiscus

plant have close botanical and physical similarities. In this test, *Malva grandiflorus* was also tested with slightly less effective results than the hibiscus.

73. Pliny, *Natural History,* 26.90.151.
74. Ibid., 20.51.139, 52.146; 27.113.139–140. I have found neither medical nor folklore reports on pennycress.
75. Scribonius Largus, *Compositiones,* 121 (Sconocchia ed., p. 64). Also included in recipe were Apollinarus' root and cinnamon, perhaps as a flavoring agent.
76. For the various plants, including mandrake (*Mandragora officinarum* L.), of the Solanaceae family (including henbane, already discussed), see Farnsworth et al. 1975, pp. 546, 553, and 574–575; Duke 1985, pp. 292, 514.
77. Scribonius, *Compositiones,* 106 (p. 57).
78. Ibid. (pp. 57–58).
79. Galen, *De simplicium medicamentorum temperamentis ac facultatibus,* 6.4.15 (Kühn ed., 11:876): the plant is called *epimēdion.*
80. Ibid., 6.4.16 (Kühn ed., 11:876).
81. Ibid., 7.10.16 (Kühn ed., 12:18).
82. Ibid., 6.8.3 (Kühn ed., 11:886).
83. Ibid., 6.8.5 (Kühn ed., 11:886–887); Varma, Vikramaditya, and Gupta 1981, p. 189, where the death carrot is reported to exert "a strong contracting effect on the uterus of guinea pigs." *Thlaspia* is probably death carrot (*Thlaspi garganica* L.), although field pennycress or shepherd's purse may be indicated as well (*T. avense* L., var. *T. burse-pastoris*).
84. Galen, *De simpl. med. temp. ac fac.,* 6.2.15 (Kühn ed., 11:854: *brathu* is probably *Juniper sabina*) and 7.10.16 (12:18).
85. Ibid., 7.11.11 (Kühn ed., 12:58–59); cf. *MM,* 3.6): *Cheiranthus cheiri* and/or *Matthiola incana.*
86. Galen, *De simpl. med. temp. ac fac.,* 7.10.17 (Kühn ed., 12:19); *MM,* 3.6).
87. Galen, *De simpl. med. temp. ac fac.,* 7.10.61 (Kühn ed., 12:50–51); *MM,* 2.165).
88. Galen, *De simpl. med. temp. ac fac.,* 8.13.7 (Kühn ed., 12:89); *MM,* 3.131.
89. Galen, *De simpl. med. temp. ac fac.,* 8.18.15 (Kühn ed.,12:122–123); *MM,*4.150, clearly as suppository.
90. Galen, *De simpl. med. temp. ac fac.,* 9.18.30–32 (Kühn ed., 12:127–128); *MM,* 1.64–65.
91. Galen, *De simpl. med. temp. ac fac.,* 8.18.37 (Kühn ed., 12:130); *MM,* 3.106, as suppository.
92. Galen, *De simpl. med. temp. ac fac.,* 8.18.37 (Kühn ed., 12:97); *MM,* 3.80 (as compound with *silphium*/Ferula).
93. Galen, *De simpl. med. temp. ac fac.,* 8.16.4 (Kühn ed., 12:95); *MM,*3.48.
94. Possibly *Polystichum filix mas* Roth. or *S. trichomanes* L. in André 1985, p. 210, or *Pteris aquilina;* Galen, *De simpl. med. temp. ac fac.,* 8.16.39 (Kühn ed., 12:109); cf. *MM,* 4.184.
95. *MM,* 4.150; Farnsworth et al. 1975, p. 549.
96. Galen, *De simpl. med. temp. ac fac.,* 7.10.1 (Kühn ed., 12:6); cf. *MM,* 3.35 (3.2).
97. Galen, *De simpl. med. temp. ac fac.,* 6.3.7 (Kühn ed., 11:857).

98. Ibid., 6.9.8 (Kühn ed., 11:891).
99. Galen, *De compositione medicamentorum secundum locus*, 9.4 (Kühn ed., 13:283–284). The second recipe Galen attributed to Scribonius Largus; I cannot find it, however, in Scribonius' text as we have it.
100. Galen, *De simpl. med. temp. ac fac.*, 7.11.777 (Kühn ed., 12:59).
101. Ibid., 8.18.16 (Kühn ed., 12:123).
102. Ibid., 5.23 (Kühn ed., 11:777); and 8.16.18 (12:101).
103. Galen, *De remediis parabilibus*, 2.20 (Kühn ed., 14:480–481): κατάπλασμα φθόριον (with aloes); 2.21 (Kühn, 14:20): κ. ὥστε φθεῖραι (with cypress leaves); 14.18 (Kühn, 14:480): πότημα ἐκβόλιον ἐμβρύου (with almonds, juniper, artemisia, and Phoenician stones); *De antidotis*, 2.9 (Kühn, 14:165)—the last two have many ingredients.
104. Galen, *De antidotis*, 2.1 (Kühn ed., 14:114–115).
105. Ibid. (Kühn ed., 14:109–110); see also 2.9 (14:152–154).
106. Galen, *De naturalibus facultatibus*, 3.12 (Brock ed. 1952); *Hippocratis Epidem. II. et Galeni in illum commentarius III*, 6.27 (Kühn ed., 17, pt. 1, p. 438); similarly the same subject is discussed in the Pseudo-Galenic treatise *Hippocratis De humoribus liber et Galeni in eum commentarii tres. I* (Kühn ed., 16:180–181).
107. *Hippocratis Epidem. II. et Galeni in illum commentarius II* (Kühn ed., 17[1]:634–636).

9. The Late Roman Empire and Early Middle Ages

1. Riddle 1987, pp. 33–61; Himes 1936, p. 100.
2. See Lacey, James, and Short 1988, p. 9.
3. Bennetts, Underwood, and Shier, (1946), pp. 2–12. See also J. B. Harborne, chap. 5, n. 39, 1977 ed., pp. 83–89.
4. Bounds and Pope 1960, pp. 3695–3705; see also Harborne 1982, p. 102.
5. Theophrastus, *Enquiry into Plants*, 9.20.3 (Hort, ed. and trans., 2:317).
6. Riddle 1984, pp. 408–429.
7. Martialis, *Medicinae ex oleribus et pomis*, 3 (Rose ed., p. 137; trans. by Tapper, p. 26).
8. Oribasius, *Books of Eunapius*, 4.114.777–778 (Raeder ed., 6, pt. 3, pp. 488–489).
9. Oribasius, *Eunapius [Euporistes]*, 2.1.Λ.3–4 (Daremberg and Bussemaker ed., 5:624–625; Raeder ed., 6, pt. 3, 370); 2.1.Σ.13–17 (D-B., 5:635; R., 6, pt. 3, 378).
10. Ibid., 2.1.A.57–61 (D-B, 5:603; R., 6, pt. 3, 352–353); 2.1.K.37 (D-B, 5:618; R., 6, pt. 3, 365); 2.1.K.59–62: ἔμβρυα ἐκβάλλειν); 2.1.A.37 (D-B, 5:618); 2.1.Σ.36–38 (D-B, 5:637; R. 6, pt. 3, 380).
11. Ibid., 2.1.K.104–105 (D-B, 5:624; R, 6, pt. 3, 369).
12. Oribasius, *Synopsis ad Eunapium*, 2.53 (Daremberg and Bussemaker ed., 5:68; Raeder ed., 6, pt. 3, p. 43).
13. Cf. *MM*, 3.86, and Galen, *De simpl. med. temp. ac fac.*, 6.3.5 (Kühn ed., 11:857).
14. *MM*, 1.16 (1.7).

15. Oribasius, *Synopsis ad Eunapium*, 2.1.K.37 (D-B, 5:618; R, 6, pt. 3, 365).
16. Ibid., 2.53 (D-B, 5:68; R, 6, pt. 3, p. 43).
17. Oribasius, *Libri ad Eunapium*, 4.116 (D-B, 5:777–778; R., 6, pt. 3, 488–489), cf. *MM*, 3.130 (1.6).
18. *Dioscoride latino Materia medica libro primo*, 1. QA (Mihäescu ed., p. 48): "Folia eius bibita post purgationem menstruorum simili modo minime conceptum admittit, . . ."
19. *MM*, 2.159 (3.4–5): ἄγει καὶ ἔμβρυα. ἀτόκιον δὲ εἶναι δοκεῖ μετὰ συνουσίαν προστιθέμενον.
20. *De materia medica*, 2.PME (Hermann Stadler, ed., *Römanische Forschungen* 10 [1897]: 233).
21. *MM*, 2.156 (2.4); Stadler, 10:232; cf. virtually the same in *De materia medica*, 2.ΠΛΓΠ (Stadler, 10:432).
22. Oribasius, *Ecologae medicamentorum*, 632 (Raeder ed., 6, pt. 2, fasc. 2, p. 302).
23. Oribasius, *Synopsis* (Mørland ed., pp. 75, 118, 148).
24. Ibid., 2. (Mørland ed., p. 148): "artemisia trita et puleiu et centauria et thimu et ruta et alia omnia qui tali sunt virtute."
25. Marcellus, *De medicamentis*, 20.10–14 et passim (Niedermann ed.).
26. Cf. *MM*, 1.11 (2.3), which says that the plant provokes menstruation.
27. Marcellus, *De medicamentis*, 20.33 (Niedermann ed., pt. 2, 340).
28. Marcellus, *De mensuris et ponderibus medicinalibus ex graeco translatus iuxta Hippocratem* (Niedermann ed., 1:10). The treatise is likely Pseudo-Marcellus.
29. Ibid., 29:11 (Niedermann ed., pt. 2, 506).
30. Quintas Serenus Sammonicus, *Liber medicinalis*, 32.618.632 (Pépin ed., p. 34). The text is corrupt at this point (see Vollmer ed., p. 31). Pépin's text reads: "At qui olim menses minus octo moratus in aluo est. Inrumpit thalamos et nexus soluit inertes. Puleium ex acido bene conuenit imbre tepenti. Cuius opem veram casus mihi saepe probarunt." Pépin translates "Inrumpit thalamos et nexus soluit inertes" as "rompt ses liens relâchés et rompt," but to me the sense of "nexus" points to a "weakened [fetus]," which is, as we have seen, a circumlocution as a reason to abort. Vivian Nutton suggests that the phrase "inrumpit thalamos" (hence, rush into the bedroom) may mean "has broken the inner chambers"—that is, the fetal sac. While he may be correct in this interpretation, it seems to me that the bursting of the sac *before eight months* is unlikely. If the condition were a premature birth, there would be no medical activity possible to the Roman to reverse the action.
31. Ibid., 32.615–618 (Pépin ed., p. 34).
32. For instance, Paul of Aegina [*Libri Medicorum*], 3.59–61 (Heiberg ed., 1:274–277); and Latin translation of bks. 1–3, in *Pauli Aeginetae libri tertii interpretation Latina antiqua*, 3.249 (Heiberg ed.).
33. Theodorus Priscianus, *Euporiston*, 3.6 (Wellmann ed., p. 240).
34. Ibid.
35. Ibid. (pp. 241–244).
36. Green 1985, pp. 156, 204–205, 227 and passim.

37. Aëtius, *Biblia iatrika*, 16.16 (Zervòs ed., p. 18); trans. by Hines 1936, p. 94: Ἀτόκιον δὲ φθορίου τὸ μὲν γὰρ ἀτόκιον οὐκ ἐᾷ γίγνεσθαι σύλληψιν, τὸ φθόριον φθείρει τὸ συλληφθὲν καὶ ἐκβάλλει.

38. Temkin, *Soranus' Gynecology* 1956, p. xliii; Ricci, *Aetios of Amida* 1950, pp. 5–6. Surviving works by Philumenos are published by Wellmann, 1907.

39. Theophrastus, *On Stones,* 62 (Caley and Richards trans. and comm., pp. 58–59).

40. André 1985, pp. 186–187.

41. Soranus, *Gynecology,* 1.62 (Ilberg ed., pp. 46–47; guided by Temkin trans., pp. 64–65).

42. Aëtius, *Biblia iatrika,* 16.17 (Zervòs ed., pp. 18–19; guided by Ricci trans. p. 25).

43. Murphy et al. 1977, p. 196.

44. On oak galls, see Sayre 1917, pp. 141–143, and *DUSA,* pp. 1772–73; *MM,* 1.107 (2.1–2).

45. *MM,* 1.26.

46. Saha 1961, pp. 149–150.

47. The use of copper is discussed in Chapter 8 above; on a connection between pregnancy and iron, see Loewit, Zambelis and Egg 1971, pp. 91–96. Dioscorides (*MM,* 5.80 [1.2]) says that iron causes inconception (ἀσυλλημψ-σίαν).

48. *MM,* 5.88; Galen, *De comp. med. per genera,* 1.12 (Kühn ed., 13:413); in *De simpl. med. temp. ac fac.,* 9.3.39 (Kühn ed., 12:243–244), Galen discussed the medicinal uses of white lead.

49. Aëtius, *Biblia iatrika,* 16.17.

50. Ibid. (Zervòs ed., p. 20)—relying on Zervòs' reading, n. 2.

51. Ibid.

52. The same sitz bath prescription is given in Soranus, *Gynaecology,* 64 (Ilberg ed., p. 48).

53. *MM,* 2.102 (1.6) on fenugreek in a vaginal suppository as a mollifying agent, and 3.113 (2.5–6) on artemisia as an emmenagogue and abortifacient. Marshmallow (3.146) has gynecology usages but none specifically for antifertility.

54. Aëtius, *Biblia iatrika,* 16.18 (Zervòs ed., pp. 21–22; Ricci trans., p. 26).

55. Ibid. (Zervòs ed., pp. 21–22; Ricci trans. pp. 26–27). With some technical changes I have followed Ricci's translation.

56. Hippocrates, *Aphorisms,* 5.31 (Jones ed., 4:166–167): Γυναικὶ ἐν γαστρὶ ἔχουσα, φλεβοτομηθεῖσα, ἐκτιτρώσκει ("A woman with child, if bled, miscarries").

57. Curiously, Dioscorides (*MM,* 4.189) said that it is a laxative and related a folk story that leaves of the female mercury boiled and eaten after menstruation ceases will cause the conception of a female; similarly, the same procedure with a male mercury plant will cause conception of a male. The attribution of sexuality to plants is common and often distinguishes species of the same plant.

58. LS, s.v., identifies this as a tree fungus (*Boletus agaricum*). The agaric in

modern (i.e., early twentieth century) pharmacy is from the fern *Polyporus officinalis* Fries (Sayre 1917, p. 82). It is also a laxative.

59. Aëtius, *Biblia iatrika,* 16.18 (Zervòs ed., p. 22; Ricci trans., p. 27—with technical changes made).

60. Hippocrates, *Aphorisms,* 5.34, 36 (Jones ed., 4:166–167).

61. The word here is γληχωνίτης, which LS, s.v., says is a wine prepared with γλήχων, which is a synonym for βλήχων (s.v.), the word used by Aristophanes for pennyroyal. But βλήχων is the male fern (= *Aspidium filix-mas*). With a possibility for confusion, the evidence points to pennyroyal here (*MM,* 4.169; André 1985, p. 36).

62. Green 1985, pp. 156–164.

63. I have used the sixteenth-century printed edition that was edited by Wolf and Gesner, in *Gynaeciorum hoc est De mulierum tum aliis* (1556), col. 28, with the chapter title "Ad absorsum proficiendum, et menstrua provocanda pessarium, quod et mortuum pecus potest foras detraher re." Early manuscripts of Cleopatra's text include Brussels, Royale De Belgique cod. 5649–67, s. 10, fols. 28v-31v, and Florence, Laurentiana, MS 73, 1, s. 9–10, fols. 149v-155r. For other manuscripts, see Augusto Beccaria 1956, s.v.

64. André 1985, p. 28, proposes three plants that the name referred to: *Psoralea bituminosa* L., *Polygnonum aviculare* L., and *Potentilla reptans* L. He believes the last of these three is the plant to which Pseudo-Apuleius referred and that Pseudo-Apuleius would have lived a little earlier, most probably, than Cleopatra but still have been close to the same time. Gunther (*Dioscorides,* p.20) believes that Dioscorides' *aspalathos* (*MM,* 1.20) is either *Cytisus lanigerus* or *Genista acanthoclad.* When identifications are so uncertain, it would be too speculative to explore possible effects.

65. Cleopatra, *Gynaecology* (Gesner-Wolf ed., cols. 28–29). The text gives one abortifacient fumigant—castoreum, applied to the nose.

66. Paul of Aegina (Paulus Aegineta), *Libri medicorum,* 3.60.12.29–34 (Heiberg ed., 1:274–275).

67. Ibid., 3.61.1–5, esp. 5.1–5 (Heiberg ed., 1:275–276).

68. Ibid., 3.61.5.26–28 (Heiberg ed., 1:276).

69. Duke 1985, pp. 408–409; Farnsworth et al. 1975, p. 737.

70. Paul, *Libri medicorum,* 7.3. s.v. (Heiberg ed., 2:251, 23–27).

71. For these emmenagogues, see ibid., 7.3., at *daucos* and *staphylinos* (both are carrots, presumably the same, *Daucus carrota*; Heiberg ed., 2:206, 14 and 2:262, 2), *elaterium* (squirting cucumber; 2:209, 6–7), *erpyllos* (wild thyme; 2:211, 22), *erythrodanon* (common madder [*Rubia tinctorum* L., fam. Rosaceae]; 2:211, 25, cf. *MM,* 3.143 [2.7–8], *thlaspi* (2:216, 6), *kapparis* (caper; 2:222, 5–6), *kassia* (*Cinnamomum cassia* L.?; 2:222, 5–6) *koris* and *hyperikon* (two species of St. John's wort, including *Hypericum coris* L. and probably *H. crispum* L.; 2:229, 20 and 2:269, 6), *costos* (costus; 2:230, 11), *crocodilium* (*Eryngium maritimum?* 2:231, 28, cf. *MM,* 3.21 [2.6–7]), *kyperos* (cyperus; 2:233,10), *leukoïon* (wall flower or stock; 2:235, 20), *ligystikon* (lovage [*Levisticum officinale* Koch]; 2:236, 22, cf. *MM,* 3.51 [2.10], as abortifacient), *melanthion* (love-in-a-mist) [*Nigella sa-*

tiva L.], 2:240, 29, cf. *MM*, 3.79 [2.8]), *mēon* (spignel [*Meum athamanti-cum* Jacq. fam Umbell., as emmenagogue]; 2:242, 19), *myrra* and *smyrna*—both myrrhs (2:244, 12 and 2:261, 10), *onosma* (2:247, 9–10), *panakes* (opoponax; 2:250,14), *polion* (hulwort) [*Teucrium polium* L. fam. Labiatae]; 2:253, 12), *selinion* (2:257, 31–32), *sisōn* (stone parsley; 2:259, 23, cf. *MM*, 2.128 [3.10?], *skammōnia* (2:260, 2—as suppository) *smyrnia* (alexanders [*Smyrnium* sp.]; 2:261, 10, cf. *MM*, 23.68 [2.8]), *stachys* (annual woundwort [*Stachys annua* L. fam. Labiatae]; 2:263, 17, cf. *MM*, 1.66 [3.2]), *styrax* (storax [*Styrax officinale* L.]; 1:96 [1. 7–8]), *philyras* (phillyrea [*Phillyrea latifolia* L., *P. medica* L. fam. Oleaceae]; 2:270, 10–11, cf. *MM*, 1.96 [1.7–8]), *chamaidrys* (2:271, 19), and *chrysokomē* (aster [*Aster linosyris* Bernh.†, 2:273, 19–20, cf. *MM*, 4.55 [1.8]). Those plants for which a reference to Dioscorides is given are encountered for the first time in this book but were specified by Dioscorides as emmenagogues and/or abortifacients.

72. Ibid., 7.3, at *kentaurion* (century plant; Heiberg ed., 2:223, 1–2), *konyza* (fleabane; 2:228, 9), *leukoïon* (wallflower or stock; 2:235, 22), *myrra* (2:244, 12), *onosma* (golden drop; 2:247, 9–10), and *pteris* (fern; 2:255, 1–2).

73. Jöchle 1974, pp. 432–433.

74. *MM*, 4.55 (1.8): πρὸς κάθαρσιν ὑστέρας.

75. Pseudo-Apuleius, *Herbarius* (Howald and Sigerist eds.), nos. 10–12 (artemisia), 19 (birthwort), 34 (great century), and 77 (filix). The fertility plants are 90 (rue), 93 (pennyroyal), 114 (squirting cucumber), and 116 (rue).

76. Ibid., nos. 83, 88, and 93.

77. Duke 1985, p. 309.

78. Farnsworth et al. 1975, p. 553.

79. Prakash et al. 1985, p. 447 (under pomegranate).

80. *Ex herbis femininis*, nos. 12, 16, 28, 45–46, and 63 (Kästner ed., pp. 578–636). Cf. *MM*, 3.4; 2.156; 3.121; 2.166; 4.176; 3.48; see Riddle 1981, pp. 43–81.

81. *Ex herbis*, no. 28 (Kästner ed., p. 608): "sucus earum cum lana genitalibus iniectus abortionem praegnantibus facit."

82. Jöchle 1974, p. 429.

83. *Ex herbis*, no. 8 (Kästner ed., p. 595): "menstrua quoque evocant et fetus e matrice mortuos." See *MM*, 3.98 (2.1).

84. Ibid., nos. 55, 58 (Kästner ed., pp. 629–630, 31); *MM*, 2:163; 3:123.

85. Cockayne (1864, 1:164–169) identifies the plant *dictamnum* as *Diptamnus alba,* but André (1985, pp. 88–89) says that in Pseudo-Apuleius it is *Organum dictamnus* L. Dioscorides' *diktamnon* is *Organum dictamnus.*

86. Pseudo-Apuleius, no. 62 (Howald-Sigerist ed., pp. 116–117); cf. *MM*, 3.32.

87. *Herbarium Apulei*, nos. 89 (Cockyne ed., 1:192), 94 (1:206), 143 (1:266), and 158 (1:286).

88. *Herbarium Apulei*, nos. 175 (Cockyne ed., 1:308); 158 (1:312); cf. *MM*, 4.36, 93.

89. Sharma et al. 1983, p. 185; for modern medical reports, see Duke 1985, p. 502.

90. Farnsworth et al. 1975, p. 559.

91. Duke 1985, p. 10.
92. Bamberg MS L.III.6, fol. 54, in Sigerist 1923, p. 25.
93. Karlsruhe, Badische Landesbibliothek MS 120, fol. 3 r&v, in Sigerist 1923, p. 43.
94. Glasgow, University Library, s. ix-x, fol. 164 (Sigerist 1923, p. 140).
95. Riddle 1965, pp. 185–198.
96. Degen 1981, p. 135; Schleifer 1926, pp. 70–122, 161–195.
97. *Book of Medicines* (Budge ed. and trans., 2:297–298).
98. Ibid., 2:485. There is a third recipe for a plaster made of euphorbium (spurge), Queen Anne's lace, seeds of gourd (*Ecballium elatarium?*), cardamom, opopanax, peppercorns, squill, and oil of nard or roses, which is said to provoke a menstrual flow (2:440–441).
99. Hrabanus Maurus, *De universo,* 19.11 (herbs), 6 (trees) (*PL,* 111, cols. 517–520, 532 passim).
100. Walafrid Strabo, *Hortulus* (*PL* 114, col. 1123 and passim).

10. The Middle Ages: The Church, Macer, and Hildegard

1. Added to the margin in another hand to Vienna MS med. gr. 16, s. xv, and several other manuscripts including Vatican Palat. Ms 77, s. xiv, and printed in the critical aparatus to *MM,* 3.45 (Wellmann ed., 2:59).
2. Peter of Padua, Gloss, printed in Latin Alphabetical Dioscorides (Colle, 1478), s.v. Asarus: "alia viridis herba ab asaros iam tacto quem autem sit ante coitum videtur ignorari."
3. Dioscorides, gloss to 2.125 (Wellmann ed., 1:198).
4. Hippocrates, *Disease of Women,* 1.75.14–15 (Littré ed., 8:166).
5. Brøndegaard 1973, p. 168.
6. Farnsworth et al. 1975, p. 544.
7. Lewin 1922, p. 85.
8. *Pactus legis salicae,* 19.4 (1962, p. 82), cited in Noonan 1986, p. 156.
9. Below 1953, pp. 126–128.
10. *Lex Alamannorum,* 91 (Lewin 1922, p. 85).
11. *Lex Bajuvariorum,* 7.18 (Lewin, p. 86).
12. *Leges Wisigothorum* (c. 600–700), 6.3.1–7 (Lewin 1922, p. 87).
13. *Lex frisionum,* 5.1 (*MGH,* 12:46).
14. Regino of Prüm, *Churchly Disciplines,* 2.89 (*PL,* 132:301, translated in Noonan 1986, p. 168).
15. Burchard, *Decretum,* 17.57 (*PL,* 140:933): "Si aliquis causa explendae libidinis, vel odii meditatione, ut non ex eo soboles nascatur, homini, aut mulieri aliquid fecerit, vel ad potandum dederit, ut non possit generare, aut concipere, ut homicida teneatur." Also, he said: "Excussisti conceptum tuum antequam vivificaretur? Si fecisti, unum annum per legitimas ferias poenitere debes: fecisti post conceptum spiritum, tres annos per legitimas ferias poenitere debes" (p. 972).
16. Noonan 1986, p. 169: "Fecisti quod quaedam mulieres facere solent, quae dum fornicantur et parus suos necare volunt, agunt ut utero conceptus excutiant suis maleficiis et suis herbis, vel si nondum conceperunt, faciunt ut non concipiant?"

17. Burchard, *Decretum* (PL, 140:972).
18. Columban, *Paenitentiale*, B6 (Bieler 1963, p. 100); cf. Noonan 1986, p. 157.
19. Columban, *Paenitentiale*, 7 (p. 110).
20. Caesarius, *Sermons*, 1.12 (Mueller, 1:13); Noonan 1986, p. 146.
21. Columban, *Paenitentiale*, B6 (p. 110).
22. Martin of Braga, *Canones*, 77 (Barlow 1950, p. 142) and attributed to Ancyra 21: "De mulieribus fornicariis et abortum facientibus. Si qua mulier fornicaverit et infantem qui exinde fuerit natus occiderit, et quae studuerit abortum facere et quod conceptum est necare aut certe ut non concipiat elaborat, sive ex adulterio sive ex legitima coniugio, has tales mulieres in mortem recipere communionem priores canones decreverunt"; cf. Noonan 1986, p. 149.
23. Noonan 1986, pp. 162–170 and passim.
24. Pseudo-Bede, *Order for Giving Penance*, 30; cited in Noonan 1986, p. 156.
25. Burchard, *Decretum*, 19 (PL, 140:972): "Nam quoties conceptum impedierat, tot homicidiorum rea erit. Se distat multum, utrum paupercula sit, et pro difficultate nutriendi, vel fornicaria causa, et pro sui sceleris caelandi faciat"; Pseudo-Bede, *Penitential*, 2.11 (ascribed by Albers to Bede and printed McNeill and Gamer 1938, p. 225); cf. Noonan 1986, p. 160.
26. Text published in Lewin 1922, p. 84, citing *Monumenta veteris liturgiae alemannicae*, ed. Gerbertus 1779, vol. 2, *Judicium poenitentis*, p. 20.
27. *Canones Hibernenses*, 1.8 (1938, p. 119).
28. *Old Irish Penitential*, 5.5–6 (1938, p. 166).
29. Dunstan trans. 1988, p. 42.
30. Noonan 1986, pp. 171–199.
31. Augustine, *De nuptiis*, 2.20 (CSEL 1986, 42:272–273).
32. Mundy 1985, 1990; Bogomils or Cathars were sometimes called Sodomites.
33. Noonan 1986, p. 171.
34. Ivo, *Decretum*, 10.55 (PL, 161; 706: "Aliquando eo usque pervenit haec libidinosa crudelitas vel libido crudelis, ut etiam sterilitatis venena procuret, et si nihil valuerint, conceptos fetus aliquo modo intra viscera exstinguat ac fundat, volendo suam prolem prius interire quam vivere, aut si in uetero vivebat, occidi antequam nasci. Prorsus si ambo [tales sibi, orig.] sunt, conjuges non sunt, et si ab initio tales fuerunt non per connubium, sed per stuprum potius convenerunt. Si autem ambo non sunt tales, audeo dicere: Aut illa est quodammodo mariti meretrix aut ille adulter uxoris."
35. Riddle 1977.
36. Macer Floridus, in *Aemilius Macer De herbarum virtutibus cum Joannis Atrociani commentariis* (1530), fol. 1: "Pellit abortuum potu, vel subdita tantum." See also Flood 1968.
37. Ibid., fols. 9v, 29v, 33v, 40, 45v, 48v, 50v, 59, 65, 66v, 77, 78v, 95, 96, 96v.
38. André 1985, p. 171, points to both species. Dioscorides (*MM*, 3.35) has *kalaminthē* as an abortifacient, but Macer's plant may not be the same plant. In any case, Macer's *nepeta* is certainly of the mint family.
39. Macer, *De herbarum virtutibus*, fol. 35.

40. Ibid., fol. 38.
41. Ibid., fols. 19, 35, 38, 47, 48, 49v, 53, 61v, 73, 76v, 81, 82, 83, 85, 86v.
42. Ibid., fols. 53, 45v.
43. Flood 1968, p. 179 and passim.
44. Facciolatus 1828, s.v. *depello, pello; OLD,* s.v.
45. To be sure, Macer was using medieval Latin, not the classical meanings. Macer used the phrase "depellit odorem" (fol. 94v), whose meaning was "to drive away an odor." Nicolaus Mutonus, the Latin translator of Serapion the Elder's work, for instance, translates "ventris lumbricos pellit" as "it drives worms from the intestines." To have it mean "it prevents worms" is too much to expect of medieval medicine. (See Ibn Serapion = Ibn Sarābi, *De simplicium medicamentorum* [Venice, 1552], fol. 20.)
46. Macer, *De herbarum virtutibus,* fol. 75v.: "Matrici succus si subditur illius ante / Quam fiat coitus mulier non concipit inde."
47. Ibid., fol. 30v.
48. Aristotle, *Historia animalium,* 7.3.583b.
49. For example, in Fischer 1927.
50. Fischer 1929, p. 261.
51. *Physica,* no. 42 *(PL,* 198:1148).
52. Ibid., 47 *(PL,* 197:1148).
53. Ibid., 111 *(PL,* 197:1174). For a report of tansy's folklore use as an emmenagogue and abortifacient, see Conway 1979, p. 257.
54. Duke 1985, p. 474. The examples of ecbolic (s.v.) given in *Taber* are cotton root, ergot, and tansy. On ecbolics, see Rall 1990, pp. 933–953.
55. *Physica,* 116 *(PL,* 197:1177). Fischer 1929, p. 264, identifies *metra* as *Pyrethrum parthenium* D.C. and *sichterwurtz alba* as white hellebore, or *Veratrum album* L. (p. 287).
56. *Physica,* 130 *(PL,* 197:183).
57. Ibid., 34, *(PL,* 197:1143): "Sed et praegnantem mulierum cum periculo corporis sui abortire facit, si eum comederit." *Hirtzswam,* or *Hirschtrüffel* in modern German, is identified supposedly as *Elacagnus angustifola* L. Hildegard's plant could also be *Polypodium singaporianum* or various varieties of ferns.

11. Salerno and Medicine through the Twelfth Century

1. Especially significant in the exaggeration of Salerno is Salvatore De Renzi, who collected and published medical documents and thereby attributed many marginal items only tangentially connected with Salerno and frequently not with a "school" (see De Renzi 1857). The assertion by Charles Homer Haskins (1957, p. 65 and passim) and often repeated that Salerno represented the first university is clearly untrue.
2. Constantine, *De coitus liber* 1536, p. 305.
3. Ibid., pp. 345–346, 348, 351.
4. Ibid., pp. 355, 358–360, 362–363, 365–366.
5. Fischer 1929, p. 269; André 1985, p. 136.
6. Constantine, *De gradibus* 1536, pp. 367–369, 371–380.

7. Ibid., pp. 382, 384, 386.
8. Ibid., p. 358.
9. Ibid., p. 359.
10. Ibid., p. 377.
11. Ibid., p. 386.
12. As noted in McLaren 1984, p. 74.
13. Green 1990, pp. 50–51. Although the translation was made by Green from the French translation by Ben Yahia, she acknowledges the translation services of El Hamel Chouki, who checked the passage in the Arabic text from Paris, BN, Ms arabe 2884.
14. Ibid., p. 51.
15. Ibid., p. 52.
16. Ibid., p. 53.
17. Saha, Savini, and Kasinathan 1961, p. 149.
18. Ibid., p. 136.
19. *MM*, 3.82, discussed various species of spurge, but he gave no antifertility usages.
20. Constantine, *De gradibus*, p. 379.
21. Kristeller 1945, p. 169.
22. *Regimen sanitatis Salernitanum*, 14 (De Renzi 1852–59, 1:462): "Pellit abortivum potu vel subdita tantum."
23. Ibid., 13–14, 16 (1:462).
24. Ibid., 72, (4:468).
25. *De aegritudinum curatione* (De Renzi 1852–59, 2:340–346).
26. Ibid. (2:348).
27. Ibid. (2:344–345).
28. Ibid. (2:332).
29. Ibid. (2:340).
30. *De secretis mulierum*, 24 (De Renzi 1852–59, 4:15).
31. *MM*, 3.62 (2.1). The identification of *Carum copticum* is by André (1985, p. 14), whereas Robert Gunther (1934, p. 304) postulates *Ammi visnaga*. The medieval plant is almost certainly *Ammi maius* (Fischer 1929, p. 259).
32. Farnsworth et al. 1975, p. 597; Jöchle 1974, p. 429.
33. Found in commentary to *De secretis mulierum* (Lyon ed. 1580). The text was supplied to me by Helen Lemay.
34. This may be a type of shrimp (as *stincus* means), or it could be an error, as I consider more likely, for *stercus tauri*, or bull shit.
35. Candidates for the medieval *polycaria* are *Plantago psyllium* L. (plantan), *Policaria dysenterica*, and *Sedum telephium* L. (See Fischer 1929, pp. 279–280, 284.)
36. Petrus Maranchus, *Tabula* (De Renzi 1852–59, 4:564). Pliny *Natural History*, 25.54.95) says that Latin writers call birthwort (*aristolochia*) "earth apples." I assume that Petrus meant the same. (Later, potatoes from the New World were called "earth apples.")
37. I am uncertain as to the meaning here. It may not be a plant but instructions for preparation (cooking) that Petrus or a scribe confused.
38. The text has *cantaris*, which is obviously an error for *centauria*.

39. Petrus Maranchus, *Tabula* (De Renzi 1852–59, 4:565).
40. Ibid.
41. Benton 1985, pp. 30–53.
42. Green 1989, pp. 434–473.
43. Trotula, [*Gynecology*] 1566, cols. 222–223.
44. Ibid., col. 223.
45. Ibid., col. 274.
46. Matthaeus Platearius, *Circa instans,* fols. 87, 92v in Erlangen MS 674, and published in Wölfel 1939, pp. 87 (opopanax), 103 (rue).
47. Ibid., fols. 58 r&v (pp. 13, 15).
48. Ibid., fols. 56v, 80v, 55v (pp. 9, 73, 7).
49. Ibid., fol. 81v (p. 74).
50. Ibid., fol. 82v (p. 77).
51. Ibid., fol. 85 (pp. 82–83).

12. Islam, Arabic Medicine, and the Late Middle Ages

1. Musallam 1983, chap. 7, n. 5, passim.
2. Ibid., p. 54.
3. Ibid., pp. 54–59.
4. Ibid., p. 77. The scientific identifications are given for plants in ibn Sina (pp. 146–147), but I am assuming that the same identifications would be found in Razi.
5. *MM,* 2.164–165 (2.6–9).
6. Maimonides, *Glossary of Drug Names,* 209 (Rosner ed., pp. 145–146). Musallam (1983, p. 147) identifies the plant as *Luffa cylindrica* without author.
7. *MM,* 2.166 (2.3–4 and 3.5). Interestingly the sixth-century Latin translation omitted abortificient qualities in this chapter but included them for another variety of arum in the preceding chapter (see *Dioscorides Longobardus,* 2. PNΓ in *Römanische Forschungen* 10 (1897): 237–238.
8. Steinegger and Hänsel 1968, p. 433 (see chap. 4, n. 82 above).
9. Himes (1936, pp. 142–43) commissioned Max Meyerhof to do a translation, which he sent to Himes from Cairo in 1924. Meyerhof introduced comments of his own and asked Himes to put his translation into readable English. In this spirit, I have taken the liberty that Meyerhof gave Himes to make changes based on a comparison of his translation with the Latin translation by Gerard of Cremona. Meyerhof was a physician who became infatuated with medieval Arabic medicine, especially pharmacy. In order to identify plants and other materials of medicine, he would go to the markets in Cairo and talk with the sellers about usages and nomenclature. Over the years, I have come to value highly Meyerhof's insights.
10. Thus, ibn Sina is accepting Galen's and Hippocrates' position that women as well as men have seed that contribute toward conception and rejects the position of Aristotle that women only provide nourishment. See discussion below in Chapter 13.
11. From Hippocrates, see Chapter 1 above.

12. Ibid.

13. Meyerhof said that the word here is *fuanaj,* a Persian loanword into Arabic for pennyroyal; Gerard of Cremona translated it as *calaminti,* or calamint.

14. Musallam 1983, pp. 67–70, 84, 146–147.

15. ʿArib ibn Saʿid, *Kitab khalq,* 7 (Jahier and Abdulkader trans., p. 50; Castro trans., p. 93).

16. Abu l-Fadl Dawud ibn Abi l-Bayan al-Israʾili, *Al-Dustur al-bimaristani fi l-adwiya al-murakkada,* 8.124 (José Luius Valverde Carmen Peña Muñoz trans. p. 87).

17. al-Samarquandi, *Medical Formulary* (Levey and al-Khaledy trans., p. 64).

18. Ibid., pp. 66–67, 85–87.

19. al-Razi (Rasis) *Ad regem mansorem,* 5.73 (Gerard of Cremona trans., p. 140).

20. al-Razi, *Antidotis,* 44 (Gerard of Cremona trans., pp. 479–480).

21. Fischer 1929, p. 269.

22. Mesuë, *Canones universales,* 2.1 (fols. 32–34).

23. Ibid., fol. 41r&v.

24. Ibid., fol. 47.

25. Ibid., fol. 52v.

26. Ibid., fol. 56v.

27. Ibid., fol. 58.

28. Yuhya ibn Sarafyun (the elder), *De simpli (cibus) medi (cinis)* (fol. 124v).

29. Ibid., fol. 133.

30. Ibid., fol. 119v.

31. Ibid.

32. Ibid., fol. 125; cf. *MM,* 1.81 (1.3).

33. Ibid., fol. 140r&v.

34. Ibid., fols. 141v, 146, 152v, 161v; cf. *MM,* 3.72 (2.6).

35. Ibid., fol. 164.

36. Ibn Sarafyun (The younger), *De simplicium medicamentorum,* 1 (fol. 8).

37. Ibid.

38. Ibid., 2, fol. 10v.

39. Ibid., 2, fol. 19: (populus albus) "creditur idem potus cum muli renibus, sterilitatem facere"; fol. 20 (brassica flowers) "faciunt sterilitatem. Semen autem in pessulis appositum sterilitatem efficit"; fol. 25 (ivy) "drachmae pondere a purgatione foeminis poti, steriliatem faciunt."

40. Ibid., 2.72, fol. 25.

41. Ibid., 2.92, fol. 30.

42. Ibid., 2.93, fol. 30v.

43. Ibid., 2.95, fol. 30v.

44. Ibid., 4.81, fol. 107.

45. Ibid., 2.201, fol. 53v.

46. Siraisi 1987.

47. Avicenna, *Canon,* bk. 3., fen. 21, tract. 1 (Gerard of Cremona trans. [1557], 2, fol. 388v).

48. Avicenna, *Canon,* bk. 3, fen. 21, tract. 1, chaps. 9–11 on sterility; tract. 2, chaps. 12–14 on abortion (chap. 12: "De regimine abortus et extractione

fetus mortui"), chapter 17 on conditions to avoid pregnancy, which includes a suppository with elephant dung. Another way in which contraceptive and abortifacient information was related is in book 2, tractatus 2, on simple drugs, for example, rue in chapter 578 (fol. 146v). Citations are to the 1507 edition.

49. Ibid., bk. 2, tract. 2, chap. 1, 2, 4 (1557 ed., 2, fols. 98v, 99; 1507 ed., fols. 88–89r).

50. Ibid., bk. 2, tract. 2, chaps. 5, 6, 50 (1557 ed., 2, fols. 99v, 102v-103; 1507 ed., fols. 89, 92v).

13. Knowledge of Birth Control in the West

1. William of Saliceto, *Summa,* chap. 175. On William, see Bullough and Brundage 1982, pp. 194–204.

2. There are many candidates presented by authorities, but there is no certainty, even about the genus. See André 1985, pp. 230–231; Fischer 1929, pp. 264, 283, 287; and Hunt 1989, p. 233.

3. William of Saliceto, *Summa,* chap. 163 (fol. 60r&v).

4. On medicine during this period, see Siraisi 1981 and Schipperges 1964. The corpus of Arnald is being published now with Michael McVaugh and García L. Ballester, editors.

5. Arnald de Villanova, *Antidotarium,* chap. 56.

6. Ibid., chap. 39, with a recipe that incites the libido (*incitat cohitum*), and chap. 232, for oil of jet that "enhances conception" (*adiuuat ad conceptum*).

7. Arnald of Villanova, *Breviarum practice,* 3.5 (no foliation).

8. Ibid., 3.6. Michael McVaugh, an editor of the Arnald text series, suggests in a letter to me of September 4, 1990, that the passage be translated "that she be made to appear a virgin" (*quasi virgo esse videatur*), but the modern meaning here is constrained. I am making a less literal translation in order to understand better what I believe the intent of its author.

9. Ibid.

10. Ibid., 3.7.

11. Peter of Spain, *Thesaurus pauperum,* 1518 ed., 46 (fol. 66v) (chap. 44, 1973 ed., p. 259).

12. Ibid., fols. 66v-67 (1973 ed., pp. 259–261).

13. Ibid., 48, fols. 68–69v (text different in chap. 40 in 1973 ed., pp. 245–251).

14. Albertus, *De mineralibus,* 2, tr. 2, chaps. 8, 13 (*Opera,* 5, 39v, 43a); also Riddle and Mulholland 1980, p. 209. Many other references to Albertus' information about herbs are given in Noonan 1986, pp. 205–206, 211 and to his theological-moral statements, in pp. 211, 233–234, 247, and passim.

15. Huby 1990, p. 115.

16. Both the reference to Maimonides on laws and the quotation from the regimen as given in Mussalam 1983, p. 66.

17. Maimonides, *On Cohabitation* (Rosner trans., pp. 169–170).

18. Maimonides, *Code.* Laws on murder and preservation of life, 1.9, cited and translated by Goodman (1990, p. 89).

19. *Juris anglicani,* 1.23.10, 12, as cited in Lewin 1922, p. 89.
20. Aristotle, *Generation of Animals,* 1.19.727a-b.
21. Hippocrates, *De semine,* 4.1 (Joly ed., pp. 46–47; see also quotation from the Hippocratic work *De natura muliebri,* 5 (Littré ed., 477), that begins Chapter 8 of this book; on Galen, see *De usu partium,* 14.11 (May trans., 2:643–645), and *De semine,* esp. 1.7 and 2.4 (Kühn ed., 4:535–539, 622–624).
22. *Placides et Timéo,* 278–288 (Thomasset ed., pp. 128–133).
23. Jacquart and Thomasset 1985, pp. 84–120; although it may not be directly relevant to the subject of male-female seed, the growth of astrological medicine and study of how the planets influence the development of the fetus may have contributed to breaking the hold of authority during the thirteenth and fourteenth centuries. See Burnett 1990, pp. 95–112.
24. Thomas' positions are examined in Noonan 1986, pp. 238–257.
25. Huby 1990, p. 119.
26. Brundage 1987, p. 358.
27. See Chapter 1 above.
28. Procopius, *Anecdota,* 9.19 (Dewing ed., 6:108).
29. *Prose Salernitan Questions,* B 10 (Lawn ed., p. 6).

14. The Renaissance

1. Ladurie 1975, p. 249.
2. Ibid., pp. 249–250.
3. Riddle 1980, p. 11; for botany during this period, see Greene 1983, 2:509–831, and a briefer and excellent account by Reeds 1975, 1976; on new drugs from the New World, see Valverde and Perez Romero 1988.
4. Hermolaus to Pontico Faccino, July 1484, translated in Reeds 1975, p. 42.
5. Hermolaus, *Dioscorides,* fol. 20.
6. Ibid., fols. 19v–20.
7. *MM,* 1.103 (2.1–2).
8. Hermolaus, *Dioscorides,* fol. 71.
9. Ibid., fol. 57v; *MM,* 2.179 (3.6).
10. Hermolaus, *Dioscorides,* fol. 92.
11. Maurice de l'Corde, p. 300.
12. Ibid., p. 309.
13. Ibid., p. 308.
14. I have used Ruel's translation as printed in the edition with Petrus Matthiolus' commentary, fol. 116.
15. *MM,* 1.104 (1.4).
16. Ruel trans., fol. 88.
17. Ibid., fol. 414; cf. *MM,* 3.134 (2.5), where Dioscorides uses ἀτόκιος for Ruel's *conceptum adimere.*
18. Ruel trans., fol. 82.
19. Ibid., fol. 247.
20. *MM,* 2.120 (3.4–5).
21. Peter of Spain, *Thesaurus pauperum,* fols. 37r&v (for regulators).

22. Peter of Spain, *Treasurie,* chap. 48 [no pagination].
23. Andrea da Belluno, [Glossary], in Avicenna, *Canon,* 3, fol. 3v.
24. Ibid.
25. Matthiolus, *Pedacio Dioscoride;* on Matthiolus, see Palmer 1985, pp. 100–117 and 303–313; and Palmer 1985a, pp. 149–157; also Reeds 1975, 1976.
26. Riddle 1980, pp. 92–97.
27. Matthiolus, *Commentarii,* fol. 349.
28. Ibid., fol. 353.
29. Ibid., fol. 88.
30. Ibid., fol. 415.
31. Ibid., fols. 530–531.
32. Ibid., fols. 115–116.
33. Friedenwald 1937, p. 622.
34. Riddle 1980, p. 61.
35. Friedenwald 1937, p. 623.
36. Amatus Lusitanus, *Commentary,* fol. 93 (printing error for 92).
37. Ibid.
38. Ibid., fols. 124–25.
39. Ibid., fol. 278.
40. Ibid., fols. 304 (pennyroyal), 307 (thyme).
41. Ibid., fol. 306.
42. Ibid.
43. Ibid., fols. 313, 324, 449.
44. Ibid., fol. 381.
45. Ibid.
46. Marcellus Vergilius, Commentary to Dioscorides, 4.15, (p. 225).
47. de l'Corde, *Hippocratis,* pp. 300, 302.
48. Ibid., p. 302.
49. Gallegos 1983, pp. 211–225. Much of vol. 31 (no. 5, May 1985) of *Contraception* is devoted to a series of articles on zoapatle. On zoapatle, see *Merck Index* 1983, p. 9994.
50. From *Every Man His Own Doctor,* quoted in Lewis and Elvin-Lewis 1977, p. 324.
51. Orta, *Coloquios,* p. 91.
52. Roys 1931, pp. 18–19.
53. Riddle 1965, pp. 189–198.
54. See especially the study by Casey (1960, pp. 590–600).
55. Needham and Gwei-Djen 1968, p. 130.
56. Burkill 1966, 1:248.
57. Ibid., 2:1955.
58. Saha, Sanini, and Kasinathan 1961, p. 140.
59. Quoted in Needham 1970, p. 323.
60. Hines 1936, pp. 108–113.
61. Stuart 1911, pp. 141–142.
62. Chaucer, *Canterbury Tales,* 604–605.
63. Stannard 1982, p. 384. The identification of *madir* is unclear. In English the

name "madder" is a term for a variety of plants including blackberry, birth-wort, and sweet flag. See Hunt 1989, p. 293.

64. *Leechbook,* no. 237, 245–250 (Dawson 1934, pp. 89, 92–95). One recipe (no. 237) is given for "cake," which Dawson says is clotting dysmenor-rhoea, but the recipe contains emmenagogic herbs: "Cake. Take parsley, sage, hyssop, wormwood [artemisia], tansy; and take a bottle of stale ale, stir the herbs therein, and seethe them from a boot to a quart; and give her at morn hot and at even cold."

65. Augustine, *Marriage and Concupiscence,* 1.15.17 (*CSEL,* 42:229–230, and translated by Noonan 1986, p. 136).

66. Soranus, *Gynaecology,* 1.10.36.

67. Sharma, Mishra, and Mehta 1988, p. 25.

68. Martialis, Gargilius *Medicinae,* 3 (Rose ed., p. 137).

69. Riddle 1980, pp. 71–74.

70. Mennell 1985, p. 53.

71. Aretino 1971, p. 130, in a context that suggests aphrodisiacs.

15. Later Developments

1. The act was passed formally as 43 Geo. III, chap. 58, in *Statutes of the Realm* 1950, pp. 203–204; cf. Mohr 1978, p. 23 and passim.

2. Taylor 1905, 2:168–169.

3. Ibid.

4. Taylor 1865, p. 786.

5. Taylor 1905, 2:168.

6. Mohr 1978, p. 276 n. 15.

7. For instance, an immensely popular eighteenth-century treatise of midwi-fery listed no contraceptives or abortifacients. It did, however, give prescrip-tions for delayed menstruation (Smellie 1752, pp. 109, 124).

8. Mauriceau, *De praegnantium,* pp. 25, 54, and passim.

9. Cited in McLaren 1984, p. 74.

10. Theodorus, *Kräuter Buch,* vol. 2, sec. 4, chap. 32, pp. 389–390, discusses rue's antifertility's qualities but hardly mentions any other plant; Gerard 1636 avoids discussing antifertility measures; see De Tournefort, *Compleat Herbal,* pp. 244, 284, 385, 433, 438, 522, 567–568, 630.

11. De Tournefort, *Compleat Herbal,* p. 149.

12. Ibid., p. 313.

13. McLaren 1984, pp. 104–105.

14. Buchan 1772, p. 656. In contrast, an early nineteenth-century guide (Jen-nings 1818, pp. 43–49) discussed menstrual stimulators—the same ones used during antiquity and the Middle Ages.

15. Sharp, *Midwives' Book,* pp. 180–181.

16. Jiu 1966, pp. 256–257; Farnsworth et al. 1975, p. 576.

17. Goris and Liot 1939, 2:1833.

18. Manske 1955, p. 199.

19. In 1991 I received a catalog from a company called Health Center for Better Living (Naples, Fl.) which advertises chamomile, rue, black cohosh, and

other herbs as stimulators of retained menses. Tansy, however, is said to be "good for the heart"; no antifertility effects are listed for it (*Useful Guide to Herbal Health Care*, pp. 8–9, 18, 20).

20. Brevitt 1810, p. 117n.
21. Ibid., pp. 45–46.
22. Woycke 1980, pp. 16–19; McLaren 1984, pp. 73–75; an earlier and thorough survey of abortifacients, including mineral and animal substances, was Lewin 1922.
23. Olivier 1760, pp. 129–131.
24. *Statutes of the Realm* 1950, p. 204.
25. Taylor 1865, pp. 786–787.
26. *Lancet* 1898, vol. 2, pp. 1723–25.
27. Whitehead 1847, pp. 143, 144.
28. Burns 1808, p. 74.
29. Meigs 1848, p. 405.
30. McLaren 1990, p. 189.
31. Whitehead 1847, p. 254.
32. Dunn 1927, 2:296; for similar positions, see p. 755 (Iowa) and p. 820 (Kansas).
33. Ibid., p. 755.
34. Ibid., pp. 923–924 (Louisiana, 1924, p. 385, Act 95 of 1920).
35. *Lancet* 1898, vol. 2, pp. 1723–24, reporting from the *Times*, March 10, 1898: *Owen v. Greenberg*.
36. Darling, *Times*, March 10, 1898, p. 13.
37. See above, Chapter 9, concerning Australian clover and sheep grazing.
38. de Gordon, *Tractabus de gradibus*, cited in Demaitre 1980, p. 128. Where Demaitre translates *in fratribus minoribus* as "on lesser brethren," I have supplied "Franciscans" as a term more familiar to moderns for this order.
39. Olivieri 1985, p. 96.
40. McLaren 1984, p. 107.
41. See, for instance, the details found in ibn Sina, *Canon*, bk. 3, fen. 21, tract. 1, 2–36.
42. Soranus, *Gynaecology*, 1.64 (Temkin trans., p. 66).
43. Oylebola 1981, pp. 777–784.
44. Kong, Xie, and But, 1986, pp. 1–44.
45. Kokwaro 1981, pp. 149–152.
46. Kharkhov and Mats 1980, pp. 291–302.
47. Weniger 1982, pp. 67–84.
48. Conway 1979, pp. 241–261.
49. Tiwari, Majumder, and Bhattacharjee 1982, p. 133.
50. Laderman 1983, esp. p. 78.
51. Casey 1960.
52. In a study of the reasons for the low fertility of the elite classes in Europe beween 1600 and 1900, S. Rayn Johansson said that the people in the class knew that eventually such rates would produce their own extinction; they were afraid, though, that high fertility would dilute their assets and thus diminish their power (Sieff 1990, pp. 40–41).

53. See above, Chapter 4.
54. Bolks 1877, pp. 270–271.
55. Crellin and Philpott 1990, 1:176; there is a report of an antiferility plant recommended by a lay herbalist in the Sudan (Estes 1989, p. 117).

⋄ BIBLIOGRAPHY ⋄

Editions of Ancient, Classical, and Medieval Sources

Abu Ḥamaid M. bn. ʿO. Najib al-Din al-Samarquandi. *The Medical Formulary of Al-Samarquandi and the Relation of Early Arabic Simples to Those Found in the Indigenous Medicine of the Near East and India*. Martin Levey and Noury al-Khaledy, trans. Philadelphia: University of Pennsylvania Press, 1967.

Abu l-Fadl Dawud ibn Abi l-Bayan al-Israîli. *Al-Dustur al-bimaristani fi l-adwiya al-murakkada*. José Luis Valverde Carmen Peña Muñoz, trans. In *El formulario de los hospitales de ibn Abi l-Baya*. Granada: Universidad, 1981.

AELIAN
On the Characteristics of Animals. A. F. Scholfield, ed. 3 vols. Cambridge, Mass.: Harvard University Press, 1959.
Varia historica. Mervin R. Dills, ed. Leipzig: B. G. Teubner, 1974.

AËTIUS
Peri ton en metrai pathon. Skévos Zervòs, ed. Leipzig: Anton. Mangkos, 1901.
Aetius of Amida: The Gynaecology and Obstretrics of the VIth Century, A.D. James V. Ricci, trans. Philadelphia: Blakiston Company, 1950.

ALBERTUS MAGNUS
De mineralibus. In *Opera omnia*, vol. 5. Auguste Borgnet, ed. Aschendorff: Monastery, 1951–.

ʾARID IBN ṢAʾID AL-KATIB AL-QURTʾUBI
Kitab Khalq al-Janin wa-Tadbit al-Hʾabale waʾl-Mawludin. French trans. by Henri Jahier and Noureddine Abdelkader, *Le livre de la Génération du foetus et le traitement des femmes enceintes et des nouveau-néd*. Algiers: Librairie Ferraris, 1956. Spanish trans. by Antonio Arjona Castro, *"El libro de la generación del feto, el tratamiento de las mujeres embarazadas y de los*

recien nacidos" de 'Arib ibn Sa'id. Cordoba: Publicaciones de la Excma, 1983.

ARISTOPHANES
Knights. Lysistrata. Peace. Benjamin Bickley Rogers, ed. and trans. 3 vols. Cambridge: Harvard University Press, 1946–1950.
Scholia in Aristophanes. 4 vols. D. Holwerda, ed. Groningen: Bouma's Boekhuis, 1960-.

ARISTOTLE
Opera. Immanuel Bekker, ed. 5 vols. Berlin: W. De Gruyter, 1960–1987.
Politics. H. Rackham, trans. New York: G. P. Putnam's Sons, 1932.

Babylonian Laws. 2 vols. G. R. Driver and John C. Miles, eds. Oxford: Clarendon Press,1952.

BIBLE
The Septuagint with Apocrypha: Greek and English. Sir Lancelot, C. L. Benton, ed. 1st ed. 1851. Rept. Grand Rapids, Mich.: Zondervan, 1980.
Exodus. J. J. Owens, ed. New York: Harper and Row, 1977. In Hebrew.

Celsus. *De medicina.* W. G. Spencer, ed. 3 vols. Cambridge: Harvard University Press, 1938.

CICERO
Pro Clentio. H. Grose Hodge, trans. Cambridge: Harvard University Press, 1952.
De divinatione. William A. Falconer, trans. Cambridge: Harvard University Press, 1964.

Cleopatra. *Gynaecologia.* In *Gynaeciorum hoc est De mulierum tum aliis.* Conrad Gesner and Caspar Wolf, eds. Basel: Thomas Guarinus, 1566.
Columba. In *The Irish Penitentials.* Ludwig Bieler, ed. Dublin: Dublin Institute for Advanced Studies, 1963.
Columella. *De arboribus. On Agriculture and Trees.* 3 vols. Harrison Boyd Ash, trans. E. S. Forster and Edward H. Heffner, eds. Cambridge: Harvard University Press, 1941–55.

Corpus Juris Civilis. Theodor Mommsen, ed. English trans. by Alan Watson. 4 vols. Philadelphia: Pennsylvania Press, 1985.
S. P. Scott, trans. 17 vols. In *Civil Code.* Cincinnati: Control Trust, 1932.

DIOSCORIDES
De materia medica. Max Wellmann, ed. 3 vols. Berlin: Weidmann, 1958. In Greek.
"Dioscorides Longobardus." In *Römanische Forschungen.* T. M. Aurachers et al., eds., 1 (1882): 49–105; 10 (1896): 181–247, 369–466; 11 (1899): 1–121; 13 (1902): 161–243; 14 (1903): 601–637. Sixth-century Latin translation.

Dioscoride Latino. Materia Medica. Libro Primo. H. Mihàescu, trans. Iasi, Romania: Alexander Terek, 1938.

Dioscorides. Colle: Per Johanem Allemanum de Medemblick. 1478. Alphabetized redaction.

[Pseudo-Dioscorides]. *Ex herbis femininis.* Heinrich Kästner, ed. *Hermes* 31:578–636.

Des Pedanios Dioskurides aus Anazarbos Arzneimittellehre in fünf Buchern. Julius Berendes, trans. Stuttgart: F. Enke, 1902.

The Greek Herbal of Dioscorides: Illustrated by a Byzantine A.D. 512. Englished by John Goodyer A.D. 1655. Robert T. Gunther, ed. New York: Hafner, 1959.

GALEN

Claudii Galeni Opera omnia. Karl Gottlob Kühn, ed. 22 vols. Medicorum opera quae exstant. Hildesheim: Olms, 1821–33, repr. 1964–65.

De usu partium. In *Galen: On the Usefulness of the Parts of the Body.* Margaret Tallmadge May, trans. 2 vols. Ithaca: Cornell University Press, 1968.

Hammurabi. *Laws.* In *The Ancient Near East: An Anthology of Texts and Pictures.* James B. Pritchard, ed. Princeton: Princeton University Press, 1958.

Herodotus. *Histories.* A. D. Godley, ed. 4 vols. Cambridge: Harvard University Press, 1946.

HIPPOCRATES

Oeuvres complètes d'Hippocrate: traduction nouvelle avec le texte grec en regard. Emile Littré, ed. 10 vols. Paris: Baillière, 1839–1861. Repr. Amsterdam: Hakkert, 1973.

Hippocrates. W. H. S. Jones, ed. 6 vols. Cambridge: Harvard University Press, 1934–88.

Hippocrate. Robert Joly, ed. Paris: Les belles lettres, 1970.

Hippocratic Writings. J. Chadwick and W. N. Mann, trans. Harmondsworth: Penguin, 1978.

De la génération. Robert Joly, ed. Paris: Collection des universités de France, 1970.

Isidore of Seville. *Origines.* W. M. Lindsay, ed. 2 vols. Oxford: Clarendon Press, 1957.

Juvenal. *Satirae.* Peter Green, trans. Baltimore: Penguin Books, 1967.

Lex frisionum. In *Monumenta Germaniae Historica: Fontes Iuris Germanici Antiqui,* vol. 12. Karl August Eckhardt and Albrecht Eckhard, eds. Hannover: Hahnsche Buchhandlung, 1982.

Lucretius. *De rerum natura.* W. H. D. Rouse, ed. Cambridge: Harvard University Press, 1953.

Macer Floridus [Marbode of Rennes?]. In *Aemilius Macer De herbarum virtutibus cum Joannis Atrociani commentariis.* Apud Friburgum Brisgoicum, 1530.

MAIMONIDES
Glossary of Drug Names. Fred Rosner, trans. Philadelphia: American Philosophical Association, 1979.
Maimonides: Treatises on Poisons, Hemorrhoids, and Cohabitation. Fred Rosner, trans. Haifa: Maimonides Research Institute, 1984.

Maranchus, Petrus. *Tabula.* In *Collectio Salernitana.* Salvatore de Renzi, ed. Bologna: Forni, 1967.
Marcellus. *De medicamentis.* Max Neidermann, ed. In *Corpus Medicorum Graecorum.* 2 vols. Berlin: Akademie-Verlag, 1968.
Marcus Aurelius. *Meditations.* C. R. Haines, ed. Cambridge and London: Heinemann, 1953.

MARTIALIS, GARGILIUS
Medicinae ex oleribus et pomis. Valentin Rose, ed. Leipzig: Teubner, 1875.
Materia Medica of Gargilius Martialis. Ruth Melicent Tapper, trans. Diss. University of Wisconsin, 1980.

Mishnah. Herbert Danby, trans. Oxford: Oxford University Press, 1933.

ORIBASIUS
Oeuvres. Charles Daremberg and C. Bussemaker, eds. 6 vols. Paris, 1851–79.
Oribasii collectionum medicarum reliquiae. Johannes Raeder, ed. 5 vols. Leipzig and Berlin: Teubner, 1928–33. Repr. Amsterdam, 1964.
Oribasius Latinus. Henning Mørland, ed. Oslo: A. W. Brøgger, 1940.

Ovid. *Metamorphoses.* Frank Justus Miller, ed. and trans. Cambridge: Harvard University Press, 1951.

PAPYRI
Ancient Egyptian Medicine: The Papyrus Ebers. Trans. from German by Cyril P. Bryan. London: G. Bles. 1930.
Five Ramesseum Papyri. John W. B. Barns, ed. Oxford: Oxford University Press, 1956.
Grundriss der Medizin der alten Ägypter. Hildegard von Deines, Herman Grapow, and Wolfhart Westendorf, eds. 7 vols. Berlin: Akademie Verlag, 1954–1962.
The Leyden Papyrus. An Egyptian Magical Book. F. Ll. Griffith and Herbert Thompson, eds. New York: Dover, 1974.
Oxyrhynchus Papyri. In *Roman Civilization,* 2 vols. Naphtali Lewis and Meyer Reinhold, eds. New York: Harper and Row, 1955.
Papyrus Ebers: Das älteste Buch über Heilkunde. H. Joachim, ed. Berlin: DeGruyter, 1973.

PAUL OF AEGINA (PAULUS AEGINETA)
Libri Medicorum. I. L. Heiberg, ed. *Corpus Medicorum Graecorum* IX, 2 vols. Leipzig: Teubner, 1921.

Pauli Aeginetae liber tertii interpretatio Latina antiqua. I. L. Heiberg, ed. Leipzig: Teubner, 1912.
Seven Books of Paulus Aegineta. Francis Adams, trans. London: C. & J. Adlard, 1844–47.

Philo. *Opera*. Thomas Manqucy, ed. 5 vols. Erlangen: Heyderiana, 1820.
Placides et Timéo; ou, Li secrés as philosophes. Claude Alexandre Thomasset, ed. Paris: Droz, 1980.

PLATO
Plato: The Laws. Trevor J. Saunders, trans. Harmondsworth: Penguin Books, 1970.
Theaetetus. In *Plato*. Harold North Fowler, ed. Cambridge: Harvard University Press, 1952.

Plautus. *Plautus*. Paul Nixon, ed. and trans. 5 vols. Cambridge: Harvard University Press, 1950–60.

PLINY
Natural History. W. H. S. Jones et al., eds. and trans. 10 vols. Cambridge: Harvard University Press, 1929–71.
Pline l'Ancien Histoire Naturelle livre XXI. Jacques André, ed. Paris: Belle Lettres, 1947–85.
Gaio Plinio secundo storia naturale. 5 vols. Pisa: Giardini, 1985.

Plutarch. *Opera*. Harold Cherniss et al. ed. 13 vols. Cambridge: Harvard University Press, 1976.
Pollux. *Onomasticon*. Ericus Bethe, ed. In *Lexicographia graeci*, vol. 10. Stuttgart: Teubner, 1967.
Polybius. *Histories*. W. R. Patton, ed. 6 vols. Cambridge: Harvard University Press, 1960.
Procopius. *Anecdota*. H. B. Dewing, ed. 7 vols. Cambridge, Mass.: Harvard University Press, 1914–40.
Pseudo-Apuleius. *Herbarius*. Ernest Howald and Henry Sigerist, eds. In *Corpus Medicorum Graecorum*, 4 vols. Leipzig: Teubner, 1927.
Pseudo-Bede. *The Order of Giving Penance*. In *The Irish Penitentials*. Ludwig Bieler, ed. Dublin: Dublin Institute for Advanced Studies, 1963.
Rocheus, Nicolaus. *De morbis mulierum curandis liber*. In *Gynaeciorum hoc est De mulierum tum aliis*. Conrad Gesner and Caspar Wolf, eds. Basel: Thomas Guarinus, 1566.
al-Samarquandi. See Abu.

Sammonicus, Quintas Serenus. *Liber Medicinalis*. R. Pépin, ed. Paris: Presses Universitaires de France, 1950.
Scholia Aristophanes. *Scholia in Aristophanes*. Vol. 2, *Pacem*, D. Holwerda, ed. Groningen: Bouma's Boekhuis, 1982.

SCRIBONIUS LARGUS
Conpositiones [sic]. George Helmreich, ed. Leipzig: Teubner, 1887.
Compositiones. S. Sconocchia, ed. Leipzig: Teubner, 1983.

Seneca. *Fragments*. Friedrich G. Haase, ed. Leipzig: Teubner, 1884 (?)–1892.

SORANUS
Sorani Gynaeciorum. Valentin Rose, ed. Leipzig: Teubner, 1882.
Sorani Gynaeciorum libri IV. De signis fracturarum. De fasciis. Vita Hippocratis secudum Soranum. Johannes Ilberg, ed. *Corpus Medicorum Graecorum*, vol. 4. Leipzig and Berlin: Teubner, 1927.
Soranos d'Éphèse maladies des femmes. Paul Burguière, Danielle Gourevitch, and Yves Malinas, eds. Paris: Belles Lettres, 1988. With French translation.
Gynaecology. Oswei Temkin, ed. and trans. Baltimore: Johns Hopkins University Press, 1956.

Syrian Anatomy, Pathology and Therapeutics, or, "The Book of Medicines." 2 vols. E. A. Wallis Budge, trans. London: Oxford University Press, 1913.
Tacitus. *Germania*. Rodney P. Robinson, ed. Middletown, Conn.: American Philological Association, 1935.

TALMUD
The Babylonian Talmud. Jerusalem: Institute for the Complete Israeli Talmud, 1972. In Hebrew.
The Babylonian Talmud. Isidore Epstein, trans. London: Soncino Press, 1935–52.
The Talmud of the Land of Israel: A Preliminary Translation and Explanation. Jacob Neusner, trans. 35 vols. Chicago: University of Chicago Press, 1987.

Tertullian. *De anima*. J. H. Waszink, ed. Amsterdam: J. M. Muellenhoff, 1947.

THEODORUS PRISCIANUS
Euporiston. In *Römische Medizin*. Theodor Meyer-Steineg, ed. Jena: Gustav Fischer, 1909.
Theodoris Prisciani Euporiston Libri III. Valentine Rose, ed. Leipzig: Teubner, 1894.

THEOPHRASTUS
Enquiry into Plants and Minor Works on Odours and Weather Signs. Sir Arthur Hort, ed. 2 vols. Cambridge: Harvard University Press, 1961.
On Stones. Earle R. Caley and John F. C. Richards, eds. and trans. Columbus: Ohio State University Press, 1956.

Trotula. [*Gynaecology*]. In *Gynaeciorum hoc est De mulierum tum aliis*. Conrad Gesner and Caspar Wolf, eds. Basel: Thomas Guarinus, 1566.

◆ REFERENCES ◆

Abdul-Ghani, A. S., R. Amin, and M. S. Suleiman. 1987. "Hypotensive Effect of *Crataegus oxyacantha.*" *International Journal of Crude Drug Research* 25:216–220.

Achari, Busudeb, Krishnakali Basu, and Satyesh C. Pakrashi. 1984. "Chemical Investigation of *Malvaviscus conzattii.*" *Journal of Natural Products* 47:751.

Al-Razi (Rasis), Muhammad ibn Zakariya. 1544. *Abubertri Rhazae Maohethi, ob usum experientiamque multiplicem . . .* Gerard of Cremona, trans. Basel: Henrichus Petrus.

Albert-Puleo, Michael. 1979. "The Obstetrical Use in Ancient and Early Modern Times of *Convolvulus scammonia* or Scammony: Another Non-fungal Source of Ergot Alkaloids." *Journal of Ethnopharmacology* 1:193–195.

Amatus Lusitanus. 1553. Commentary, in *In Dioscoridis Anazarbei de medica materia libros quinque enarrationes.* Venice: Gualterus Scotus.

Amundsen, D. W., and C. J. Diers. 1969. "The Age of Menarche in Classical Greece and Rome." *Human Biology* 41:125–132.

Anderson, John E., and John G. Cleland. 1984. "The World Fertility Survey and Contraceptives Prevalence Survey: A Comparison of Substantive Results." *Studies in Family Planning* 15:1–13.

André, Jacques. 1985. *Les noms de plantes dans la Rome antique.* Paris: Société d'Edition, Les Belles Lettres.

Andrews, Alfred C. 1941–42. "The Silphium of the Ancients: A Lesson in Crop Control." *Isis* 33:232–236.

Angel, John Lawrence. 1969. "The Bases of Paleodemography." *American Journal of Physical Anthropology,* n.s. 30.427–438.

———— 1972. "Ecology and Population in the Eastern Mediterranean." *World Archaeology* 4:88–105.

———— 1979. Bibliography. *American Journal of Physical Anthropology* 51:509–516.

Angeles, L. T., et al. 1970. "Toxicity Studies on Aristolochic Acid Isolated from *Aristolochia tagala* Cham." *Acta Medica Philippina* 6:139–148.

Arenas, P., and R. Moreno Azorero. 1977. "Plants Used as Means of Abortion, Contraception, Sterilization and Fecundation by Paraguayan Indigenous People." *Economic Botany* 31:302–306.

Arends, G., and H. Zörnig, eds. 1949. *Hager's Handbuch der pharmazeutischen Praxis.* 2 vols. Berlin: Springer Verlag.

Ariès, Philippe. 1948. *Histoire des populations françaises et de leurs attitudes devant la vie depuis le XVIIIe siècle.* Paris: Editions Self.

——— 1953. "Sur les origines de la contraception en France." *Population* 8:465–472.

Arnald de Villanova. 1495. *Antidotarum.* Valencia: Nicolas Spindeler. Facsimile rept., Burriana: Castellon, 1985.

——— [pseud.]. 1483. *Breviarium practice.* In *Articella.* Venice: Herman von Lichtenstein.

Atal, C. K., Usha Zutshi, and P. G. Rao. 1981. "Scientific Evidence on the Role of Ayurvedic Herbals on Bioavailabilty of Drugs." *Journal of Ethnopharmacology* 4:229–232.

Avicenna. *Canon.* 1557. Gerard of Cremona, trans. 3 vols. Venice: Junta. Previously pub. Venice, 1507. Facsimile reproduction, Hildesheim: George Olms, 1964.

Azad Chowdhury, A. K., R. A. Kaleque, and S. K. Chakder. 1984. "Antifertility Activity of the Traditional Contraceptive Pill Comprising *Acacia catechu, A. arabia* and *Tragia involucerta.*" *Indian Journal of Medical Research* 80: 372–374.

Beccaria, Augusto. 1956. *I codici di medicina del periodo presalernitano (secoli IX, X et XI).* Rome: Edizione di Storia e Letterature.

Below, Karl-Heinz. 1953. *Der Arzt im römischen Recht.* Munich: Beck.

Bembrose, Stephen. 1990. "'Come d'animal divegna fante': The Animation of the Human Embryo in Dante." In *The Human Embryo.* G. R. Dunstan, ed. Exeter: University of Exeter Press, pp. 123–135.

Bennetts, H. W., E. J. Underwood, and F. L. Shier. 1946. "A Specific Breeding Problem of Sheep on Subterranean Clover Pastures in Western Australia." *The Australian Veterinary Journal* 22:2–12.

Benton, John F. 1985. "Trotula, Women's Problems, and the Professionalization of Medicine in the Middle Ages." *Bulletin of the History of Medicine* 59:30–53.

Biller, P. P. A. 1982. "Birth-Control in the West in the Thirteenth and Early Fourteenth Centuries." *Past and Present* 94:3–26.

Bingel, Audrey A., and Harry H. S. Fong. 1988. "Potential Fertility-Regulating Agents from Plants." *Economic and Medicine Plant Research* 2:73–118.

Bolks, W. P. 1877. "Cases with Autopsies." *Medical and Surgical Reports of the Boston City Hospital.* Series Boston. Boston City Hospital.

Boswell, John. 1988. *The Kindness of Strangers: The Abandonment of Children in Western Europe from Late Antiquity to the Renaissance.* New York: Pantheon Books.

Bounds, D. B., and G. S. Pope. 1960. "Light-absorption and Chemical Properties of Miroestrol, the Oestrogenic Substance of *Pueraria mirificia.*" *Journal of the Chemical Society,* Part 3:3695–3705.

Boylan, Michael. 1984. "The Galenic and Hippocratic Challenges to Aristotle's Conception Theory." *Journal of the History of Biology* 17:83–112.

Braude, Peter R., and Martin H. Johnson. 1990. "The Embryo in Contemporary Medical Science." In Dunstan 1990, pp. 208–221.

Braudel, Fernand. 1979. *Civilization and Capitalism, 15th-18th Century.* Vol. 1, *The Structures of Everyday Life: The Limits of the Possible.* Siân Reynolds, trans. New York: Harper and Row.

Brevitt, John. 1810. *The Female Medical Repository, to Which Is Added a Treatise on the Primary Diseases of Infants Adapted to the Use of the Female Practitioners and Intelligent Mothers.* Baltimore: Hunter and Robinson.

Brissaud, Yves. 1972. "L'infanticide à la fin du moyen âge, ses motivations psychologiques et sa répression." *Revue historique de droit français et étranger* 50:229–256.

Brockliss, L. W. B. 1990. "The Embryological Revolution in the France of Louis XIV: The Dominance of Ideology." In Dunstan 1990, pp. 158–186.

Brøndegaard, V. J. 1964. "Der Sadebaum als Abortivum." *Sudhoffs Archiv für Geschichte der Medizin und der Naturwissenschaften* 48:331–351.

——— 1973. "Contraceptive Plant Drugs." *Planta Medica* 23:167–172.

Brothwell, Don. 1972. "Paleodemography and Earlier British Populations." *World Archaeology* 4:75–87.

Brown, Peter Robert Lamont. 1982. *The Making of Late Antiquity.* Berkeley: University of California Press, 1982.

——— 1988. *The Body and Society: Men, Women and Sexual Renunciation in Early Christianity.* New York: Columbia University Press.

Brundage, James A. 1987. *Law, Sex, and Christian Society in Medieval Europe.* Chicago: University of Chicago Press.

Brunt, P. A. 1971. *Italian Manpower, 225 B.C.-A.D. 14.* London: Oxford University Press.

Bubio, Boris, et al. 1970. "A New Postcoital Oral Contraceptive." *Contraception* 1:303–14.

Buchan, William. 1772. *Domestic Medicine; or, A Treatise on the Prevention and Cure of Diseases by Regimen and Simple Medicines.* London: Strahan.

Bulfinch's Mythology: The Age of Fable. 1894. E. E. Hale, ed. Boston: S. W. Tilton.

Bull, Arthur W., et al. 1987. "Copper-Containing IUD's Are Not Associated with an Increase of Malondialdehyde Levels in Cervical Muscus." *Contraception* 35:49–55.

Bullough, Vern, and James Brundage. 1982. *Sexual Practices and the Medieval Church.* Buffalo: Prometheus Books.

Bullough, Vern, and Bonnie Bullough. 1990. *Contraception: A Guide to Birth Control Methods.* Buffalo: Prometheus Books.

Bullough, Vern, and C. Campbell. 1980. "Female Longevity and Diet in the Middle Ages." *Speculum* 55:317–325.

Burkill, I. H. 1966. *A Dictionary of the Economic Products of the Malay Peninsula.* 2 vols. Kuala Lumpur: Governments of Malaysia and Singapore.

Burnett, C. S. F. 1990. "The Planets and the Development of the Embryo." In Dunstan 1990, pp. 95–112.

Burns, John. 1808. *Observations on Abortion Containing an Account of the Manner in Which It Takes Place, the Causes Which Produce It, and the Method of Preventing or Treating It.* 1st American ed. Troy, N.Y.: Wright, Goodenow and Stockwell.

Butenandt, A., and H. Jacobi. 1933. "Über die Darstellung eines krystallisierten pflanzlichen Tokokinins (Thelykinins) und seine Identifizierung mit dem α-Follikelhormon." *Zeitschrift für Physiologische Chemie* 218:104–112.

Bydeman, Marc. 1981. "Prostaglandins in Fertility Regulation." In *Recent Advances in Fertility Regulation* (Symposium, Being, 2–5 September 1980), Chang Chai Fen, David Griffin, and Aubrey Woolman, eds. Geneva: Atar.

Cameron, Averil. 1986. "Redrawing the Map: Early Christian Territory after Foucault." *Journal of Roman Studies* 76:266–271.

Carnoy, A. 1959. *Dictionnaire étymologique des noms grecs de plantes.* Louvain: Publications universitaires.

Casey, R. C. D. 1960. "Alleged Anti-fertility Plants of India." *Indian Journal of Medical Sciences* 14:590–600.

Chaddock, Robert E. 1956. "The Age and Sex in Population Analysis," In *Demographic Analysis,* Joseph J. Spengler and Otis Dudley Duncan, eds. Glencoe, Ill.: Free Press, pp. 443–451.

Chaudhury, R. R. 1966. "Plants with Possible Antifertility Activity." *Indian Council for Medical Research: Special Reports Series* 55:1–19.

Che, Chung-Tao, et al. 1984. "Studies on *Aristolochia* III: Isolation and Biological Evaluation of Constituents of *Aristolochia indica* Roots for Fertility-Regulating Activity." *Journal of Natural Products* 47:331–341.

Chen, Lincoln C., Emdadul Qua, and Stan D'Souza. 1981. "Sex Bias in the Family Allocation of Food and Health Care in Rural Bangladesh." *Population and Development Review* 7:55–70.

Chinese Herbal Medicine: Materia Medica. 1986. Dan Bensky and Andrew Gamble, comp. and trans. Seattle: Eastland Press.

Cockayne, Thomas Oswald. 1864. *Leechdoms, Wortcunning and Starcraft of Early England.* 3 vols. Rept. London: Kraus, 1965.

Coleman, Emily R. 1974. "L'infanticide dans le haut moyen age." *Annales economies-sociétés-civilisations* 29:315–335.

Compadre, César, Eugene F. Robbins, and A. Douglas Kinghorn. 1986. "The Intensely Sweet Herb, *Lippa dulcis* Trev.: Historical Uses, Field Inquiries, and Constituents." *Journal of Ethnopharmacy* 15:89–106.

Constantine the African (Constantinus Africanus). 1536. *De coitus liber* and *De gradibus.* In *Opera.* Basel: Henricus Petrus.

Conway, George A., and John C. Slocumb. 1979. "Plants Used as Abortifacients and Emmenagogues by Spanish New Mexicans." *Journal of Ethnopharmacology* 1:241–261.

Corde, Maurice de l'. 1585. (Mauricus Cordaeus). Translation and commentary to *Hippocratis Coi, medicorum principis, Liber prior de morbis mulierum.* Paris: Dionysius Duvallis.

Crellin, John, and Jane Philpott. 1990. *Herbal Medicine Past and Present.* 2 vols. Durham: Duke University Press.

Crutchfield, Larry V. 1989. "Abortion as the Early Church Fathers Saw It." *All about Issues* (Nov.-Dec.): 34–38.

Csapo, A. I. 1976. "Prostaglandin Impact." In *Advances in Prostaglandin and Thromboxane Research,* B. Samuelsson and R. Paoletti, eds. New York: Raven Press, vol. 2, pp. 705–718.

Darling, Justice. 1898. "Owen v. Greenberg." *London Times* (March 10), p. 13.

Das Gupta, Manka. 1987. "Selective Discrimination against Female Children in Rural Punjab, India." *Population and Development Review* 13:77–100.

Dawson, Warren R. 1934. *A Leechbook or Collection of Medical Recipes of the Fifteenth Century.* London: Macmillan.

de Bennett, Raymond, Shui-Tze Ko, and Eric Heftmann. 1966. "Isolation of Estrone and Cholesterol from the Date Palm, *Phoenix dactylifera* L." *Phytochemistry* 5:231–235.

de Laszlo, Henry, and Paul S. Henshaw. 1954. "Plants Used by Primitive Peoples to Affect Fertility." *Science* 119:626–631.

De Renzi, Salvatore, ed. 1857. *Storia documentata della scuola di Salerno [Collection Salernitana].* 5 vols. Naples; rept. Milan: Ferro Edizioni, 1967.

Dean, P. D. G., D. Exeley, and T. W. Goodwin. 1971. "Steroid Oestrogens in Plants: Re-estimation of Oestrone in Pomegranate Seeds." *Phytochemistry* 10:2215–2216.

Dean-Jones, Lesley. 1989. "Menstrual Bleeding According to the Hippocratics and Aristotle." *Transactions of the American Philological Association* 119:177–192.

Defoe, Daniel. 1727. *Conjugal Lewdness; or, Matrimonial Whoredom.* Rept. Menston, England: Scholar Press, 1970.

Degen, Rainer. 1981. "Galen im Syrischen: Eine Überlieferung der Werke Galens." In *Galen: Problems and Prospects. A Collection of Papers Submitted at the 1979 Cambridge Conference.* London: Wellcome Institute for the History of Medicine, pp. 131–166.

Demaitre, Luke E. 1980. *Doctor Bernard de Gordon: Professor and Practitioner.* Toronto: Pontifical Institute.

Devereux, George. 1976. *A Study of Abortion in Primitive Societies.* Rev. ed. New York: International Universities Press.

Dhawan, B. N., and P. N. Saxena. 1958. "Evaluation of Some Indigenous Drugs for Stimulant Effect on the Rat Uterus: A Preliminary Report." *Indian Journal of Medical Research* 46:808–811.

Dickison, Sheila K. 1973. "Abortion in Antiquity." *Arethusa* 6:159–166.

Dierbach, Johann Heinrich. 1824. *Die Arzneimittel des Hippokrates.* Rept. Heidelberg: George Olms, 1969.

Dittenberger, Wilhelm. 1920. *Sylloge inscriptionum Graecum.* In *Aktualisierende Konkordanzen zu Dittenbergers Orientis Graeci in scriptiones selectae (OGIS) und zur dritten Auflage der von ihm begründeten Sylloge inscrip-*

tionum Graecarum (Syll. 3). Wilfried Gawanthka, ed. Rept. Hildesheim and New York: George Olms, 1977.

Dixon, Suzanne. 1988. *The Roman Mother.* Norman: Oklahoma University Press.

Duke, James A. 1985. *CRC Handbook of Medicinal Herbs.* Boca Raton, Fla.: CRC Press.

Duke, James A., and E. S. Ayensu. 1985. *Medicinal Plants of China.* 1st ed., 2 vols. Algonac, Mich.: Reference Publications.

Duncan-Jones, Richard. 1974. *The Economy of the Roman Empire: Quantitative Studies.* Cambridge: Cambridge University Press.

Dunn, Charles Wesley. 1927. *Dunn's Food and Drug Laws: Federal and States.* 3 vols. New York: United States Corporation.

Dunstan, G. R. 1988. "The Human Embryo in the Western Moral Tradition." In *The Status of the Human Embryo: Perspectives from Moral Tradition,* G. R. Dunstan and Mary J. Seller, eds. London: King Edward's Hospital Fund for London, pp. 39–61.

—— ed. 1990. *The Human Embryo: Aristotle and the Arabic and European Traditions.* Exeter: University of Exeter Press.

Duquénois, Pierre. 1972. "*Salvia officinalis* L. antique panacée et condiment de choix." *Quarterly Journal of Crude Drug Research* 12:1841–1849.

East, June. 1955a. "The Effect of Certain Plant Preparations on the Fertility of Laboratory Mammals. 3. *Capsella Bursa Pastoris* L." *Journal of Endocrinology* 12:267–72.

—— 1955b. "The Effect of Certain Plant Preparations on the Fertility of Laboratory Mammals. 1. *Polygonum hydropiper* L." *Journal of Endocrinology* 12:252–262.

Edelstein, Ludwig. 1967. "The Hippocratic Oath: Text, Translation and Interpretaiton." In *Ancient Medicine: Select Papers of Ludwig Edelstein,* Oswei Temkin and Lilian Temkin, eds. Baltimore: Johns Hopkins University Press, pp. 4–63.

Elujoba, Anthony A., Stella O. Olagbende, and Simeon K. Adesina. 1985. "Antiimplantation Activity of the Fruit of *Legenaria breriflora* Robert." *Journal of Ethnopharmacology* 13:281–288.

Engels, Donald. 1980. "The Problem of Female Infanticide in the Greco-Roman World." *Classical Philology* 75:112–120.

—— 1984. "The Use of Historical Demography in Ancient History." *Classical Quarterly* 34:386–393.

Estes, J. Worth. 1989. *The Medical Skills of Ancient Egypt.* Canton, Mass.: Science History Publications.

Facciolatus, Jacobus, and Aegidius Forcellinus. 1828. *Totius latinitatis lexicon.* 2 vols. London: Baldwin and Credock.

Farnsworth, Norman P., et al. 1975. "Potential Value of Plants as Sources of New Antifertility Agents." Part I, *Journal of Pharmaceutical Sciences* 64 (April): 535–598. Part II, 64 (May): 717–754.

Farnsworth, Norman P., et al. 1981. "Prospects for Higher Plants as a Source of Useful Fertility Regulating Agents for Human Use." In *Recent Advances in*

Fertility Regulation (Proceedings of a Symposium, Beijing, 2–5 September 1980), Chang Chai Fen, David Griffin, and Aubrey Woolman, eds. Geneva: Atar, pp. 330–364.

Feen, Richard. 1983. "Abortion and Exposure in Ancient Greece: Assessing the Status of the Fetus and 'Newborn' from Classical Sources." In *Abortion and the Status of the Fetus,* William B. Bondeson et al., eds. Dordrecht: Reidel.

Feng, P. C., et al. 1962. "Pharmacological Screening of Some West Indian Medicinal Plants." *Journal of Pharmacy and Pharmacology* 14:556–561.

Fischer, Hermann. 1927. *Die Heilige Hildegard von Bingen: Die Erste Deutsche Naturforscherin und Ärztin.* Munich: Verlag der München Drucke.

———— 1929. *Mittelalterliche Pflanzenkunde.* Munich: Verlag der München Drucke.

Fischer, Ioannes. 1927. *Die Gynäkologie bei Dioskurides und Plinius.* Vienna: Julius Springer.

Flandrin, Jean-Louis. 1969. "Contraception, mariage et relations amoureuses dans l'occident chrétien." *Annales economies, sociétés, civilisations* 24:1370–1390.

———— 1985. "Sex in Married Life in the Early Middle Ages." In *Western Sexuality: Practice and Precept in Past and Present Times,* Philippe Ariès and André Béjin, eds. Oxford and New York: B. Blackwell.

Flood, Bruce. 1968. *Macer Floridus: A Medieval Herbalism.* Diss., University of Colorado.

Flückiger, Friedrich A., and Daniel Hanbury. 1879. *Pharmacographia: A History of the Principal Drugs of Vegetable Origin Met with in Great Britain and British India.* 2nd ed. London: Macmillan.

Fontán-Candella, J. L. 1960. "Neuvas fuentes de estrógenos (Ensayos en fanerogamas)." *Revista Española de Fisiologia* 16:7–16.

Fontanille, Marie-Thérèse. 1977. *Abortement et contraception dans la médecine grèco-romaîne.* Paris: Laboratoires Searle.

Foucault, Michel. 1984. *Histoire de la sexualité.* Vol. 2, *L'usage des plaisirs;* vol. 3, *Le souci de soi.* Paris: Gallimard.

Frazer, James George. 1935. *The Golden Bough; A Study in Magic and Religion.* 3rd ed. 12 vols. New York: Macmillan.

Frey, Emil F. 1985–86. "The Earliest Medical Text." *Clio Medica* 20:79–90.

Friedenwald, Harry. 1937. "Amatus Lusitanus." *Bulletin of the Institute of the History of Medicine* 5:603–653.

Gallegos, Alfredo J. 1983. "The Zoapatle I—A Traditional Remedy from Mexico Emerges to Modern Times." *Contraception* 27:211–225.

Garg, S. K., and G. P. Garg. 1971. "Antifertility Screening of Plants. Part VII: Effect of Five Indigenous Plants on Early Pregnancy." *Indian Journal of Medical Research* 59:302–306.

Garg, S. K., and V. S. Mathur. 1970. "Effect of Chromatographic Fractions of *Polygonum hydropiper* Linn. (Roots) on Fertility in Female Albino Rats." *Journal of Reproduction and Fertility* 29:421–423.

Gemmill, Chalmers L. 1966. "Silphium." *Bulletin of the History of Medicine* 40:295–313.

Gerard, John. 1636. *The Herball, or General Historie of Plants.* London.

Gies, Frances, and Joseph Gies. 1987. *Marriage and the Family in the Middle Ages.* New York: Harper and Row.

Gildemeister, E., and Fr. Hoffmann. 1900. *The Volatile Oils.* Edward Kremers, trans. Milwaukee: Pharmaceutical Review Publ. Co.

Golden, Mark. 1981. "Demography and the Exposure of Girls at Athens." *Phoenix* 35:316–331.

Goodman, L. E. 1990. "The Fetus as a Natural Miracle: The Maimonidean View." In Dunstan 1990, pp. 79–94.

Goodman, Louis, and Alfred Gilman. 1941. *The Pharmacological Basis of Therapeutics.* New York: Macmillan.

Gopinath, K., and K. Raghunathan. 1985. "Historical Significance of Contraception." *Bulletin of the Indian Institute for the History of Medicine* (Hyderabad) 15:17–45.

Goris, A., and A. Liot. 1939. *Pharmacie Galénique.* 2 vols. Paris: Masson.

Gorman, Michael J. 1982. *Abortion and the Early Church: Christian, Jewish and Pagan Attitudes in the Greco-Roman World.* Downers Grove, Ill.: Inter-Varsity Press.

Goswami, H. K. 1978. "Effect of Oral Contraceptives on Plant Chromosomes." *Current Science* 47:515–516.

Gourevitch, Danielle 1984. *Le mal d'être femme: la femme et la médecine dans la Rome antique.* Paris: Société d'édition "Les Belles Lettres".

Green, Monica. 1985. *Transmission of Ancient Theories of Female Physiology and Disease through the Early Middle Ages.* Diss., Princeton University. Distributed by University Microfilms International.

——— 1989. "Women's Medical Practice and Health Care in Medieval Europe." *Signs: Journal of Women in Cultures and Society* 14:434–73.

——— 1990. "Constantinus Africanus and the Conflict between Religion and Science." In Dunstan 1990, pp. 47–69.

Greene, Edward Lee. 1983. *Landmarks of Botanical History.* Frank N. Egerton, ed. 2 vols. Stanford: Stanford University Press.

Grensemann, Hermann. 1982. *Hippokratische Gynäkologie.* Wiesbaden: F. Steiner.

——— 1987. *Knidische medizin.* Part 2: *Versuch einer weiteren Analyse der Schicht A in den pseudohippokratischen "Da natura muliebri" und "Da muliebribus I und II."* Supp. *Hermes,* no. 51. Stuttgart: F. Steiner.

Grmek, Mirko D. 1989. *Disease in the Ancient Greek World.* Mireille Muellner and Leonard Muellner, trans. Baltimore: Johns Hopkins University Press.

Guerra, M. O., and A. T. L. Andrade. 1974. "Contraceptive Effects of Native Plants in Rats." *Contraception* 18:191–199.

Gujral, M. L., D. R. Varma, and K. N. Sareen. 1960. "Oral Contraceptives. Part I: Preliminary Observations on the Antifertility Effect of Some Indigenous Drugs." *Indian Journal of Medical Research* 48:46–51.

Gupta, I., and P. K. Devi. 1975. "Studies on Immediate Post-abortion Copper 'T' Device." *Indian Journal of Medical Research* 63:736–739.

Gupta, I., Rita Tank, and V. P. Dixit. 1985. "Fertility Regulation in Males: Effect of *Hibiscus rosa-sinensis* and *Malvaviscus* Flower Extract on Male Albino

Rats." *Proceedings of the National Academy of Sciences, India,* Section B 55 (4):262–267, through Chemical Abstracts CA107 (9):70981x.

Hagenfeldt, Kerstin. 1972. "Intrauterine Contraception with the Copper-T Device." *Contraception* 6:37–54.

Hager's Handbuch. See Arends and Zörnig, and List and Horhammer.

Hanawalt, Barbara. 1977. "Childrearing among the Lower Classes of Late Medieval England." *Journal of Interdisciplinary History* 7:1–22.

—— 1986. *The Ties That Bound: Peasant Families in Medieval England.* New York: Oxford University Press.

Hanson, Ann. 1989. "Greco-Roman Gynecology." *Society for Ancient Medicine and Pharmacy Newsletter* 17:83–92.

Harborne, J. B. 1982. *Introduction to Ecological Biochemistry.* 2nd ed. London: Academic Press.

Harris, Marvin. 1977. *Cannibals and Kings: The Origins of Cultures.* New York: Random House.

Harris, William V. 1982. "The Theoretical Possibility of Extensive Infanticide in the Greco-Roman World." *Classical Quarterly* 32:114–116.

Haskins, Charles Homer. 1957. *The Renaissance of the Twelfth Century.* New York: Meridan Books.

Hawley, Amos H. 1959. "Population Composition." In *The Study of Population,* Philip M. Hauser and Otis Dudley Duncan, eds. Chicago: University of Chicago Press, pp. 361–382.

Heftmann, Erich, Shui-Tze Ko, and Raymond D. Bennett. 1966. "Identification of Estrone in Pomegranate Seeds." *Phytochemistry* 5:1337–1339.

Helmholtz, Richard H. 1975. "Infanticide in the Provinces of Canterbury during the Fifteenth Century." *History of Childhood Quarterly* 2:382–390.

Herlihy, David. 1965. "Population, Plague and Social Change in Rural Pistoria, 1201–1430." *Economic History Review* 18, 2nd ser.:225–244.

—— 1969. "Vieillir à Florence au Quattro-centro." *Annales economies, societas, civilisations* 24:1338–1352.

—— 1970. "The Tuscan Town in the Quattro-centro: A Demographic Profile." *Medievalia et humanistica,* n.s. 1:81–109.

—— 1972. "Mapping Households in Medieval Italy." *Catholic Historical Review* 58:1–24.

—— 1973. "The Population of Verona in the First Century of Venetian Rule." In *Renaissance Venice,* J. Hale, ed. London: Rowman and Littlefield.

—— 1974. "Ecological Conditions and Demographic Change." In *One Thousand Years: Western Europe in the Middle Ages,* Richard L. DeMolen, ed. Boston: Houghton Mifflin.

—— 1985. *Medieval Households.* Cambridge: Harvard University Press.

Hermolaus Barbarus. 1516. *Pedacii Dioscorides Anazarbei de medicanale materia.* Venice.

Himes, Norman Edwin. 1936. *Medical History of Contraception.* Baltimore: Williams and Wilkins. Reprt. New York: Gamut Press, 1963.

Hollingsworth, T. H. 1969. *Historical Demography.* Ithaca: Cornell University Press.

Hopkins, Keith. 1964–65. "The Age of Roman Girls at Marriage." *Population Studies* 18:309–327.

—— 1965. "A Textual Emendation in a Fragment of Musonius Rufus." *Classical Quarterly* 15:72–74.

—— 1965–66. "Contraception in the Roman Empire." *Comparative Studies in Society and History* 8:124–151.

Huby, Pamela M. 1990. "Soul, Life, Sense, Intellect: Some Thirteenth-Century Problems." In Dunstan 1990, pp. 113–122.

Hunt, Tony. 1989. *Plant Names of Medieval England.* Cambridge: D. S. Brewer.

Ibn Sarafyun (the younger). 1552. *De simplicium medicamentorum historia libri septem.* Venice: Andrea Arrivabenius.

Ibn Sarafyun, Yuhya (the elder). 1525. *De simpli[cibus] medi[cinis] sumpta a plantis, mineralibus, et animalibus.* Lyons: Jacobi Myt.

Indira, M., et al. 1956. "The Occurrence of Some Estrogenic Substances in Plants. Part I: Estrogenic Activity of *Cyperus rotundus* (Linn.)." *Journal of Scientific and Industrial Research* 15C:202–204.

Jackson, Ralph. 1988. *Doctors and Diseases in the Roman Empire.* London: British Museum Publications.

Jacquart, Danielle, and Claude Thomasset. 1985. *Sexualité et savoir médical au moyen âge.* Paris: Presses universitaires de France.

Jennings, Samuel K. 1808. *The Married Lady's Companion; or, Poor Man's Friend.* 2nd rev. ed. New York: Lorenzo Dow.

Jiu, J. 1966. "A Survey of Some Medicinal Plants of Mexico for Selected Biological Activities." *Lloydia* 29:250–259.

Jöchle, Wolfgang. 1971. "Biology and Pathology of Reproduction in Greek Mythology." *Contraception* 4:1–13.

—— 1974. "Menses-Inducing Drugs: Their Role in Antique, Medieval and Renaissance Gynecology and Birth Control." *Contraception* 10:425–439.

Jones, W. H. S. 1924. *The Doctor's Oath: An Essay in the History of Medicine.* Cambridge: Cambridge University Press.

Joshi, B. C., et al. 1981. "Antifertility Effects of Chronically Administered *Malvaviscus conzattii* Flower Extract on Male Albino Mice." *Planta Medica* 41:274–280.

Kaliwal, B. B., R. Nazeer Ahamed, and M. Appaswomy Rao. 1984. "Abortifacient Effect of Carrot Seed (*Daucus carota*) Extract and Its Reversal by Progesterone in Albino Rats." *Comparative Physiology and Ecology* 9:70–74.

Kamboj, V. P., and B. N. Dhawan. 1982. "Research on Plants for Fertility Regulation in India." *Journal of Ethnopharmacology* 6:191–226.

Kanjanapothi, Duangta, et al. 1981. "Postcoital Antifertility Effect of *Mentha arvensis.*" *Contraception* 24:559–567.

Kant, Ashwini, Dennis Jacob, and N. K. Lohiya. 1986. "The Oestrogenic Efficacy of Carrot (*Daucus carota*) Seeds." *Journal of Advanced Zoology* 7:36–41.

Keil, C. F., and F. Delitzsch. 1983. *Commentary on the Old Testament.* 10 vols. Grand Rapids: Eerdmans.

Kekkey, Marc A. 1979. "Parturition and Pelvic Changes." *American Journal of Physical Anthropology,* n.s. 51:541–545.

Keller, Achim. 1988. *Die Abortiva in der römischen Kaiserzeit.* Stuttgart: Deutscher Apoteker Verlag.

Kellum, Barbara. 1973–74. "Infanticide in England in the Later Middle Ages." *History of Childhood Quarterly* 1:367–388.

Kharkhov, V. V., and M. N. Mats. 1980. "Plants as a Potential Source of Contraceptive Drugs" (in Russian). *Rasttite 'nye resursy* 17:291–302.

Kholkute, S. D., V. Mudgal, and K. N. Udupa. 1977. "Studies on the Antifertility Potentiality of *Hibiscus rosa sinensis.*" *Planta Medica* 31:35–39.

King, Helen. 1990. "Making a Man: Becoming Human in Early Greek Medicine." In Dunstan 1990, pp. 10–19.

Knodel, J., and E. van de Walle. 1979. "Lessons from the Past: Policy Implications of Historical Fertility Studies." *Population and Development Review* 5:217–245.

Ko, Shui-Tze, and Eric Heftmann. 1966. "Isolation of Estrone and Cholesterol from the Date Palm, *Phoenix dactylifera* L." *Phytochemistry* 5:231–235.

Kong, Yun Cheung, Jing-Xi Xie, and Paul Pui-Hay But. 1986. "Fertility Regulating Agents from Traditional Chinese Medicines." *Journal of Ethnopharmacology* 15:1–44.

Kong, Yun Cheung, et al. 1985. "Yuehchukene, a Novel Anti-implantation Indole Alkaloid from *Murraya paniculata.*" *Planta Medica* 51:304–307.

Kopcewicz, Jan. 1971. "Estrogens in Developing Bean (*Phaseolus vulgaris*) Plants." *Phytochemistry* 10:1423–27.

Kristeller, Paul O. 1945. "The School of Salerno." *Bulletin of the History of Medicine* 17:138–194.

Ku, Savita Sharma, Shashwat Mishra, and B. K. Mehta. 1988. "Antifertility Activity of *Echinops Echinatus* in Albino Rats." *Indian Journal of Medical Sciences* 42:23–26.

Lacey, John R., Lynn F. James, and Robert E. Short. 1980. *The Ecology and Economic Impact of Poisonous Plants on Livestock Production.* Boulder, Colo., and London: Westview Press.

Lachs, Jan. 1949. *Ginekologia u Dioskuridesa.* Polska Akademia Umiejetonosci Prace Komisji Historii Medycynyinauk matematyczno-przrodniczych, vol. 3, no. 1. Krakow: Nakladem Polskiej Adademii Umiejetnosci. 32 pp.

Laderman, Carol. 1983. *Wives and Midwives. Childbirth and Nutrition in Rural Malaysia.* Berkeley: University of California Press.

Ladurie, Emmanuel Le Roy. 1973. "Demographie et 'funestes secrets' le Languedoc (fin XVIIIe–début XIXe siècle)." In *Le territoire de l'historien.* 2 vols. Paris: Gallimard, vol. 1, pp. 316–330.

―――― 1975. *Montaillou: village occitan de 1294 à 1324.* Paris: Gallimard.

Lehner, Ernest, and Johanna Lehner, 1960. *Folklore and Symbolism of Flowers, Plants and Trees.* New York: Tudor.

Leung, A. Y. 1980. *Encyclopedia of Common Natural Ingredients Used in Food, Drugs, and Cosmetics.* New York: Wiley.

Levinson, Warren. 1978. "Contraceptive Action of Copper." *New England Journal of Medicine* 299:779.

Lewin, L. 1922. *Die Fruchtabtreibung durch Gifte und andere Mittel: ein Handbuch für Ärzte und Juristen.* Berlin: Julius Springer.

Lewis, Naphtali. 1983. *Life in Egypt under Roman Rule*. Oxford: Clarendon Press.

Lewis, Walter H., and Memory P. F. Elvin-Lewis. 1977. *Medical Botany: Plants Affecting Man's Health*. New York: Wiley.

Lichtenthaeler, Charles. 1984. *Der Eid des Hippokrates: Ursprung und Bedeutung*. Cologne: Deutscher Ärzte-Verlag.

Lin, Zhong-Min, et al. 1981. "Some Pharmacology Studies of Two Abortifacient Diperpenoids, Yuanhuacine and Yuanhuadine." In *Recent Advances in Fertility Regulation* (Symposium, Beijing, 2–5 September 1980), Chang Chai Fen, David Griffin, and Aubrey Woolman, eds. Geneva: Atar.

List, P. H., and L. Horhammer. 1969–79. *Hager's Handbuch der pharmazeutischen Praxis*, vols. 2–6. Berlin: Springer.

Loewit, K., N. Zambelis, and D. Egg. 1971. "Contraceptive Effect of Iron Reduced Fertility after Vaginal Application of Iron Chloride in Rats." *Contraception* 4:92–96.

Lorimer, Frank. 1959. "The Development of Demography." In *The Study of Population: An Inventory and Appraisal*, Philip M. Hauser and Otis Dudley Duncan, eds. Chicago: University of Chicago Press, pp. 124–179.

Löw, Immanuel. 1934. *Die Flora der Juden*. 3 vols. Vienna: Kohut-Foundation.

Mabberley, D. J. 1987. *The Plant-Book*. Cambridge: Cambridge University Press.

Malhi, B. S., and V. P. Trivedi. 1972. "Vegetable Antifertility Drugs of India." *Quarterly Journal of Crude Drug Research* 12:1922–1928.

Manniche, Lise, 1989. *An Ancient Egyptian Herbal*. Austin: University of Texas Press.

Marcellus Vergilius. 1518. Commentary to Dioscorides, in *Dioscorides: De medica materia libri sex*. Florence: Philippi Juntae.

Martin of Braga. 1950. *Opera omnia*. Claude W. Barlow, ed. Papers and Monographs of the American Academy in Rome. New Haven: Yale University Press.

Matossian, Mary Kilbourne, 1989. *Poisons of the Past: Molds, Epidemics, and History*. New Haven: Yale University Press.

Matsui, Adelina de S., et al. 1971. "A Survey of Natural Products from Hawaii and Other Areas of the Pacific for an Antifertility Effect in Mice." *Internationale Zeitschrift für klinische Pharmakologie, Therapie, und Toxikologie* 5:65–69.

Matthaeus Platearius. 1939. *Circa instans*. In *Das Arzneidrogenbuch Circa Instans in einer Fassung des XIII. Jahrhunderts aus der Universitätsbibliothek Erlangen*. Hans Wölfel, ed. Diss., Berlin.

Matthiolus, Petrus (Matthioli Petri). 1554. *Commentarii in libros sex Pedacii Dioscoridis*. Jean Ruel, trans. Venice: Vincentius Valgrisium.

——— 1544. *Di Pedacio Dioscoride Anazarebo libri cinque della historia et materia medicinale tradotta in lingua volgare italiana*. Venice: Nicolo de Bascarinia da Pavone di Brescia.

Mauriceau, Francis. 1681. *De praegnantium et partiurientium et puerperarum morbis tractatus*. Paris.

——— 1718. *The Diseases of Women with Child*. Hugh Chamberlen, trans. London: A. Bell.

Mazur, Mieczaslaw, et al. 1966. "Pharmacology of Lupanine and 130 Hydroxy-lupanine." *Acta Physiologiae Polononica* 17, no. 2:299–309, reported through *Chemical Absracts* 65:11163q.

McLaren, Angus. 1984. *Reproductive Rituals: Perceptions of Fertility in England from the Sixteenth Century to the Nineteenth Century.* London and New York: Methuen.

—— 1990. "Policing Pregnancies: Changes in Nineteenth-Century Criminal and Canon Law." In Dunstan 1990, pp. 187–207.

Meigs, C. D. 1848. *Females and Their Diseases.* Philadelphia: Lea and Blanchard.

Mennell, Stephen. 1985. *All Manners of Food, Eating and Taste in England and France from the Middle Ages to the Present.* Oxford: Blackwell.

Merck Index of Chemicals and Drugs. 1976. 19th ed. Rahway, N.J.: Merck.

Mesuë. 1525. *Canones unversales.* Lyons: Jacobi Myt.

Milne, J. S. 1907. *Surgical Instruments in Greek and Roman Times.* Chicago: Ares.

Mohr, James C. 1978. *Abortion in America: The Origins and Evolution of National Policy.* New York: Oxford University Press.

Moïssidés, M. 1922. "Contribution à l'étude de l'abortement dans l'antiquité grecque." *Janus* 26:59–85.

Mols, Robert. 1955. *Introduction à la démographie historique des villes d'Europe du XIVe au XVIIIe siècle.* 3 vols. Louvain: Publications universitaires.

Murphy, James C., et al. 1977. "Evaluation of an Aqueous Extract of Pine Needles Utilizing the Rat Reproductive System." *Quarterly Journal of Crude Drug Research* 15:193–197.

Murthy, R. S. R., D. K. Basu, and V. V. S. Muri. 1984. "Anti-implantation Activity of Isoadiantone." *Indian Drugs* 21 (4):141–144, reported through *Chemical Abstracts* CA101(3):17582t.

Musallam, B. F. 1983. *Sex and Society in Islam: Birth Control before the Nineteenth Century.* Cambridge: Cambridge University Press.

Nakai, Yasuo, and Sadao Sakamoto. 1977. "Variation and Distribution of Esterase Isozymes in *Heteranthelium* and *Taeniatherum* of the Tribe Triticeae, Gramineae." *Botanical Magazine* (Tokyo) 90:269–276.

Nardi, Enzo. 1971. *Procurato aborto nel mondo greco romano.* Milan: Dott. A. Giuffré.

Needham, Joseph. 1970. *Clerks and Craftsmen in China and the West.* Cambridge: Harvard University Press.

Needham, Joseph, and Lu Gwei-Djen. 1968. "Sex Hormones in the Middle Ages." *Endeavor* 27:130–132.

Newmeyer, Stephen. 1988. "Antonius and Rabbi on the Soul: Stoic Elements of a Puzzling Encounter." *Koroth* 9:108–123.

Noonan, John Thomas, Jr. 1986. *Contraception: A History of Its Treatment by the Catholic Theologians and Canonists.* Rev. ed. Cambridge: Harvard University Press.

Nutton, Vivian. 1990. "The Anatomy of the Soul in Early Renaissance Medicine." In Dunstan 1990, pp. 136–157.

—— ed. 1981. *Galen: Problems and Prospects. A Collection of Papers Submit-*

ted to the *1979 Cambridge Conference*. London: Wellcome Institute for the History of Medicine.

Oldenziel, Ruth. 1987. "The Historiography of Infanticide in Antiquity." In *Sexual Asymmetry: Studies in Ancient Society*, Josine Blok and Peter Mason, eds. Amsterdam: J. C. Gieben.

Olivier, M. 1760. "Observation." *Journal de médecine, chirurgie, pharmacie* 12:129–131.

Olivieri, Achillo. 1985. "Eroticism and Social Groups in Sixteenth-Century Venice: The Courtesan." In *Western Sexuality: Practice and Precept in Past and Present Times*, Philippe Ariès and André Béjin, eds. Anthony Forster, trans. Oxford: Blackwell, pp. 95–113.

Orta, Garcia d'. 1567. *Coloquios dos simples e grogas e cousas medicinais da India*. Charles L'Ecluse (Carolus Clusius), trans., in *Aromatum, et simplicium aliquot medicamentorum apud indos nascentium historia*. Antwerp: Christophorus Plantinus. Facsimile reproduction, Nieuwkoop: B. De Graaf, 1963.

Oster, Gerald, and Miklos P. Salgo. 1975. "The Copper Intrauterine Device and its Mode of Action." *New England Journal of Medicine* 293:432–438.

Oylebola, D. D. O. 1981. "Yoruba Traditional Healers' Knowledge of Contraception, Abortion, and Infertility." *East African Medical Journal* 58:777–784.

Palma, L. 1964. *Le piante medicinali d'Italia: botanica, chimica, farmacodinamica, terapia*. Rome: Societá Editrice Internazionale.

Palmer, Richard. 1985a. "Medical Botany in Northern Italy in the Renaissance." *Journal of the Royal Society of Medicine* 78:149–157.

———— 1985b. "Pharmacy in the Republic of Venice in the Sixteenth Century." In *The Medical Renaissance of the Sixteenth Century*. Cambridge: Cambridge University Press, pp. 100–117, 303–312.

Pavlík, Adeněk. 1990. Reply to Daniel F. Sieff. *Current Anthropology* 31:41.

Pellegrino, Edmund D., and Alice A. Pellegrino. 1988. "Humanism and Ethics in Roman Medicine: Translation and Commentary on a Text of Scribonius Largus." *Literature and Medicine* 7:22–38.

Peter of Spain (Pope John XXI). 1973. *Obras médicas de Pedro Hispano*. Acta Universitatis Conibrigensis. Coimbra, Portugal: University of Coimbra, 1973. Latin text with Portuguese translation.

———— 1518. *Thesaurus pauperum*. Venice: Georgio di Rusconi. In Italian translation.

———— 1560(?). *The Treasurie of Health Contayning Many Profitable Medicines* . . . [London: William Copland].

Pirenne, Henri. 1937. *Mahomet et Charlemagne*. Paris: F. Alcan.

———— 1946. *Medieval Cities: Their Origins and Revival of Trade*. Princeton: Princeton University Press.

Polgar, Steven. 1972. "Population History and Population Policies from an Anthropolgoical Perspective." *Current Anthropology* 13:203–211.

Polunin, Oleg. 1969. *Flowers of Europe: A Field Guide*. London: Oxford University Press.

Pomeroy, S. 1975. *Goddesses, Whores, Wives, and Slaves: Women in Classical Antiquity*. New York: Schocken Books.

—— 1984. *Women in Hellenistic Egypt: From Alexander to Cleopatra.* New York: Schocken Books.

—— 1985. "The Family in Classical and Hellenistic Greece." *Trends in History* 3:19–26.

—— 1988. "Greek Marriage." In *Civilization of the Ancient Mediterranean: Greece and Rome,* Michael Grant and Rachel Kitzinger, eds., 3 vols. New York: Scribner's.

Prakash, Anand O. 1986. "Potentialities of Some Indigenous Plants for Antifertility Activity." *International Journal of Crude Drug Research* 24:19–24.

Prakash, Anand O., et al. 1985. "Anti-implantation Activity of Some Indigenous Plants in Rats." *Acta Europaea Fertilitatis* 16:441–448.

Preuss, Julius. 1978. *Biblical and Talmudic Medicine.* Fred Rosner, ed. and trans. New York: Sanhedrin Press.

Price, R. 1965. *Symposium on Agents Affecting Sterility.* C. R. Austin and J. S. Perry, eds. London: J. A. Churchill.

Prose Salernitan Questions. 1979. In *Auctores Britannici Medii Aevi.* Brian Lawn, ed. London: Oxford University Press.

Pschera, H., et al. 1988. "The Influence of Copper Intrauterine Device on Fatty Acid Composition of Cervical Mucus Lecithin." *Contraception* 38:341–48.

Qian, Y. X., et al. 1986. "Spermicidal Effect in Vitro by the Active Principle of Garlic." *Contraception* 34:295–302.

"Quacks and Abortion: A Critical and Analytical Inquiry." 1988. *Lancet* 2 (Dec. 24,): 1723–25.

Rall, Theodore W. 1990. "Oxytocin, Prostaglandins, Ergot Alkaloids, and Other Drugs: Tocolytic Agents." In *Goodman and Gilman's Pharmacological Basis of Therapeutics.* 8th ed. New York: Pergamon Press, pp. 933–953.

Reeds, Karen. 1975. "Botany in Medieval and Renaissance Universities." Diss., Harvard University.

—— 1976. "Renaissance Humanism and Botany." *Annals of Science* 33:519–542.

Reiners, W. 1966. "7-Hydroxy-4'-methoxy-isoflavon (Formononetin) aus Süssholzwurzel: über Inhaltssotoffe der Süssholzwurzel. II." *Experientia* 22:359.

Reynolds, A. K. 1955. "Uterine Stimulants." *Alkaloids Chemistry and Physiology* 5:163–209.

Riddle, John M. 1965. "The Introduction and Use of Eastern Drugs in the Early Middle Ages." *Sudhoffs Archiv* 49:185–198.

—— 1977. *Marbode of Rennes' (1035–1123) De lapidibus. Sudhoffs Archiv,* vol. 20. Wiesbaden: Franz Steiner Verlag.

—— 1980. "Dioscorides." In *Catalogus Translationum et Commentariorum,* Paul Oskar Kristeller, ed. Washington: Catholic University Press, pp. 1–143.

—— 1981. "Pseudo-Dioscorides' *Ex herbis femininis* and Early Medieval Medical Botany." *Journal of the History of Botany* 14:43–81.

—— 1984. "Gargilius Martialis as a Medical Writer." *Journal of the History of Medicine and Allied Science* 39:408–429.

—— 1985. *Dioscorides on Pharmacy and Medicine.* Austin: University of Texas Press.

—— 1987. "Folk Tradition and Folk Medicine: Recognition of Drugs in Classical Antiquity." In *Folklore and Folk Medicines,* John Scarborough, ed. Madison: American Institute for the History of Pharmacy, pp. 33–61.

Riddle, John M., and James Mulholland. 1980. "Albert on Stones and Minerals." In *Albertus Magnus and the Sciences,* James A. Weishepl, ed. Toronto: Pontifical Institute, pp. 203–234.

Riquet, R. P. 1949. "Christianisme et population." *Population* 4:615–630.

Ritner, Robert K. 1984. "A Uterine Amulet in the Oriental Institute Collection." *Journal of Near Eastern Studies* 43:209–221.

Robson, J. M., J. R. Trounce, and K. A. H. Didcock. 1954. "Factors Affecting the Response of the Uterus to Serotoine." *Journal of Endocrinology* 10:129–132.

Rouche, Michel. 1987. "The Early Middle Ages in the West." In *A History of Private Life,* vol. 1, Paul Veyne, ed. Cambridge: Harvard University Press.

Roys, Ralph L. 1931. *The Ethno-Botany of the Maya.* New Orleans: Tulane University. Rept. Philadelphia: ISHI, 1976.

Russell, Jeffrey. 1972. *Witchcraft in the Middle Ages.* Ithaca: Cornell University Press.

Russell, Josiah Cox. 1948. *British Medieval Population.* Albuquerque: University of New Mexico Press, 1948.

———— 1956. "Demographic Pattern in History." In *Demographic Analysis: Selected Readings,* Joseph J. Spengler and Otis Dudley Duncan, eds. Glencoe, Ill.: Free Press, pp. 52–68.

———— 1976. "The Earlier Medieval Plague in the British Isles." *Viator* 7:64–78.

———— 1985. *The Control of Late Ancient and Medieval Population.* Philadelphia: American Philosophical Society.

Saha, J. C., E. C. Savini, and S. Kasinathan. 1961. "Ecobolic Properties of Indian Medicinal Plants." *Indian Journal of Medical Research* 49:130–151.

Sandbach, F. H. 1940. "Plutarch on the Stoics." *Classical Quarterly* 34:20–25.

Sayre, Lucius E. 1917. *A Manual of Organic Materia Medica and Pharmacognosy . . .* 4th ed. Philadelphia: P. Blakiston.

Scarborough, John. 1979. "Nicander's Toxicology II: Spiders, Scorpions, Insects and Myriapods." *Pharmacy in History* 21:3–34.

———— 1984. *Pharmacy's Ancient Heritage: Theophrastus, Nicander, and Dioscorides.* Lexington, Ky.: College of Pharmacy.

Schipperges, Heinrich. 1964. *Die Assimilation der arabischen Medizin durch das lateinisches Mittelalter.* Sudhoffs Archiv, vol. 3. Wiesbaden: Franz Steiner.

Schleifer, J. 1926. "Zum Syrischen Medizinbuch." *Zeitschrift für Semitistik und verwandte Gebiete* 4:70–122, 161–195.

Scrimshaw, Susan C. M. 1978. "Infant Mortality and Behavior in the Regulation of Family Size." *Population and Development Review* 4:383–399.

Sharaf, A., and N. Goma. 1965. "Phytoestrogens and Their Antagonism to Progesterone and Testosterone." *Journal of Endocrinology* 31:289–290.

Sharma, B. B., et al. 1983. "Antifertility Screening of Plants. Part I: Effect of Ten Indigenous Plants on Early Pregnancy in Albino Rats." *International Journal of Crude Drug Research* 21:183–187.

Sharma, M. M., Gopal Lel, and Dennis Jacob. 1976. "Estrogenic and Pregnancy Interceptory Effects of Carrot *Daucus carota* Seeds." *Indian Journal of Experimental Biology* 14:506–508.

Sharp, Jane. 1671. *Midwives' Book*. Facsimile reproduction, 1985.

Shaw, Brent D. 1987. "The Age of Roman Girls at Marriage." *The Journal of Roman Studies* 77:30–46.

Sieff, Daniela F. 1990. "Explaining Biased Sex Ratios in Human Populations: A Critique of Recent Studies." *Current Anthropology* 31:25–48; with replies.

Singh, M. M., et al. 1985. "Contraceptive Efficacy and Hormonal Profile of Ferujol: A New Coumarin from *Ferula jaeschkeana*." *Planta Medica* 51:268–270.

Siraisi, Nancy G. 1981. *Taddeo Alderotti and His Pupils: Two Generations of Italian Medical Learning*. Princeton: Princeton University Press.

—— 1987. *Avicenna in Renaissance Italy: The Canon and Medical Training in Italian Universities after 1500*. Princeton: Princeton University Press.

—— 1990. *Medieval and Early Renaissance Medicine: An Introduction to Knowledge and Practice*. Chicago: University of Chicago Press.

Sizov, P. I. 1969. "Experimental Parturifacient Action of Pachycarpine Brevicolline and Thalictrimine." *Zdravookhranenie Belorusii* 15:44–46, reported through *Chemical Abstracts* 72 (1970):119957u.

Skarzynski, Boleslaw. 1933a. "An Oestrogenic Substitute from Plant Materials." *Nature* 131:766.

—— 1933b. "Recherches sur les corps oestrogènes d'origine végétale." *Zoologischer Bericht* 35:323.

Smellie, William. 1752. *A Treatise on the Theory and Practice of Midwifery*. London: D. Wilson.

Smith, Wesley. 1988. Review of H. Grensemann, *Knidische medizin*. *Bulletin of the History of Medicine* 62:649–651.

Sokolowski, Francisziek. 1955. *Lois sacrées de l'asie mineure*. Paris: Boccard.

—— 1962. *Lois sacrées des cités grecques*. Suppl. no. 115. Paris.

Soloway, Richard Allen. 1982. *Birth Control and the Population Question in England, 1877–1930*. Chapel Hill: University of North Carolina Press.

Stannard, Jerry. 1982. "Botanical Data and Late Mediaeval Rezeptliteratur." In *Fachprosa-Studien: Beiträge zur mittelalterlichen Wissenschafts- und Geistesgeschichte*. Berlin: Erich Schmidt Verlag, pp. 371–395.

Statutes of the Realm. Annon regni quadragesimo tertio Georgii III. 1950. London: Stationery Off.

Steele, D. Gentry, and Claud A. Bramblett. 1988. *The Anatomy and Biology of the Human Skeleton*. College Station: Texas A&M University Press.

Steinegger, E., and R. Hänsel. 1963. *Lehrbuch der allgemeinen Pharmakognosie*. Berlin: Springer.

—— 1968. *Lehrbuch der Pharmakognosie auf phytochemischer Grundlage*. Berlin: Springer.

Stewart, T. Dale. 1970. "J. Lawrence Angel." *American Journal of Physical Anthropology* 51:509–516.

Stuart, G. A. 1911. *Chinese Materia Medica: Vegetable Kingdom*. Shanghai: American Presbyterian Mission.

Suchey, Judy Myers, et al. 1979. "Analysis of Dorsal Pitting in the Os Pubis in an Extensive Sample of Modern American Females." *American Journal of Physical Anthropology* 51:517–540.

Suder, W. 1988. "A partu, utraque filiam envia decessit: mortalité maternelle dans l'empire romain." In *Mémoires VIII: Études de médicine romaine,* Guy Sabbah, ed. Saint-Étienne: Publications de l'université.

Taylor, Alfred Swaine. 1865. *The Principles and Practice of Medical Jurisprudence.* London: John Churchill. 5th ed., 2 vols. Frederick J. Smith, ed. London: 1905.

Terra, M. 1980. *The Way of Herbs.* Santa Cruz: United Press.

Te Velde, H. 1967. *Seth, God of Confusion: A Study of His Role in Egyptian Mythology and Religion.* Leiden: Brill.

Theodorus, Jacobus. 1664. *New vollkommen Kräuter Buch.* Basel: Jacob Werenfels.

Thomlinson, Ralph. 1965 *Population Dynamics: Causes and Consequences of World Demographic Change.* New York: Random House.

Thrupp, S. L. 1965. "Plague Effects in Medieval Europe." *Economic History Review* 18:101–119.

Tiwari, K. C., R. Majumder, and S. Bhattacharjee. 1982. "Folklore Information from Assam for Family Planning and Birth Control." *International Journal of Crude Drug Research* 20:133–137.

Tomin, Julius. 1987. "Socratic Midwifery." *Classical Quarterly* 37:97–102.

Tournefourt, Joseph Pitton de. 1719. *The Compleat Herbal; or, The Botanical Institutions of Mr. Tournefourt . . .* 2 vols. London: R. Bonwicke et al.

Trease, G. E., and W. C. Evans. 1966. *A Textbook of Pharmacognosy.* 9th ed. London: Ballière, Tindall and Cassell.

Tuskaev, A. K. 1971. "Estrogennaia aktivnost 'nekotorykh kormovykh rasteni severnoi osetii" (The Estrogenic Activity of Certain Fodder Crops of Northern Ossetia). *Rastiyrl'nyr Resurdy* 7:295–298.

Tyler, Varro E., Lynn R. Brady, and James E. Robbers. 1981. *Pharmacognosy.* 8th ed. Philadelphia: Lea and Febiger.

Ullsperger, R. 1953. "Die Entwickung der Crataegusforschung." *Planta Medica* 1:43–50.

United Nations. 1953. *The Determinants and Consequences of Population Trends.* Population Studies, no. 17. Department of Social Affairs, Population Division. New York: United Nations.

Useful Guide to Herbal Health Care. N.d. Naples, Fla.: Health Center for Better Living.

Usher, George. 1974. *A Dictionary of Plants Used by Man.* London: Constable.

Vague, J., et al. 1957. "Note sur l'action oestrogène de divers corps gras." *Annales d'Endocrinologie* 18:745–751.

Valverde, Jose Luis, and Jose A. Perez Romero. 1988. *Drogas americanas en fuentes de escritores franciscanos y dominicos.* Granada: Universidad de Granada.

Van Kampen, K. R., and L. C. Ellis. 1972. "Prolonged Gestation in Ewes Ingesting Veratrum Californicum: Morphological Changes and 'Ev3 Steriod Biosynthesis in the Endocrine Organs of Cyclopic Lambs." *Journal of Endocrinology* 52:549–560.

Varma, Paras Nath, Vikramaditya, and Harish Chandra Gupta. 1981. "Pharmacognostic Studies on Drug of *Thlapsi bursa-pastoris* Moenhch." *Quarterly Journal of Crude Drug Research* 19:189–196.

Verma, O. P., et al. 1980. "Antifertility Effects of *Malvaviscus conzattii* Green Flower Extract (sc) on Male Albino Mice." *Indian Journal of Experimental Biology* 18:561–564.

Veyne, Paul. 1987. "The Roman Empire." In *A History of Private Life*, vol. 1. Paul Veyne, ed. Cambridge: Harvard University Press, 9–233.

Voland, Eckart, and Eva Siegelkow. 1990. Reply to Daniel F. Sieff, "Explaining Biased Sex Ratios in Human Populations." *Current Anthropology* 31:42–43.

Wagler, P. 1894. "Agnos." *Real Encyclopädie der classischen Altertumswissenschaft.* Stuttgart: Metzlerscher Verlag, col. 832–834.

Wang, W. H., and J. H. Zheng. 1984. "The Pregnancy Terminating Effect and Toxicity of an Active Constituent of *Aristolochia mollissima* Hance, Aristolochic Acid α" (in Chinese). *Yao Hsueh Hseuh Pao* 19:405–409.

Waszink, J. H. 1950. "Abtreibung." *Reallexikon für Antike und Christentum.* Stuttgart: Hiersemann.

Watt, J. M., and M. G. Breyer-Brandwijk. 1962. *The Medicinal and Poisonous Plants of Southern and Eastern Africa.* 2nd ed. Edinburgh: E. & S. Livingstone.

Weniger, B., M. Haag-Berrurier, and R. Anton. 1982. "Plants of Haiti Used as Antifertility Agents." *Journal of Ethnopharmacology* 6:67–84.

Whitehead, James. 1847. *On the Causes and Treatment of Abortion and Sterility.* London: John Churchill.

William of Saliceto. 1502. *Summa conservationis et curationis.* Venice.

Willigan, J. Dennis, and Katherine A. Lynch. 1982. *Sources and Methods of Historical Demography.* New York: Academic Press.

Woom, Wan Sick, et al. 1987. "Antifertility Principle of *Dictamnus albus* Root Bark." *Planta Medica* 53:399–401.

Woycke, James. 1988. *Birth Control in Germany 1871–1933.* London and New York: Routledge.

Zhu, Shou-Min. 1981. "The Copper Intrauterine Device: Copper Corrosion in Uterus and the Effects of the Copper Ion on Some Enzyme Activities." In *Recent Advances in Fertility Regulation* (Symposium, Beijing, 2–5 September 1980), Chang Chai Fen, David Griffin, and Aubrey Wollman, eds. Geneva: Atar, pp. 248–264.

Zohary, Michael. 1966. *Flora Palaestina.* 2 vols. Jerusalem: Israel Academy of Sciences and Humanities.

—— 1982. *Plants of the Bible.* Cambridge: Cambridge University Press.